Family Medical Care

Family Medical Care

A REPORT ON THE FAMILY HEALTH
MAINTENANCE DEMONSTRATION

GEORGE A. SILVER, M.D.

HARVARD UNIVERSITY PRESS

Cambridge, Massachusetts

1 9 6 3

Distributed in Great Britain by Oxford University Press, London

Library of Congress Catalog Card Number 62–20250
Printed in the United States of America

To: Bailey B. Burritt and

Albert G. Milbank

Bailey B. Burritt (1872–1954) was the "onlie beget-ter" of this project and of this book; it was a privilege to follow in his path. Family Health Maintenance was an idea he hoped to see applied in pursuit of his ideals.

Albert G. Milbank (1873–1949) embodied a lofty philanthropic spirit combined with a practical approach to solution of social problems. His spirit and skill made the Family Health Maintenance Demonstration a reality.

PREFACE

"I am particularly interested in fostering preventive and constructive social measures for the welfare of the poor of this city, as distinguished from relief measures affecting particular individuals and families." The Family Health Maintenance Demonstration really began with this letter written in 1913 by Mrs. Elizabeth Milbank Anderson.

Local history and individuals play an important role in any community program. Early public health interest in the Western world centered on New York City's reform which by the turn of the century had reached significant proportions. Leaders of the Sanitary Revolution even then were looking ahead from disease prevention to health promotion.

In the succeeding years public health reform in New York spread to include improvement of health organization and health practices. The movement was accelerated by various community agencies and health-centered philanthropic foundations such as the Committee for Neighborhood Health Development and the Milbank Memorial Fund. Individuals — John Kingsbury and Edgar Sydenstricker, Mayor Fiorello La Guardia, Health Commissioner S. S. Goldwater, philanthropists Livingston Farrand and Albert G. Milbank — played a large part.

London's Peckham experiment had attracted the attention of Bailey B. Burritt who propagandized the Community Service Society and the Milbank Memorial Fund to consider introducing a similar program into the United States. Urged by Albert G. Milbank, Dr. Frank G. Boudreau and Dr. George Baehr outlined a program offering complete medical care (which Peckham did not) to the family with the addition of preventive services, and contributed the idea of "Family Health Maintenance." Mr. Milbank, who was not only president of the Milbank Memorial Fund but a director of the Community Service Society and Chairman of their Health Committee, formed a subcommittee on Family Health Maintenance of the Health Committee of the Community

Service Society in 1943. This consisted of: Albert G. Milbank, Chairman; Dr. George Baehr, Vice-Chairman; Dr. Frank G. Boudreau; Stanley P. Davies; Homer Folks; Bailey B. Burritt, Executive Secretary.

Because of the Second World War the development of a family health maintenance program was delayed until 1947. By this time group practice was achieving status, and the Health Insurance Plan of Greater New York (a creation of Mayor La Guardia and Dr. Baehr) was in operation. Dr. Baehr suggested that the comprehensive medical care envisioned in Mr. Burritt's proposal be provided by the newly developed Health Insurance Plan, using a university medical group to take advantage of its learning and teaching opportunities and developing the family health maintenance aspects from that base.

By 1943, Bailey Burritt had issued a memorandum outlining a health maintenance project for the Community Service Society. He saw this as an opportunity for offering "positive robust health" (which was the goal to be attained) with medical, nursing, and social services directed to this end. An important additional objective would be the utilization of such a program for the training of medical students, nurses, and social workers in health services by affording opportunities for field work in preventive medical practice.

Cooperative but not unified services were envisioned: nursing and social work from Community Service Society, out of their own offices; medical care from a medical group center in some other place — no single location for the combined services, no single unit for health and welfare services. In a postwar memorandum, "Proposed Experiment in the Prevention of Sickness and the Maintenance of Health," Mr. Burritt delineated the Family Health Maintenance Demonstration in what came to be very much its final form: group medical practice affiliated with a medical school; prepayment for medical care; the family as the unit of health (and of service), "with educational nursing and social case staff work that will make possible the best health guidance and preventive treatment that the skills of the medical, educational nursing, and case work professions can provide." A month later, in January 1949 ("Proposed Experimental Approach to Determining of Direction of Future Health and Welfare Services"), he added, ". . ." the proposed Demonstration in the pooling of skills of these professions is primarily a demonstration in the art of teaching. This would help to give reality to the title of *educational* nurse and suggest the fact that caseworkers and physicians practicing preventive medicine are also *educational*."

Thus, the pattern was set. March 31, 1950, in a final memorandum prior to the establishment of the Demonstration ("An Experimental Demonstration in Health Maintenance"), Mr. Burritt reported the basic concepts, and the funds Community Service Society obligated itself to provide and suggested an Operating Board to supervise the project, Montefiore Hospital to carry out the plan, and the Columbia University College of Physicians and Surgeons as the affiliated university medical school.

Between 1943 and 1950 the Health Maintenance Committee, stimulated by Mr. Burritt and with the active interest of Mr. Milbank, of Dr. Baehr and Dr. Boudreau, had had time to flesh out its ideas. Dr. Thomas Dublin and Dr. Marta Fraenkel prepared a careful and detailed report to the Committee in 1948 outlining objectives and some research procedures. Montefiore Hospital (affiliated with the Columbia University College of Physicians) had a going medical group-practice unit with an excellent reputation and the Montefiore Hospital under the enlightened leadership of Dr. E. M. Bluestone was anxious to become involved in other community health activities. The Committee was able to move into action.

Many more than can be named here played a part in bringing about the Demonstration or in carrying it on. Some small tribute has been paid to Albert Milbank and Bailey Burritt. They were supported by the Operating Board and principally by Dr. George Baehr. The generous grant of the Community Service Society provided the initial base on which the Demonstration operated.

For Dr. Frank G. Boudreau's help enough thanks cannot be given. Besides providing additional monies each year for statistical research, he arranged that the 1953 annual meeting of the Milbank Memorial Fund be devoted to the Family Health Maintenance Demonstration and furnished two years' additional financial support from the Milbank Memorial Fund when the Community Service Society was unable to continue its support of the Demonstration after 1957.

Dr. Martin Cherkasky, presently Director of the Montefiore Hospital, was the first Director of the Family Health Maintenance Demonstration. He has remained a critical and helpful consultant and friend.

Dr. Donald Young of the Russell Sage Foundation provided a residency stipend for the social scientists who contributed important concepts to the Demonstration's work. The interest and advice of Dr. Esther Brown and Dr. Leonard Cottrell, of the Russell Sage Foundation, broadened the scope of the program. Dr. John Clausen of the National Institute of Mental Health (now at the University of California) offered patient counsel over the years.

The United States Public Health Service (Hospital and Medical Facilities Research Grant Committee) supplied the grant (W-95) which made it possible to report this program and its results.

A deep debt is owed to the physicians, social workers, and nurses who made the observations and carried out the field work. In a real sense they are co-authors.

The criticisms of Dr. Eliot Freidson helped greatly in the actual writing of the report. Mr. A. B. Siegelaub's recording, collection, and tabulation of information were basic to the development of the results and evaluations, and Mr. Monroe Lerner's resetting of the tables and analyses was vital in the preparation of the data. Appreciation is due Mrs. Edith Pais who did the I.B.M. machine operations, Miss Helen Schulman and Mrs. Gladys Hubler who did the typing and preparation of the manuscript. I want to thank also Mr. Joseph Axelrod, Medical Group Administrator, and Dr. Shirley Grossman, Deputy Medical Director, of the Montefiore Medical Group who relieved me of administrative obligations in the Medical Group during the time I was involved in the writing of this report.

Errors, omissions, inaccuracies, or infelicities of expression are entirely my responsibility.

Contents

CONTENTS

APPENDIXES

Tables

PART ONE

ORGANIZATION OF THE HEALTH TEAM

- I -

BEGINNINGS

I think it is only right to discourage at the very beginning, those dilettante readers who are searching for an unbiassed dissertation.

— William James, *The Will To Believe*

The roots of the Family Health Maintenance Demonstration go deep. The program's development was affected by changing social factors in disease and in medicine and changing attitudes toward health and toward medical care throughout the world. The fact that in 1948 community leaders could accept as feasible an experiment in providing a comprehensive family medical service is in itself an important statement about the climate of the time. Equally significant is the emphasis on health maintenance rather than sickness care, combining prevention and treatment of both physical and emotional disorder.[1]

Four major developments gave impetus to the idea of Family Health Maintenance, readied the minds of community leaders to accept such a conception, and prepared the framework on which a program could be built. First and most important was the recognition of the importance of prevention in disease and professional dedication to the concept of prevention. Second was the changing nature of medical practice deriving from the fact that chronic illness and psychiatric problems with their social implications increased in relative importance. Third was the growing conviction that mental and physical health were interrelated and that emotions had some part to play in disease causation and maintenance. Fourth was the changing role of professional work-

3

ers in the medical field, as a result of altered technology, the clashing expectations of patient and doctor, and the growing importance of paramedical workers in number and function.

Edgar Sydenstricker years ago laid out the problems of change and indicated the direction medical-care services should take, pointing out that the method of practice influenced access to medical care, partly through economics (the efficiency of group practice) and partly through improved quality of the services. He recognized the changing environmental contribution to health and disease, listing the factors that predisposed to sickness and the steps even then in process to arrest these evil effects. Growing urbanization and poor working and living conditions were offset by improved standards of living and working, greater diversity in diet, and more leisure and recreation. Health he saw as being in dynamic equilibrium with the environment, the changed needs inviting change in solutions. A part of this was the profound transformation imposed by the sanitary revolution of the early twentieth century, with new solutions unfolding as new problems arose.[2]

Since 1933 the changes Sydenstricker saw have become intensified, and diseases have appeared that were previously unknown or unrecognized. Urbanization, mechanization, and increasing mobility have isolated the family from the protection of community bonds, magnifying the peril to individual members as the family broke down or weakened in influence.[3] "Anomie" * is either increasing, or at any rate is increasingly an explanation of the psychological depression and anxiety of urban and civilized man.

These social changes were augmented by the changes in medical knowledge and treatment. One such development in recent years was largely the result of the conquest of epidemic and infectious disease. In 1900, with a population of 75,000,000, over 30,000 people died of infectious disease in the United States. In 1953, with the population at 160,000,000, only 9,000 died of infectious disease. More people survived to reach the older age

---

* Dürkheim invented this term to describe a specific social state. It is equated with a feeling of rootlessness and not belonging. More commonly now, anomie is applied to the state of mind or attitude of individuals suffering the result of this social situation (see his *Suicide*). Changing the rules of the game while maintaining the fiction that the old rules obtain, thereby creating frustrating frictions as the ideal and the real come into conflict is another definition of anomie.

groups, and these were more susceptible to, or eventually succumbed to, chronic diseases. The rank order of the causes of death changed radically. As tuberculosis, "the Captain of the Men of Death," fell into tenth place, heart disease and cancer rose to first and second place.[4] Chronic diseases usually require less dramatic medical attention, but more frequent, longer lasting, services; more important, they require the services of paramedical workers to a greater degree. Thus, another characteristic of changing need resulted from the changing rates and types of illness which required supervision in a continuous fashion, not episodically or only when grave illness occurred.

Other significant developments appeared after the Second World War: specialism in medical practice; a decreasing number of family doctors; increasing costs of medical care due to improvements in technology and increasing numbers of technicians; the central place of the hospital in teaching, research, and medical service; the increasingly psychiatric orientation of social work, coupled with the increasingly educational orientation of public health nursing. Obviously, a new plan for medical care had to include the family as the unit of service, a way of family doctoring that would involve paramedical workers along with the physician, prevention as well as treatment, group practice, and emphasis on emotional as well as physical health.

<h3 style="text-align:center">SOME PRECURSORS</h3>

While radical experimentation was indicated, precedents did exist. As far back as 1926, a "family club" was opened in South London by Williamson and Pearse which, while not so elaborate as the later Pioneer Health Centre (commonly referred to as "Peckham") established a basic pattern that became crucial in our own Family Health Maintenance Demonstration. Improvement of health was conditional on modification of the environment.[5] The early club offered only an annual physical examination, a room for social purposes, and a small day-care unit for children. The later center had extensive recreational facilities which helped to alter the milieu in which the people lived.[6]

The spirit, ideology, and goal of the Peckham Experiment informed the Family Health Maintenance Demonstration to a significant degree. Aware of the conclusions of Williamson and

5

Pearse, the Operating Board of the Family Health Maintenance Demonstration chose to provide comprehensive continuous medical care with health promotion added, as the contribution to modification of the environment.

The most striking similarity between the two programs was the family consultation. After the annual physical examination, the family met with the Peckham "biologists" and were informed of the defects and disorders discovered. "Information without advice" was the policy, and the families were expected to solve their own problems.[7] In the Family Health Maintenance Demonstration, the family conference was adopted as a major technique for health education and health promotion, but a schedule and plan for correction of defects was offered as well.

The idea of comprehensive family health service was also germinating in South Africa, in Sidney Kark's Institute of Family and Community Health.[8] This Institute Health Center developed principles of "health bookkeeping," health education, and health promotion which are similar to the physical examination records of Peckham and our own continuous records and activities. But the remoteness of South Africa prevented the information from circulating widely in the United States until after the Family Health Maintenance Demonstration was well under way. The disparity of problems in the rural locations, the differences in professional role, and the wide cultural gap also diluted the effect.[9]

THE FAMILY HEALTH TEAM OPERATION

The wide employment of the team concept in industry, government, and research made it seem reasonable to undertake to yoke together separate but interlinked professional skills in health services. However, when for thousands of years medicine had been identified with the individually practicing doctor, why did medical service in this age suddenly demand a team?

The four factors responsible for this trend to a team arrangement for the provision of medical care are: social change; changes in medical science; specialism and the changing doctor's role; and increasing costs of medical care.

Changes in living conditions and family patterns in the United States are clearly recognizable. We are all aware of the spectacular changes in disease prevalence and incidence and increased life expectancy.[10] Medicine is practiced in a complex social environment. Social needs modify medical practice. In the heyday of the Industrial Revolution, the blossoming industries needed more hands all the time. Illness, with its consequent loss of time or inefficiency, was intolerable. Interference with production was a social disaster, and public health development as an aspect of social reform owes its existence to the need to stem epidemics lest they interrupt production. At the same time society itself became an instrument for helping masses of people to get and keep jobs, funneling them into cities, and into tenements within cities, designing new goals of success and achievement, fragmenting family life, remolding character and personality to fit the new social demands. The new proletariat had to work hard and for long hours — women and children as well as men. Family life was weakened in other ways. More people, more crowding, and eventually, as transportation improved, more mobility, ruptured family linkages and made the individual uncomfortably independent. Industrialization and urbanization seriously threatened the supportive values of family life. Mutual help became more necessary but less socially acceptable. The goal of man had become independence, the struggle an individual one. Economic philosophy centered on laissez faire, on the individual. At the same time, the individual who suffered the consequences of social, emotional, and physical dislocation and who needed help, had nowhere to turn.

Those who suffered from this conflict tended to panic in the face of symptoms that might formerly have been dealt with by the family without a physician's attention. From the standpoint of medical practice, the effect of this new social situation was increased medical demand.[11] Furthermore, as the patient was educated into a social concept of medical care, he developed a new *expectation* of medical service. He saw the doctor as a friendly and knowledgeable professional person, an advisor in health and family problems, a neighbor easily available in times of emergency. He gave advice in a way acceptable to the patient, and whatever he ordered or devised for his care was realistic and feasible.

This is the Golden-Age doctor archetype of a century ago

7

whose pervasive image colors all modern thinking about medical care. With further social change, shifting family responsibility, increased medical demand, this image of the physician began to take on heroic dimensions.[12]

While social developments increased the need for a friendly family advisor type of doctor, American professional development was heading in the direction of specialism and away from family doctoring. The huge number of physicians who poured out of proprietary medical schools[13] in the nineteenth century, and apprentice training, as well as university teaching centers, reinforced the American image of the readily available family doctor. The competition inherent in such large numbers, however, laid the groundwork for specialism.[14]

The United States entered the twentieth century with an abundance of physicians, in higher proportion to the population than had ever existed anywhere before at any time. As a consequence, the rigid caste system which had developed in Europe because of the scarcity of physicians — where the wealthy had private doctors and the masses had a "poor" doctor — was nonexistent in the United States, where everyone could have a personal physician. This conformed with the egalitarian aspects of American life generally. But, once the scientific revolution made it possible to learn more about a certain medical subject, many physicians wanted to, and were able to, specialize. Unlike the European experience, it was not only possible for doctors to specialize, it was actually desirable in communities that were already crowded with physicians. In the beginning, specialists were self-trained. Very soon, however, medical education in the United States took its cue from Europe, the schools became more scientific and laboratory-oriented, and specialism began to follow the university pattern.[15]

Specialism could grow because of the large number of physicians and their desire to specialize, because training opportunities became increasingly available, and because specialism as an epitome of scientific medicine gained in prestige. It has grown so rapidly that, between 1910 and the present day, the percentage of specialists has increased from 20 percent to over 60 percent.[16] At present over 25,000 physicians are in training for specialties. Since most medical school graduates specialize, the day is ap-

8

proaching when there will be very few, if any, general practitioners.

The growth of medical knowledge with concentration on narrower fields within medical practice has had repercussions. Not too long ago a doctor went to school for three or four years, read a few books and kept copies of these in his library so that the sum total of medical knowledge was always available to him. What he learned about human relations or disease by the acuteness of his observation over the years of practice may have helped to make him a better doctor; but he didn't have to go back to school to learn more or different things, and there were few other books he had to read in his lifetime. Few journals came out with new observations or new findings to modify the old knowledge, increase the new, or change radically the base on which he was practicing.

Today it is quite otherwise.[17] Medicine undergoes almost revolutionary shifts in concept (Stress), emphasis (Psychosomatics), or etiology (Viruses). And there is a staggering inflow of new drugs and equipment. Today's doctor is constantly in danger of becoming obsolete. If he continues to practice only what he learned in medical school, in a very short time he must become a poorer physician. Unless he keeps up with changes he is not capable of providing modern medical care to his patients. This is true of specialists as well as general practitioners. The lack of organized liaison, or communication in daily medical practice is a serious defect which tends to make the doctor less a physician than a technician. Once the physician was responsible for all medical aspects of the patient's illness. Then specialism narrowed the range of his interest, apportioning elements of medical practice to different specialists, and "integration" was to be the generalist's role. Since the generalist is disappearing, who is to integrate the specialized activities in the patient's interest?

One of the solutions to this problem — integrating the fragments specialism has created — has been the development of group practice. Group practice has been growing at a slow but continuing rate.[18] Some of its increasing popularity is undoubtedly economic — shared space, facilities, and technical help are more efficient and offer financial advantage — but part of the growth derives from professional considerations of cooperative

9

medicine, sharing information, and more readily available consultations.[19] For patients group practice has gained in prestige from association with scientific medicine (The Mayo Clinic, for example), and criticism, though not rare, tends to be minimal.

ORGANIZATION OF THE MONTEFIORE MEDICAL GROUP

It was natural therefore for a new program of medical care such as the Family Health Maintenance Demonstration to be a part of group practice. The Montefiore Medical Group, on which the Family Health Maintenance Demonstration was based, is a somewhat unique type of group structure.[20]

The Group Practice Unit at the Montefiore Hospital was invited to participate in the Demonstration partly because of the university affiliation (Columbia University College of Physicians and Surgeons) and partly because of the standards that it had established for itself and was aiming to carry out as a participant group of the Health Insurance Plan of Greater New York.[21]

When the Health Insurance Plan started, it was felt that some model group (preferably hospital-based) was necessary in which standards of group practice could be developed. The Montefiore Medical Group was planned as a yardstick.

The following conditions were laid down:

(1) The Group was to use only internists* as family doctors. Since the general practitioner was not qualified for the complexity of modern practice, and declining in numbers anyway, his professional replacement might reasonably be expected to be found among the growing number of internists. The internist had sufficient training so that he could be at ease with his specialist colleagues, and the high degree of visibility of his work in group practice would not be a source of embarrassment.

(2) All the other specialists affiliated with the Group would have to be equally qualified (Board members or Board eligible), drawn from the staff of the hospital, or eligible for hospital staff service.

(3) The Group was to operate out of a single center. With-

---

* Eligible for or qualified by the American Board of Internal Medicine. His concern is adult medicine — everything that goes on inside the skin. He does not attempt to deal with pediatrics, obstetrics, dermatology, ophthalmology, or surgery, a smattering of each of which is needed by the generalist.

10

out unified quarters, group practice may be a nominal association of physicians, but in reality it is merely a series of solo practices.

(4) Division of income was to be arranged on a salary basis, with a job description and agreement of what constituted full-time work and full-time salary, and a proviso for equal pay for equal training, experience, and seniority. This scheme abolished any incentive for full-time people to compete for patients, and abolished the differential income between operating and non-operating specialists which exists in ordinary practice.[22]

(5) Supervision was applied through conferences, record review, and physician committee activities. The process of supervision in the Group may be somewhat less formal than in the hospital itself, but the necessity for registration of diagnoses through the hospital record room and the periodic conferences of the various clinical divisions mean that the doctor's work in the Group comes up for constant review within the hospital.

The nature of the "yardstick" that the Montefiore Medical Group offered has something of the nature of a hospital teaching unit: physicians of high quality in close physical proximity of practice, under formal economic and practice arrangements, with a considerable degree of hospital supervision, providing medical care to subscribers of the Health Insurance Plan. Within such a structure, where physicians could practice untrammeled by financial considerations, it was expected that there would be satisfaction for patients and doctors as well as opportunities for study of patients, doctors, and medical practice.

Family Practice

Nevertheless, a missing element made it impossible for group practice to provide the family medical care envisioned for the Family Health Maintenance Demonstration. A barrier prevented the internist from carrying out the role of family guide and advisor despite the cohesive tendency of group practice. Bringing together the fragmented elements of practice is useful, but what if family practice is neither emphasized nor highly respected in medical school, and already other professional groups have accepted responsibility for some of the fragments?

It is fruitless to look for family orientation in the internist, a specialist, when even the small number of generalists turned out lack it because nonlaboratory interests are deemphasized in medical training. Yet the patient demands "family doctoring." There may be a higher degree of sophistication in health matters among patients than ever before — assuming that more schooling and more exposure to magazine, newspaper, radio, and TV health education lead to more sophistication — but basic patient attitudes toward physicians do not seem to change. The patient's view of the doctor's role stubbornly retains its traditional features.[23] But doctors no longer see themselves this way. Medical schools bend their efforts to turn out laboratory scientists. If patients expect to have pain relieved, or discomfort allayed, or fear warded off, and expect this of the practitioner, he sees himself diagnosing and treating illness, exercises in which relief of discomfort or pain or fear are desirable but secondary. How the doctor visualizes himself has an important bearing on what he does, and therefore on whether the patient will be satisfied.[24] Our Group doctors were like other doctors in this regard, removed from the popular understanding of medical practice, laboratory-oriented, and enthusiastically interested in their specialties. They were bedeviled by this lost liaison to the needs of the patient, and bewildered by the patients' criticism.

As specialism increased, some components of general practice gravitated out of medicine entirely, and were absorbed into other disciplines. Since these continued to be important aspects of satisfactory medical care, responsibility for them had to be established by introducing these other disciplines into daily medical practice. The most noticeable change has occurred in technology where technicians do laboratory, radiologic, and therapeutic tasks the physician himself disdains. But even in the area of patient care, the physician has yielded some responsibilities.

The medical social worker dealing with emotional problems of individuals and disputed family relations and the nurse taking on preventive services and family advisor functions relieve the doctor in precisely those areas which medical education has tended to exclude. As a corollary, increasing numbers of non-physicians have become concerned with the practice of medicine.[25] The very number of physicians engaged in specialized practice, although increasing the doctor's knowledge and power in a limited field, decreases his ability to control the field of medicine in general.

Integration of medical care *and* family service were the hall-marks of the generalist, and for the internist of a group practice to replace him as family doctor, he had to be encouraged to adopt the integrative approach to family care while using his more advanced medical skills. This really required a different type of doctor, a product of a different type of medical education. A host of new educational approaches and curriculum content changes are being leveled against the scientism of most medical schools. Western Reserve and Cornell have launched revolutionary programs of medical education that will undoubtedly provide differently (and from this viewpoint *better*) prepared doctors. Other schools are engaged in a variety of experimental changes in the curriculum to encourage family practice. Psychiatric course content in many schools is directed at helping provide such interest and skills. The development of preceptorships which will allow medical students to see family problems is also encouraging. Attacking from another angle, the earnest solicitation of practicing physicians to acquire psychiatric orientation so as to want to, and know how to, deal with family problems is being attempted.[26]

Family orientation and concern for problems formerly disregarded or relegated to paramedical workers may restore the doctor of tomorrow to a central place in family medical service, and realign the doctor's image of himself with the patient's image of him. But for the purpose of the Demonstration at the time it was being organized, the use of nurse and social worker to augment the doctor's role in patient care seemed obligatory.

-II-

PROBLEMS OF EMOTIONAL HEALTH
AND TREATMENT

> Happy families are all alike; every unhappy family is unhappy in its own way.
>
> — Leo Tolstoy, *Anna Karenina*

A series of related assumptions underlay the design of the Family Health Maintenance Demonstration. The leading assumption was, of course, that "something" could be done (and observed) that would favorably influence the health of families concerned.[1] It will be useful to look at the conception of "health" operative in the Demonstration, but first the chain of assumptions should be outlined:

(1) Behavior, sick or well, is predicated upon early conditioning.

(2) The family is the main source of early conditioning.

(3) In this conditioning, the mother is the most important family figure.

(4) Modification of behavior necessitates modifying maternal child-rearing practices.

(5) The milieu and interaction of family members influence maternal attitudes, and so family attitudes must be modified as well. In addition to these assumptions — or "axioms" — other socially current maxims were applied: that health education and health promotion as well as treatment of existing defects are valuable instruments for modification of both interpersonal problems and child-rearing practices; and that such modification can

14

be stimulated by advice and guidance in daily medical practice. To these was added our own unique Demonstration assumption — that a health team, substituting for the family doctor, is an appropriate device for carrying on these daily health services.

At the risk of engaging in too broad a philosophical discourse, I would like to examine a few of our working hypotheses.

BEHAVIOR AND EARLY CONDITIONING

A great deal of information, some derived from studies and observations, some from impressions and speculations, is available in the area of behavior and early conditioning. Probably the clearest compilation from the psychoanalytic viewpoint is *Maternal Care and Mental Health* by J. Bowlby who states: "our relationships with friends, acquaintances and professional colleagues are in great measure colored by our relationships within our families — relationships which carry . . . emotional significance for us . . . The form our family relationships take when we are grown up is to a high degree dependent on the form they took in our early years, and the very first relationship we made — that with our mothers — is the most important of all."[2]

Not only psychoanalysts emphasize the role of the family in molding character. Social scientists underline the fact that "the family . . . is the major transmission belt for the diffusion of cultural standards to the oncoming generation." Merton places the emphasis somewhat differently from Bowlby when he says, further: "*The projection of parental ambitions* onto the child is also centrally relevant."[3] It is clear that parental attitudes and values are formative of the child's, and later adult's, character and behavior. Piaget writes "Society is nothing but a series . . . of generations each exercising pressure on the one which follows it."[4]

From this premise arises the emphasis on child care and the concern with the child as the central figure in the Family Health Maintenance Demonstration, a corollary of the assumption that health and healthy functioning in adult life could be ordered most effectively through improving the physical and emotional health of children.

Those who have had an opportunity to observe family development in other parts of the world uphold the point of view that

15

there is a basic human pattern, and a common quality of childhood behavior, childhood needs, and childhood responses.[5]

If this is true, defective mothering must be considered dangerous to wholesome childhood development. Gross defects such as absolute deprivation of love, "hospitalism" (Spitz's excellent phrase), or institutional care generally are quite easily recognizable.[6]

The Critical Phase. Early conditioning may have a time element; that is, traumata will not always produce the same, or any, effects unless they are introduced at some significant juncture. This theory, termed by Bowlby "the critical phase," presumes that an emotion-provoking event or stressful situation will have more effect at one point in the developmental history than in another.[7] A tissue or organ is "ready" at a certain moment to be damaged. Lack of vitamins in childhood is pathogenic of defects that lack of the same vitamins in adult life will not induce. So, if vitamin and mineral lack in childhood and oxygen deprivation or infection in utero may have an impact on the growing child varying as the stage of development of that child, why not emotional traumata?

Cultural Factors. Concepts such as "social isolation," as it affects parental behavior and children's emotional reactions, enter into consideration. There is a logical possibility that prolonged dependency may produce a crippled personality in the psychosexual area.

Another cultural influence derives from parental behavior's differing from the child's expectations — as in the children of immigrant families. If "Personality develops in the child and the adult through interaction with their culture," defective behavior patterns might reflect disturbances in the family pattern because of such cultural incompatibility.[8]

The Marital Relation

The self-perpetuating nature of conditioning factors is curious. Cottrell said, "Marriage adjustment may be regarded as a process in which marriage partners attempt to re-enact certain relational systems or situations which obtain in their own earlier family groups. Or in other words, marriage partners tend to play the habitual roles they evolve in their childhood and adolescence."[9] The overwhelmingly important maternal figure, carving the child's character, has herself been shaped (predestined?) by similar forces. For this reason we concerned ourselves intensively with the nature of marital relations. Because sexual activity gave us a clue about the person, we were interested in his sex life.[10] Life behavior and sexual behavior are so related that it is impossible to determine whether sexual difficulties are causes or results of family problems. Although one can obtain histories of impotent men and frigid women, of disturbed or distorted sexual relationships, and disturbed or distorted patterns of behavior in the children in such households, cause and effect were unclear. Sexual behavior was evidence of the *type* of interpersonal behavior that could be expected of the individual, and as such was observed and noted. Furthermore, since the children would take the parents as models, evidences of affection, or lack of it, in the parental relationship would be conditioning factors in the future course of the child's life.[11]

The Influence of the Milieu

Parental attitudes, various elements in the family relationship, cultural values, and social pressures, all play a part in forming character,[12] but a word of caution is in order as to how rigidly the formulation of the effects of child-rearing practices on personality or disordered action can be applied.[13] None of the evidence favors a one-to-one relation; it seems to be a matter of the totality of influences — the milieu itself.

Within the milieu, factors that condition parents condition the children as well. The parents' social view of the world may interfere with or facilitate guidance. Where parental behavior and the social norm conflict, the child's milieu will not be consistent and difficulties may develop in his behavior pattern. At the same time, parental behavior consistent with the social norm may be pathogenic of behavior disorder in a specific child.[14] Looking at these factors from the standpoint of health promotion — for example, what might be done to influence parents to modify child-rearing practices so as to reduce the conflict — the obstacles become apparent. Yet the need for retaining a perspective on social attitudes and the need for modifying parental attitudes had to be worked into the program.

17

The milieu and the family mold behavior by exercising controls. As we examined parental influences, the emphasis was on the power of love and affection on future behavior. At the same time, children have to learn to do without, to accept frustration, to share and help and give as well as take. "Permissiveness," which is assumed as "good" in child-rearing practice, does not imply "without limits."

A child may require parental control to feel protected. Without such control he may feel abandoned and insecure, "unwanted." Anna Freud says that children have to be deprived, that this deprivation and frustration is part of emotional development. This is the way the child matures, by learning to delay gratification.[15] Again two apparently contradictory approaches to child-rearing must be reconciled. Our assumption was that in each family the presence and type of control in child-rearing was a formative influence on later behavior.[16]

Conclusions

First, early conditioning, particularly the mother's affectionate care, is very important in healthy child-rearing. Too much affection, smothering the child, not allowing him to assert his independence or find the limits of acceptable social behavior seems to be a bad form of early conditioning.

Second, sexual satisfaction and the marital relation are important components of the mother's satisfaction and therefore of her maternal role.

Third, social and cultural factors influence children's character — both directly, and indirectly through a molding of parental character.

And, finally, parental attitudes and the other influences are more or less important, depending on the phase of child development during which crucial events take place.

From these it is but a step to the designation of the preventive role of any family health program as focusing on childhood. In a child-centered culture it is easier to get action from a family if what is to be done is related to the welfare of the children. Further, childhood is the time in which the greatest amount of preventive service can be done, in which the greatest amount of visible progress might be noted, and in which preventive services might have the most lasting effects.

HEALTH — QUESTING FOR A DEFINITION

It is hard to quarrel with anyone in favor of health, and it seems almost unfriendly to seek precise knowledge of what health is. Yet, in order for the Demonstration to draw any meaningful conclusions in the research area, health had to be defined. To say a family "improved," implied a point before and a point after, or at least a direction. The dictionary definition of health is periphrastic ("physical and mental well-being"), and that of the World Health Organization is hardly less so ("a state of complete physical, mental and social well-being").[17] Neither measures "well-being." We sought unsuccessfully for a definition which would enable us to devise a numerical scale of health.

Very early, it became clear that health as a substance to be measured was an illusion. There were actions, feelings, attitudes, and physical states that could be judged "healthy," but none of these was a simple measurable quantity. Health was really a series of *attributes* of behavior. It is important to see health as an attribute of function, a description of functioning in which a human being accomplishes (or fails) according to his nature. So, for our purposes, we tried to assess appropriate functioning in those areas in which a human being demonstrates his humanity: work, play, sex, and family life.

As far as physical condition is concerned, healthy functioning is not too difficult to recognize or score. We can recognize disease, gauge its seriousness, and measure the degree to which activity is hampered. We can know and measure the range of chemical constituents in the blood and body fluids and what their superabundance or deficit may imply.

Emotional health, the crucial "feeling" and social reaction that is "healthy," is far more difficult to pin down. Yet it is really the health of the whole person, not just physical health that we had in mind when we defined healthy functioning.[18] It was to the concept of healthy functioning that we turned next.

Alcmeon of Crotona over two milleniums ago defined health as harmony. If by harmony we mean a dynamic, changing relationship to meet changing situations the definition is hard to improve

19

on. Disease and decompensation become synonymous.[19] The definition is attractive too because it portrays healthy functioning as a range of activities and allows for the appearance of apparently unhealthy activity within healthy individuals. It helps to visualize people and families as composed of disparate elements, healthy and unhealthy, so that the appearance of unhealthy signs or symptoms may be anticipated. Wide fluctuations of behavior may be neither serious nor dangerous. And prevention may be defined as damping the oscillation to help maintain a steady state with lesser fluctuation.

"Healthy" versus "Normal"

Ross and Van den Haag eliminate "normal" as an attribute synonymous with healthy by defining norm as conformity to a socially accepted rule.[20] On this basis, both sick and healthy may be conformists, and therefore normal. Conversely, neither conformity nor rebelliousness may be considered a sign of either health or sickness.[21]

In this connection, note must be taken of the widespread use of the word "sick" to describe behavior judged not normal or not healthy. The word is used so carelessly (by professional people as well as laymen) that one becomes uncomfortable in its presence. We must distinguish between the sickness of decompensation and sickness of symptomatology in an otherwise well compensated person. "Sick" refers only to the symptom. Just as a headache may be trivial in origin or most ominous, one cannot judge from the symptom alone. Whatever one thinks or feels about the patterns of behavior, unless they are disruptive of functioning, they cannot be considered unhealthy.

As a corollary in this rather tenuous area of health and emotional symptoms it was necessary to develop standards of what constituted clear evidence of sickness.[22] For our purposes, it was assumed that behavior characteristics of children such as nail biting, enuresis, and nightmares were evidences of malfunctioning. We did not conclude that these were permanent evidences of malfunction, nor that they had any predictive value, but they were to be noted and considered.

Summing up, health is a word difficult to define and not measurable as a substance. As an attribute, "healthy" can be applied to functioning; and in human beings the functions of work, sex, play, and family life can show visible, measurable evidences of healthy or unhealthy functioning. "Normal" (as average) is not synonymous with healthy, and the harmonious balance which is healthy may contain unhealthy elements in a moment in time or swing through unhealthy behavior periods without rendering the whole of the behavior pattern unhealthy. It is not surprising therefore to find symptomatic or "unhealthy" traits in "normal" families.

ANXIETY — A BRIEF NOTE

Among the very first observations made, while the program was still in the process of formation, was the prevalence of anxiety in the family members. The physician noted "anxiety" or "tension" in his observations as part of the physical examination in, if not the majority, at least a large number of cases. This was disconcerting because we had previously decided to include "anxiety" as an emotional defect. By implication, a large number of people would have to be marked down automatically in the evaluation, because of the presence of anxiety. Examination of the literature showed that there was no lack of literary sources for discussion, but scientific investigation was very meager. Some scales had been developed [23] but they avoided the real issue: is anxiety abnormal, or conversely, is there such a thing as normal anxiety? [24] There seems to be no agreement among physicians as to what anxiety is, let alone whether it is an evidence of an abnormal or unhealthy state. Some psychiatrists have divided anxiety into two types — precursor of adjustment and consequence of breakdown of adjustment. Others conceive of it as a feeling associated with bodily disorders, and deny that it is either a cause or manifestation of emotional disorder. [25] Anxiety is a general, pervasive phenomenon, historically associated with human behavior under stress and not necessarily evidence of emotional illness. [26] It is not anxiety itself that is abnormal but the degree of anxiety and its appropriateness.

For our purposes anxiety as such was not measured. We had to determine whether the anxiety was based on real events and real possibilities or on psychological constructions which might be called figments; then, given a stressful situation, whether the degree of anxiety was appropriate. It is futile to try to establish a standard of wellness in which an individual would be completely free of anxiety or one in which anxiety would be an indicator of illness. If the person was anxious, it was considered within the context of his whole functioning. If he functioned poorly or there was interference in the areas of work, play, sex, and family life, and if anxiety were a contributing factor in the development of this malfunctioning, the anxiety would be mentioned or scored.

THE HEALTH OF THE FAMILY

The key word in the title of our Demonstration is "family." Much of the emphasis of our program and the focus of the research design derives from the assumption that the family is the basic unit and primary source of learning social behavior. But even superficial observation provides an amazing variety of patterns of family living, arising in part from the origins of the individual family members, ethnic and cultural diversity, kinds of work, and amount of education. The burdens and stresses of economic and social life, the problems of politics and international relations, the destructive potential of nuclear weapons, the death throes of colonialism, and the rise of virulent types of nationalism, all have an impact on the family. While the family is conceived of as playing a part in fostering these various social and political phenomena, the relation is clearly reciprocal. So, we are faced with an ambiguous reality; while we are concerned with measuring the effectiveness of the family in socializing the individual and thereby serving society, at the same time society may be modifying family structure and family attitudes so as to impair this effectiveness. Therefore, measurements of healthy functioning in individuals must be correlated with reference to forces outside the family. However, the assumption mentioned earlier, of the powerful effect of the early maternal relation leads to the conception of the family unit as largest in influence on the formation of character — with society (the neighborhood and the world outside) of lesser importance. It was reassuring to recall that control families were involved in the measurement, balancing the effect of society; as we worked with and measured the study families, we could expect that extrafamilial influences, however great, were working equally on study and control families.

The Job of The Family

What was a "healthy" family? How could it be described, and what criteria were to be used in evaluating the success of the family in meeting its obligations? By and large, "healthy family" is defined in descriptive terms, like the embodiment of "good" qualities (socially desirable) in a children's tale.[27] The statements are so general as to be useless as criteria; they have no substantive or predictive value. As goals, the attitudes may be valuable, but as living standards they are hopeless.

A recent publication of the Community Service Society answers the question, "What is a family for?," by outlining general functions. The family's basic biological function is reproduction, not only of human life but as a transmitter of our heritage and culture, transferring from one generation to another the special way of life that makes up a civilization.[28] It provides physical security, protection, and material opportunities for living and for growth. It is a place where enduring and deep emotional satisfactions can be achieved, and where adults and children are given opportunities for emotional, intellectual, spiritual, and social development so that they may acquire a feeling of usefulness, self-respect, and belonging. Socially desirable character traits can be instilled in the members by the family, and sound relations between the members of the family and the outside community can be fostered.[29]

While these functions lend themselves better to classification and measurement they still lack dynamism. The family today is in a transitional state. Many personal needs are met from outside the family. Not only are clothing and food purchased, but welfare services have become agency functions. More income has resulted from additional family members working but this has created other stresses.[30]

This transitional state may be seen in the ambivalent public attitudes toward child care. There is no single "right" way of dealing with children, and it is important that the "right" thing be done for them. All definitions of a "good" marriage include common goals, satisfactory sexual relationship, and favorable atmosphere for individual personality development, but emphasize the child as the cement of the family.[31] Since our culture is so child-oriented, many people become unduly concerned about child-rearing practices. With a wealth of contradictory advice in popular publications, disquiet and conflict are engendered by the compulsion to do more than what one is already doing for children.

There may also be public acceptance and private rejection of cultural norms. What mothers say at P.T.A. meetings as opposed to what they do in the privacy of their homes may arouse conflict in the children, and in them. Many mothers go through great anguish at the inability to do the "right" thing or to keep from doing the "wrong" thing, conditioned on the one hand by their background and on the other by the pressures of school and society.

Changing function and changing structure unsettle family attitudes. But taken together, we do care about what will become of our children. The pilot study of the Family Health Maintenance Demonstration supports this contention. Before we started on the full 150-family study, we wanted to know if we could obtain participation by simply inviting random families to come into the program. Of the families invited, those with children were more cooperative. The families with children who refused to participate did so because of unwillingness to separate themselves from a familiar doctor, or unwillingness to put themselves in the hands of an unfamiliar one. Again medical concern for the children, rather than disinterest, dictated the refusal. This fact was underscored in final program interviews, when parents admitted that their satisfaction stemmed in some part from the better care for their children in the Demonstration.

Family Stability

There are gaps in our knowledge of what the best family may be and a suspicion that the features of the family are changing, as well as evidence that the family may not always do what is best for children, but there is no question about the fact that children need families. They need mothers at any rate, and mothering is a family trait.[32]

Families are important because of what happens to people in them, and without them. Not only is the traumatic separation of an institution, or total absence of the mother, harmful, but even

24

the more subtle separation of an ever-changing sequence of maids, governesses, and so on may result in emotional deprivation.[33] Maternal love seems to be a necessity for healthy growth. So compelling is the relation of cherishing mother to sound child that the public health successes of the recent century are mourned by some as emotionally pathogenic while physically salutary. Mildred Creak writes that children were prized in earlier times because of the appalling death rates of the young. Now, "Parents no longer cherish a large family, hoping to keep some of their children alive: instead they are engaged in a competitive attempt to produce perfection out of a relatively small number of children." [34]

In carrying on a study like the Family Health Maintenance Demonstration we had to be aware of implicit threats to family stability and maternal attitudes. It was considered desirable to know about a parent's childhood in order to get a perspective on attitudes and values used by parents in indoctrinating their children. Social events and catastrophes have their effect and enter into consideration of child-rearing practices. Life experiences had to be evaluated. Illness in a family member has a disruptive effect and may seriously interfere with family stability and effective mothering.[35] It is evident that a medical care service has a large, if ill-defined, impact on family health which evolves from more than simply treating disease in a family member.

The health of the family has to be seen from the standpoint of family function and particularly from the needs of the children. A balance of forces exists within the family structure. In fostering healthy functioning in the children the mother plays the key role in this balance. But she, like the other family members, is a product of past events and conditioning. Parents are blamed (or blame themselves) for the difficulties of their children, and the children grow up to blame their parents (or to feel guilty for what they are doing to their own children). It seems inevitably circular, and if anything is to be done for the family in the way of preventive medicine, it would have to be in the breaking of the circle. It seems desirable to concentrate on one generation, introducing a feeling of health and security there so that, hopefully, the next generation will grow up with a little better insight. Then, they as parents will feel a little less guilty and be able to give their chil-

25

dren a little more security and satisfaction. This constitutes the program of the Family Health Maintenance Demonstration: To concentrate on the children and on health promotional activities.[36]

~ III ~

AIMS AND METHODS OF THE STUDY DESIGN

The objective of medicine is the preservation of life, the complete and perfect exercise of all its functions or the restoration of health which is seen in three different states: Sustained in full vigor; endangered and in jeopardy; or finally, broken and destroyed.

— François Joseph Callot, *The Concept and Triumph of Medicine*

Callot continues: "When there is health and vigor, medicine is concerned to safeguard and maintain it by virtue of a knowledge of all the factors which favor well-being . . . If health is in jeopardy, then it is the task of medicine to foresee the danger and to devise precautionary steps to ward off the menace and put the enemy to flight. But if health and vigor have been lost, whether because of the onslaught of the powerful enemy or as a consequence of neglect, then medicine should redouble its efforts to secure a capitulation on the best possible terms." [1]

ORGANIZATION AND DEFINITION OF OBJECTIVES

Despite the 200-year gap between Callot and the architects of the Family Health Maintenance Demonstration, there is congruence of views. Only the possibilities of attainment have improved markedly in our time. "Preservation of life" and "restoration of health," objectives toward which we have moved clearly and strongly in the twentieth century, epitomize the Demonstration. "Complete and perfect exercise of functions" represents a more complicated and less easily defined conception, and one of whose

27

achievement we must be more uncertain, as in our struggle to define "health." Could we "foresee the danger?" Did we even know it? How were we to "devise precautionary steps to ward off the menace and put the enemy to flight?"

In the Family Health Maintenance Demonstration, while a path was being marked out toward the attainment of objectives, the objectives themselves had to be clarified. We were charged with providing an organized service to maintain and improve family health, but we had to pose and answer questions about what we were doing. This dual role of investigation and provision of service was difficult since assessment of results had to be part of the effort. Our objectives reflect this duality and underline the difficulties. The design of the program required novel methods, flexibility, and predisposition to change; yet research design demanded consistency and invariance for the sake of comparability. Objectives to meet service *and* research needs had to be defined.

Cherkasky summarized the broad objectives succinctly:

1. To determine how best the family can be motivated or their known motivations utilized to make them see health.
2. To determine what range and kind of services are necessary in the encouragement and maintenance of health.
3. To systematically record observations about a family in a manner which will be susceptible to scientific evaluation and analysis.
4. To determine objectively the difference in health of those families receiving such care as compared to the control groups.
5. To provide Family Health Maintenance on so realistic a basis that it is reproducible elsewhere.[2]

Dublin and Fraenkel had catalogued similar objectives although with more of the research aims in mind. Their original projection of a program was very close to what we finally undertook.[3]

Methodology followed upon the heels of these objectives. Cherkasky outlined the procedures to be followed: a health team; a health inventory as a baseline for family evaluations; family conferences; team conferences; team care, group health education and health promotion.[4]

It would be hard to match the blithe confidence with which the organization of the Demonstration was begun. The decision to locate the program at the Montefiore Hospital was made late in 1949, and by the end of 1950 a staff had been assembled so that a pilot investigation of 20 families could be undertaken early in 1951. This pilot group was to provide a methodological sample initially, furnish information both about family interest in such a health endeavor and family motivation toward the pursuit of health. It was at this point that the magnitude of the undertaking and the vastness of the uncharted area upon which this Demonstration was entering became more apparent.

First, even in putting the staff together the composition of the team and interaction between members had to be weighed, assumptions made, and professional interrelationships justified. What is a "team"? Given the job to be done, is there only one specific kind of worker to do it? Should one worker be trained to do a number of jobs or should we concentrate on specialists? In brief, do we accept existing medical care organizations, personnel, job descriptions? If not, what do we construct in their place?

Second, how many families can we take as a continuing responsibility and what shall we define as a family? How shall they be selected, for comparability, statistical purposes, and even geographical area of service? What about controls?

Third, what sorts of forms will be necessary to maintain service records and utilization and evaluation records? Can one source be used for all of them? Or must each be gathered separately? Can research needs be met by a code so objective that it is unnecessary that the records be continuously maintained? Or are subjective experiences to be noted while still fresh?

Fourth, could we arrive at agreement rapidly on objective and useful criteria for the standard content of the examinations, interviews and evaluation data of the "health inventory"? Last, and unfortunately not the least, what about definitions? Health, for example, what was to be its criterion in measurement? How would anxiety be measured?

We came to terms with some of the questions quickly (if not perfectly) and accepted certain definitions as guides for the program. With the help of an expert in the field * we developed a set of record forms for daily staff reporting of services, and the

* Mr. Louis Feldman, registrar of the Health Insurance Plan of Greater New York.

accumulation of service data. An evaluation form was worked out to include all the areas in which family members would be scored, and an appropriate scoring system was devised. A good deal of discussion went on for almost a year as to the values inherent in scoring systems of 3, 4, 5, and 7 steps and odd versus even steps. Since there seem to be arguments of equal weight for all, eventually it was decided arbitrarily in favor of a 4-step scoring system, with fairly elaborate definitions of the steps to try to avoid the "shading" which is the bane of most such scales. This scale did not prove satisfactory in the long run, for it was mostly used as a 2-step or 3-step scale, and had value primarily in that the scores indicated direction of change rather than absolute value of the changes marked in the families.[5]

The content of the "health inventory" was fairly soon agreed upon and schedules completed. In addition to customary history, physical examination, laboratory work, and tests of visual and auditory acuity, a dental evaluation was completed on each person. The direction of questioning in the social work interview (on which scoring was based) and the content of the housing and nutrition forms obtained by the nurse (also used in scoring) can be seen in the appended instruction sheets.

It was decided to postpone coding and punching of service data necessary for research. This turned out to be an unwise decision that proved very costly in time at the end of the program. Instead of the staff people providing daily material for coding, service records were kept in continuous essay form, like ordinary medical records, and used as such. It was time-consuming, tedious, and difficult to sort these out 5 and more years later and record them separately for quantitative purposes.

SELECTION OF FAMILIES

For the purposes of the study, a family was defined as a group of people living together in a single establishment, related by blood or marriage. This enabled us to take into account and under our care parents of a Health Insurance Plan subscriber (otherwise not covered by the contract) or other relatives boarding with the family. Families were selected according to the following criteria: members of the Health Insurance Plan belonging to the Montefiore Medical Group and resident in the 1951 zone of coverage;

both parents alive, and father not more than 45 years old; with a few deliberate exceptions, at least one child.

From the 5000 families belonging to the Montefiore Medical Group the Machine Records Unit of the Health Insurance Plan selected a random group of 35 families which had the first two characteristics. These families were the "pilot group" in 1951. Of the 35, only 20 agreed to participate. Of the 15 families who did not agree to participate, 3 families were not reached at all, 3 were not interested, and the others refused because of the pressure of work. Of the 20 participating families only 2 had no children, while of the 15 nonparticipating, 8 had no children. It seemed obvious that concern for the children was a prime factor in participation. In the introductory discussions, the parents were told of the examinations and interviews that would be carried out, and the amount of time that might be involved. They seemed content to accept the burden because of the value to them of help for the children.

For this reason, when it came to selecting the study group, to ensure maximum participation of families in the program we added the qualification that the family have a child. In two cases we did select young married couples without children in the hope that they might have children while under observation and so add another dimension to our information.

The pilot group was of outstanding value in that it offered a testing ground of methods and techniques that were later extended to the Demonstration. An early staff meeting report (January 1951) reads, "In summary, it was the general consensus of opinion that the first 20 families of the experimental group should be seen as soon as possible and should be used as a pilot experiment; that the results obtained from working with these families should not be incorporated as part of the total experiment; that these 20 families should be given service but their primary use should be experimental in terms of the initial approach of the staff." Because their selection was not made on the same basis as the study families, and the methods varied from later methods, this pilot group information cannot be included in the results. In the tables where there is noted "Pilot Study" and "Pilot Control"

31

figures along with or sometimes separate from "Study" and "Control" family data, "Pilot" refers to these initial 20 families.

DURATION OF STUDY

The duration of the Demonstration had to be extended as a result of experience, and in response to an unforeseen problem. When the Health Maintenance Committee budgeted for the Demonstration, the members agreed to a 5-year study. This seemed a reasonable time for observation of families, and indeed it is. However, the complexity of examining and interviewing families — what with jobs, school, and other time limitations (including procrastination on the part of families in an unfamiliar medical milieu) — created unexpected delays. Estimates of how long it might take for a complete examination, laboratory work, psychological testing, and interviews ran to 5 and 6 hours in advance of the study. This turned out to be quite accurate, but the 6 hours could not be taken concurrently or during the working day. A great deal of work had to be done nights and weekends. There occurred lapses between appointments, follow-ups, and returns. At one time 500 families had been envisioned as the study group. Using 2 teams of examiners, it took 2 years to bring less than 150 families into the study group.

When it became apparent that there would be a protracted time interval in including study families, a decision was made that each family should have at least 4 years of observation. This meant that, if 2 years were required to do an initial evaluation on 150 study families, 2 more years might be required to do final evaluations on them. If 4 years of service were provided to each family, the program would consume 8 years.

During the first 2 years, in addition to time needed for evaluations, time would be needed to provide services — both medical care and health promotional — to the increasing number of people in the study group. During the last 2 years, while final evaluations were being done on study families, time made available from services no longer required by families which had dropped out of the program would be used for final evaluations on *control* families. Therefore 2 teams would be employed continuously during the 8 years and the efficiency of the operation worked out reasonably well.

Through the generosity and sympathetic cooperation of Dr. Frank Boudreau and the Milbank Memorial Fund, additional funds were made available to complete the 8 years of Demonstration activity, after the Community Service Society could not find funds for support for more than 6 years.

SOME STATISTICAL QUESTIONS

The Sample

Some of the questions raised in developing Demonstration methodology stubbornly eluded either quick or satisfactory answers. Selecting the experimental sample from the Health Insurance Plan population presented no difficulty. Data indicated the comparability of New York City population with the Health Insurance Plan population;[6] use of a random sample of the Health Insurance Plan population of the Montefiore Medical Group could be expected to yield information applicable in some degree rather more widely than to that limited group. Since one of the objectives of the Demonstration was to apply the lessons learned, it was important that the lessons *could* be extrapolated. However, a good bit of discussion was engendered by the fact that Health Insurance Plan subscribers were to be used exclusively. One could argue (and some did) that we were actually setting ourselves an impossible task by so doing. Health Insurance Plan subscribers were entitled to comprehensive medical care within a prepayment framework — less than 5 percent of the population of the United States had such coverage. And since about one-third of the sample had been in the Health Insurance Plan for a full year prior to selection, it seemed likely that they would have had their ills cared for and be fairly near the top of the scale physically. Would we be hobbling ourselves in that improvement could not be shown? Others argued that the routine accessibility to medical care which is part of the Health Insurance Plan pattern and the group practice structure separated this group of patients sharply from comparability with the rest of the people in the United States.

33

Controls

In any case, a control group was clearly needed. Not only did we need to know if study families would change over the years of observation, but we needed to know if the change was attributable to our intervention. A control group, not exposed to the new medical-care system and the added health-promotion activities, was necessary to furnish background information on what general changes occurred in the HIP population during the study period.

This was managed easily by the device of "matched controls." As a list of 100 families was provided by the Machine Records Unit, a coin was tossed for each pair. If the coin came up heads, the first member of the pair was the study family, and the other a control. If the coin turned up tails, the first member of the pair was the control, and the other the study family. Matched control families were carried during the same period as the matched study families, and dropped simultaneously, so that the periods under review for both groups were identical.

A conference held under the auspices of the Milbank Memorial Fund in 1953 was helpful in clarifying many problems relating to the structure and direction of the Family Health Maintenance Demonstration, but nowhere more helpful than in the statistical area. It was as a direct result of this conference, for instance, that the steps were taken to get some information on the controls as *initial* data. Prior to the conference, it had been the intention to do only *final* evaluations on the control families. This had been decided out of respect for the "Hawthorne" effect,[7] that tampering with the controls in any way would alter their response, and partly on moral grounds, that to find defect or disease, or incipient disaster, and not take steps to help was in violation of human as well as professional codes of conduct. On the other hand, under such circumstances, to help would be to destroy the effectiveness of the controls. Obtaining by mail information in specific areas, enough to assure comparability, would not affect either condition.[8]

Matching did not dispose of all statistical control problems, some of which we did *not* resolve. Of the families selected as study, 85 percent agreed to participate. The control families were not actually invited to share the total experiences but were asked to fill out forms — either by mail or with the help of a program nurse. Again about 85 percent participated by filling out the forms. We did not have a detailed baseline examination on the control families as we did on the study families. Study families were seen in scheduled interviews and examinations, at the beginning, at intervals, and at the end of the study. The Demonstration teams collected the data and filled out evaluation forms. In the case of the control families, where physical examinations and histories were done (by the Health Insurance Plan family doctor) they were noted, and the Cornell Medical Index and nutrition and housing forms which the families had completed were used as initial comparisons with the study families. For the final comparisons, the control families were brought in and examined, interviewed, and evaluated by the Demonstration teams as were the study families.

There was great similarity between the study and control families, from the initial data obtained, as can be seen from Figure 1 and Table 1. This relieved anxiety on that score, even though doubt as to the reliability of such random statistics was humorously excoriated by Professor Cochran as "deviation from the statistician's party line." [9]

Losses and Nonrespondents

One of the statistical problems turned out to our advantage. The question was raised about families moving away from the area, thereby reducing the effective observations. But far fewer study families moved than control families.

Our percentage of participating families was good — excellent as a matter of fact — but we did nothing to gather information about those who refused to participate. There is certainly valuable information to be obtained from the nonrespondents, if only to find out why they refused to participate and how they differed from those who did; but this will have to wait future exploration. A study of nonrespondents under somewhat similar circumstances was made and reported by Cobb, King, and Chen.[10] Apparently our excellent returns may be attributable to the fact that the group selected was under 45, for relatively high status people under 45 are good candidates for participating in health programs of any kind.

Table 1. Comparison of study and control families.

Characteristic	Study	Control
Mean age (years):		
Father	37.0	37.5
Mother	34.6	35.0
Eldest child	8.5	8.3
Son	7.1	7.6
Daughter	6.8	6.7
Mean number of children	2.1	2.3
Occupation (percent working):		
Father	100.0	100.0
Professional and semiprofessional	41.1	37.2
Fireman and policeman	28.2	27.3
Skilled and semiskilled	16.1	16.5
Clerical and sales	11.2	15.7
Other	3.4	3.3
Mother	32.3	26.4
Professional and semiprofessional	18.5	16.0
Clerical and sales	9.7	8.0
Other	4.1	2.0
Median rental (dollars)	62.7	66.0
Education (median years completed):		
Father	13.0	13.0
Mother	12.0	12.0

Objectivity of the Data

Squarely across all other considerations of a statistical nature was manifest the concern for the reliability of the information that went into the evaluations, scorings, and numerical comparisons.[11] Some of the definitions were more precise than others. "Major illness" in the "Physical health" evaluation category had a sharp outline. The numerical designation in this evaluation area was therefore more clearly objective than in the evaluation category "Personal adjustment," where a whole series of questions pointing toward a subjective decision on the marker's part left some doubt as to the sharpness of the score. In other words, the number itself may have had no subjective qualifications, but the observations that went into the production of that number did.

There was also the possibility that, due to an element of subjectivity in some of the scoring, an additional complication might arise: a change of attitude or scoring value in the mind of the worker over the years. Granted that some of the scores had lesser or greater judgments of value in their composition, what was to

CHARACTERISTICS OF FAMILIES
STUDY and CONTROL

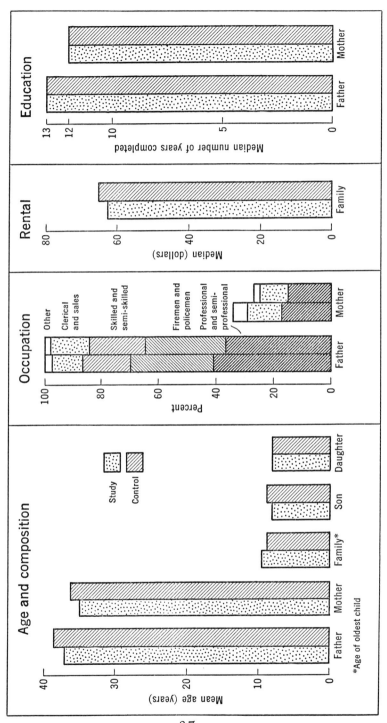

Figure 1

37

prevent these judgments from varying as the program progressed, as the workers became more sophisticated in their work?

Not all ratings could be done in a comparable period of time, so the amount of information and its comparative freshness varied in some degree from individual to individual in providing background for the judgment of the scorer. Some people came within a month for their interview and examination; others dragged it out over six months. Furthermore, as a worker piled up his interview material, he might be seriously backlogged and not dictate or score an individual until 6 months after the work had been completed. (This was true only in the beginning and affected comparatively few families.)

A parallel question raised by evaluations performed by different people was resolved by asking each team member to evaluate the individual in his area of competence. Where these overlapped, the scores were correlated, providing another helpful clue as to their validity.

All in all, there were serious limitations in reliability — the degree of subjectivity associated with the possibility of changing criteria and the delay in some instances affecting the scoring. At the same time, other factors in the nature of the study may have compensated for or offset these limitations. The very fact that control families were investigated and scored canceled out some bias, since the same bias would be expected to operate in study and control scoring. Internal checks which compared the rating of nurse with social worker and doctor in individual instances also helped balance the subjective factors. In the area of personal adjustment, with its implicit subjectivity, were the results of the Thematic Apperception Test which were applied and interpreted by a psychologist who was separated from involvement in the team observations and made appraisals independently.[12]

At the same time that the reliability of the scoring is thus called into question, we must emphasize that the value of the Demonstration does not stand or fall on the basis of objective criteria alone. One important over-all purpose of the Demonstration was to *obtain a broad range of information about families and their reaction to medical care of a new type*. That some of the data collected would be cruder than other data, or less precise, was to be expected. This initial study of family health was to provide clues, to serve as a reconnaissance from which other studies and more carefully designed research could be developed.

Scientists and statisticians are justly critical of too empirical an approach or too rigid adherence to the numerical aspects of experimental work. Hume condemns preoccupation with numbers alone in considering data, offering Bateson's ironic comment that "Though all science may be measurement, all measurement is not necessarily science." [13] MacMahon also joins in attacking the application of tests of significance and other mathematical instruments of precision to biased and heterogeneous data. "Interpretation of such data requires not detailed statistical knowledge but detailed knowledge of all aspects of the problem under investigation, a critical disposition, and acceptance and use of elementary statistical principles and techniques." [14] Reid writes, "In published accounts of clinical investigations, the gross mistakes are seldom due to the statistical test of significance being either absent or inappropriate." [15]

Statisticians recognize that social research offers complications in research design that make it imperative to risk some bias and heterogeneity in order to get data at all. Cochran, speaking directly of the Demonstration problem in this regard says, ". . . there are a great many facets of interest in this Demonstration, so that despite the difficulties of evaluation, the eggs are by no means all in one basket. Secondly, although this study is unique in a number of ways, it is far from unique in its methodological problems, and particularly in the problem of evaluation. It is, in fact, almost typical of the problem of evaluation that exists in a great deal of current research in public health and sociology. Problems of this kind will become more rather than less common. Scientists working in similar field research will be grateful to this project for the constructive ideas that it seems sure to contribute to problems of evaluation and also perhaps for advice on some pitfalls to avoid." He goes on to add that even data with recognizable bias and subjectivity may supplement narrower and more precise information in a significant way.[16]

Densen on another tack makes an analogous point. "Referring to the trend of mortality from typhoid fever since 1895, if one were to apply rigid tests of scientific proof to these data, one would be hard pressed to demonstrate unequivocally that the drop is entirely the result of public health activities. Nevertheless, the magnitude of the change, together with other evidence as laboratory data showing the influence of sanitary practices on the typhoid bacillus, leave little doubt that some of the change is the result of the application of these practices to the population at large. There are a good many well baby clinics in operation, but as far as I know, there is no quantitative evidence indicating that they are having a beneficial influence on the health of the population. It does not follow from this lack of evidence that well baby clinics are not effective. It may simply mean that we have not found the means to measure the effect, which does not manifest itself in such gross ways as a marked reduction in mortality." [17]

A judicious blend of critical and sympathetic judgment may therefore be urged upon the reader, who will balance the deficiencies of our data against the inherent difficulties so as to find herein some things of interest and value.

- IV -

SERVICE AND RESEARCH IN OPERATION

> The investigator should have a robust faith — and yet not be-
> lieve.
> — Claude Bernard, *Introduction à la médicine expérimentale*

The basic data of the Demonstration derives from what we did
and what we found. In order to weigh effects, comparable information had to be noted and events counted. For this reason a
standard sequence of activity was prescribed and standard forms
provided to describe the results of the activity. When the Machine
Records Unit and a coin toss had established that a particular
family was selected for study in the Demonstration, a definite
procedure followed.

COURSE OF A FAMILY SELECTED FOR STUDY

Invitation

The parents received a letter from me, inviting the family to
participate. The letter read, in part,

You already know some things about the medical care to which you
are entitled as Health Insurance Plan subscribers. But there is a brand
new special service which we are inviting your family and a few others
to use, *at no additional cost to you!*

This special service is part of a study of how to *prevent* illness, how
to *encourage* health, and continue comfortable living. Our doctors and
staff are pleased as you must be, that you as parents, and your children, can take advantage of this extra service.

This brief letter cannot explain the details, or answer the questions
that you must have. Dr. A will phone you soon to arrange to see you

41

in order to describe how you may enjoy these special added health benefits which can now be yours.

Instead of "Dr. A," "Miss R" or "Mrs. S" would be typed on successive letters, since each member of the team took a turn at establishing contact with new families and describing the Demonstration.[1]

Home Visit and Registration

As a follow-up to the telephone call, a visit was made at the family's convenience and the program was explained. No attempt was made to hide the fact that there were disagreeable aspects to participation; the number of visits and the duration of the interviews was painstakingly defined and the possible inconvenience was in no way minimized. However, positive aspects of participation were emphasized as well: added service from the team, dental care for the children, health education.

Most of those approached favored the program and the rate of participation was very high. Refusal to participate stemmed from two main sources: work conditions (two jobs, or both parents working) which made cooperation extremely difficult, or attachment to a Group physician (or non-Group physician) which generated reluctance to begin a new medical relationship.

Baseline Evaluation

Once a family had agreed to participate, appointments were made for its members to undergo examination and study. The total time allotted ranged from 5½ to 7½ hours.

Fill out Cornell Medical Index (each parent)	½ hour
History and physical examination by physician (each family member)	1 hour
Interview with Social Worker (each member over six years of age)	1 or 2 hours
Nursing visit to the home, completion of nutrition and housing form	1 or 2 hours
Psychological testing (each family member over six years of age)	1 hour
Laboratory and X-ray examinations	½ hour
Dental survey	½ hour

The nature of the various examinations and content of the interviews appear in the Appendix.

42

The actual time involved in getting this work done for a family may be seen in a typical schedule.

Intake Process for Typical Study Family

1. *Jan. 15–21*
   - Jan. 15: Nurse interview with parents to discuss program and entry.
   - Jan. 18: Parents accept program.
2. *Jan. 22–28*
   - Jan. 28: Physical examination of eldest son.
3. *Jan. 29–Feb. 4*
   - Feb. 3: Laboratory examination, eldest son.
     Physical examination and laboratory examination, second son.
     Physical examination and laboratory examination, daughter.
     Physical examination and laboratory examination, mother.
4. *Feb. 5–11*
   - Feb. 8: Social Worker interview of mother.
   - Feb. 9: Home visit by nurse.
     Laboratory examination, eldest son.
   - Feb. 10: Laboratory examination, eldest son.
5. *Feb. 12–18*
   - Feb. 15: Social worker interview of mother.
     Laboratory examination, eldest son.
     Laboratory examination, daughter.
     Laboratory examination, mother.
6. *Feb. 19–25*
   - Feb. 23: Psychological test, second son.
7. *Feb. 26–March 3*
   - March 2: Psychological test, mother.
     Psychological test, eldest son.
8. *March 4–10*
   - March 8: Psychological test, second son.
   - March 10: Nurse interview of father.
     Physical examination, father.
   - March 17: Social worker interview of father.
9. *March 11–17*

43

10. *March 18–24*
11. *March 25–31*
12. *Apr. 1–7*
13. *Apr. 8–14*
    Apr. 12: Family conference.
14. *Apr. 15–21*
15. *Apr. 22–28*
16. *Apr. 29–May 5*
17. *May 6–12*
18. *May 13–19*
19. *May 20–26*
    May 21: Nurse school visit re second son.
    May 25: Nurse school visit re eldest son and daughter.

Not shown are the occasions the 3 staff members spent checking records and judging evaluation ratings in the various areas for each of the 5 family members. The delay was occasioned mostly by the need for suiting the time to the family's convenience, but also by the staff worker's needs for spreading the intake examination over a period of time. The staff had to continue service and health promotional activities, keep up with the dictation and records, hold conferences and perform associated jobs such as school visits.

The Team Conference

After all the information on a family had been gathered, the team held a conference at which the findings were discussed, diagnoses exchanged, and a plan for the family laid out. Here are two typical summaries (on different families) of a team conference. The format varies because team members took turns keeping minutes.

TEAM CONFERENCE — 9/27/54

Family Name: Z
  Present: Dr. A (Family Doctor)
          Dr. E (Pediatrician)
          Miss R (Public Health Nurse)
          Mrs. S (Psychiatric Social Worker)
Mr. Z
  1. Essentially healthy
  2. Congenital right sided aortic arch

44

Recommendations:
1. Electro-cardiogram (never done)
2. Laboratory work (never done)

Mrs. Z
1. Chronic duodenal ulcer
2. Bilateral cystic mastitis
3. Obesity
4. External hemorrhoids
5. Anxiety
6. Fibroids of uterus

Recommendations:
1. Lose weight
2. Sigmoidoscopy for hemorrhoids
3. Watch fibroid tumors of uterus and cystic mastitis

Oldest child (son)
1. Atopic eczema
2. Enuresis
3. Personality disturbance

Recommendation:
1. Psychiatric help — ? Adolescent clinic at Mt. Sinai

Second child (son)
1. Rheumatic fever
2. Allergic

Recommendations:
1. Prophylactic bicillin once a month
2. Reassure as to heart status — no change

Third child (daughter)
1. Heart murmur — functional
2. Feeding problem — finicky eater
3. Enuresis
4. New experience upsetting

Recommendations:
1. EKG
2. More relaxed attitude to be encouraged
3. Part of general personality difficulty is that mother is not so eager to do anything re her and feels it more important to concentrate on oldest child. To be discussed with mother.
4. Play therapy — Mrs. S.

TEAM CONFERENCE — 10/8/53

Family Name: X

The X family consists of Mr. X a 39-year-old (type of employment deleted); Mrs. X age 35, and four children — oldest child (daughter), 5; second child (son), 3; third child (daughter), 2; and fourth child (son), ½ year old.

Medical Findings:

Mr. X has acne with retention cysts in his face. He also has varicose veins and small external hemorrhoids.

Mrs. X is mildly obese and has small varicose veins. Special shoes have been recommended for her by the Orthopedist.

Oldest child is healthy.

Second child is healthy except for pronation of the feet for which corrective shoes were recommended.

Third child is healthy.

Fourth child had a mild skin rash at time of examination. Since coming on Family Health Maintenance he has had a hernia operation.

Social and Psychological Findings:

The X family appears to be a rather close-knit one, Mrs. X being the more dominant parent. She appears to be quite dependent on her own mother who is living with the family. Mrs. X is very tense and nervous and cries very easily. She feels that this has begun only since she is married and that before she was a very easygoing person. Mrs. X was a very compulsive housekeeper, and she allows her children to play only in their own room so that they will not upset the apartment.

Mr. X gets much satisfaction out of his work, and appears to be a rather warm, easygoing person. He does, however, have a lot of covered up hostility toward his wife and has some recognition of the difficulty he has in accepting responsibility. He feels that at times he has to run away from these responsibilities, and, because of this, drinks quite excessively. Although he has cut down somewhat recently, his drinking continues to be the main problem in the family. Both Mr. and Mrs. X have expressed their feeling that this is not going to change; therefore, in their opinion there is no sense in getting any help around this problem. Mr. X also talked about the difficulty he has always had in handling money. Mrs. X is the one who handles the family income. She is also paying back a sum of money borrowed by Mr. X in the past, in order to have enough money to spend on his drinking.

Both Mr. and Mrs. X are interested in their children, but Mr. X finds it easier than does his wife to play with them and take them places. Mrs. X has some difficulty in deciding how much control she should exercise over the children. Conformity to rules is very important to her, and she tends to be quite disturbed by the fact that (oldest child) and (third child) "both have a mind of their own." Actually the two girls seem to be getting along very well and have no particular difficulties. (Second child), on the other hand, appears to be too compliant and conforming and also was found to be rather fearful when coming for his examination.

46

Recommendations:

1. Review of medical findings and follow-ups.
2. Mrs. X to see Miss B (social worker) to talk about the problems with (second child) and her ambivalence about how much freedom to give the children.
3. The question of whether to discuss the question of Mr. X's drinking was taken up with Dr. S. (psychiatrist) who felt that this could be mentioned in the course of conversation, but that it should be left up to Mr. and Mrs. X to discuss this further if they were interested. The reason for this decision was that while Mr. X's drinking is a problem, they both seem to have accepted it and to feel that there is no sense in working on this.

This is the "team conference" referred to in the text. Suggestions were made for each family member if necessary. If individual therapeutic visits were recommended, a notation was made of the team members who were to guide the family members. Depending on what the defect or difficulty was, the appropriate worker was assigned to look after a particular family member. However, if the problem was related to an area in which more than one was competent, then the team member with whom the family had developed the greatest rapport was to take on the responsibility for care and follow-up. (This refers to an area such as child-rearing practices, in which the pediatrician, social worker, and public health nurse all had training and interest.)

The Family Conference

Next the team held a conference with the parents, referred to as the "family conference." The same material that had been reviewed at the team conference was gone over, with perhaps more judicious language, approach, and emphasis. A course of action was laid out for the family to follow, treating illness that had been discovered, shoring up weaknesses suspected, and taking active preventive measures where possible to prevent illness from occurring. At this conference, appointments would be made for future individual visits to team members. If the team's decision as to which member should work with a family member was disputed, the family's request or decision was followed. If the team suggested a social worker and the family preferred the nurse or doctor for advisor or therapist, the matter was discussed, but the

47

family's request was honored. A transcript of a report of a typical conference follows.

FAMILY CONFERENCE — 10/29/53

Family Name: X

Present:

Right from the beginning of the conference, some tension between Mr. and Mrs. X was apparent. At the same time they were calling each other "dear" in what seemed to be a rather guarded uncomfortable way. The medical findings were discussed, and there was some discussion about Mr. X's facial cysts which Dr. A felt should be taken care of. Mr. X went along with this and Mrs. X was pleased that he did. There was also a discussion of his hemorrhoids, and the question of what should be done about these. Mrs. X is very anxious for him to have these taken care of, whereas he has not been too ready to do so. He hesitated somewhat when Dr. A asked him when he gets these, but then said they occur mainly after he drinks beer. Mrs. X got obvious satisfaction out of his having to say this, but she at this point did not say anything further. There was discussion of her being overweight, and here Mr. X was the one who seemed glad that this was brought up. Mrs. X spoke of feeling hungry all the time, and there was then some explanation of the reasons for this kind of feeling and its being actually due to tension.

There was a good deal of conversation concerning Mrs. X's being very tense, and while she agreed that she had a problem, she felt that it would get better as the children would get older and as her husband would too "grow up." After having said this she turned to him and asked him, "Shall we talk?" and she then made him talk about his need to drink. They began to blame each other and the team attempted to get the conversation away from the question of who was to blame and to concentrate on the question of what could be done. Mrs. X said that she is too cooped up at home and does not get out enough, and Mr. X pointed out that he is trying to get her to go away from home more, but feels that she wants to go only with him instead of getting out alone or with some of her friends. As this was discussed further, Mrs. X's compulsiveness and her always having things to do around the house were brought up. Gradually Mrs. X agreed that if she were to get some help with this she would be able to get out more and would not have as great a need to eat all the time.

Both Mr. and Mrs. X were at this point ready to involve themselves in a discussion of the causation of problems like theirs, and the fact that it was not a question of blaming one another, but of considering what each one's part in it was and working it out on that basis. They recognized that by their yelling at each other they could not really come to any understanding, and felt that after this conference they would want to go home and consider these things more between themselves. Mrs. X thought she might come in to see Miss B around the problem of her compulsiveness, and there was also a question of (second child's) nightmares and where these come from. Mrs. X will also try to go on a diet and will discuss this with Miss K and Mr. X will see Dr. A about his cysts and hemorrhoids. No definite appointment was made by Mrs. X since she felt that she was too busy right now to make a definite appointment.

No sanctions were employed against families which refused to follow the plan or would not cooperate. Efforts were made to encourage cooperation, and a worker meeting an uncooperative mother or father in the Group building would comment or reiterate a recommendation for a service or visit, but there was no threat of loss of service, of being dropped from the program or losing some part of the benefits. The families had been "invited" to cooperate, and participation remained on this basis throughout their 4 years of involvement.

Medical-Care Services

All medical services customarily rendered in the Montefiore Medical Group by the family internist were rendered by the Family Health Maintenance team. Services customarily rendered by other specialists of the Medical Group were made available. When the patient wanted care he made contact with the Demonstration. He could ask to speak to, or be referred to the doctor, the nurse, or the social worker. He could come into the Center or bring his child in, or he could have someone come to the house if necessary. If there was urgent need, an ambulance and access to the hospital were available. In any case, the comprehensive medical aspect of the Demonstration was within the same framework as the comprehensive medical care of the Montefiore Medical Group and all group services were equally available to all Demonstration members. Over a period of 4 years, the patients could have medical care when they wanted it, when they asked for it or needed it, and in addition they were the focus of a complex preventive and therapeutic service offered by the health team. The additional services available to study families through the team combined family guidance and emotional support short of actual psychotherapy with an active health promotional program. The latter included literature distributed at the Center, meetings, films, and small group conferences.

Preventive and Health-Promotion Activities

Certain preventive measures in the area of emotional health along lines generally considered beneficial by health educators and psychiatrists were an integral part of the Demonstration. There were individual conferences with the physician, nurse, or social worker when there was a recognition of a problem on the part of the patient. Sometimes invitations to conferences were made even when the patient saw no problems. These could be disguised as "study" conferences. Several types of literature were distributed. This included general material helpful to parents raising children or watching their children grow into puberty or adolescence. There was reading focused on some special problems such as obesity, heart disease or diabetes, or family problems such as the emotionally disturbed child. Beside the individual conferences and the reading materials, there was emphasis on preventive aspects in the daily medical service. In addition, an effort was made to develop discussion groups as a health promotional activity (not "group therapy"), simply by arranging for people with some common interest to come together to discuss this common interest. Subjects for discussion tended to be the same as those selected in the literature: raising children, family problems, and chronic illness. A significant contribution to the health-promotion activity was made through the availability of the nurse and social worker who were present when patients came to see the doctor for medical reasons. Through friendly and informal contacts they could use their professional skills to advise and guide, underlining or emphasizing health practices. Another significant health promotional aspect derived from the simple fact that the doctors could spend more time with patients and so had more opportunity to hear as well as to speak.

Annual Evaluations

Each year the study families were examined and interviewed according to the schedule and reevaluated. There were rare lapses from this. Of the 209 parents present during the whole 4 years of the Demonstration experience, 65 percent had all 4 examinations. Only 6 people missed more than one examination!

The last examination was a final evaluation. A final conference with the family was held to assist in their transfer to the routine care of the Montefiore Medical Group. Health problems the families brought up at this final conference or matters the team felt were important to follow up were included in the letter written to the Group physician into whose care the patient was to be placed. The medical chart was returned to him, and he was also informed of the existence of the Demonstration family records, containing the social work, nursing, and conference notes, psychological test results, nutrition and housing information.

RESEARCH PROCEDURES

Essentially the research design involved measurement of movement ("improvement" or "deterioration" in health or interpersonal relationships). Lacking sufficient precedents, we decided at the outset to devise a series of categories measuring health, to establish grades within these categories, and to score or mark the family members at the beginning and end of the study. This turned out to be far from simple. The difficulty of establishing clean-cut categories, or of defining terms within the categories, and of maintaining objectivity in scoring rapidly became obvious. However, we proceeded with the plan, attempting to minimize the bias where possible. The forms and instructions for completing them are in the Appendix. While some of the evaluation criteria and procedures need no interpretation, it may be of interest to examine a number of these to explain their use and limitations.

Parts I and II of the Evaluation Form, "Family History" and "Physical Condition," are self-evident. Parts IV and IX, "Sleep and Rest" and "Recreation," are also self-explanatory. Parts V and VI, "Personal Adjustment," derive from the social worker's interview schedule and from the Cornell Medical Index. Part III, "Nutrition," Part X, "Housing," and Parts VII and VIII, "Occupational Adjustment" and "Education," require some elucidation, as does the Psychological Test which played a part in the evaluations.

51

Psychological Testing

One of the questions raised when we discussed methods was: what kind of psychological testing should we do — if any? Psychological testing was decided upon for two reasons. First, information about character or personality not obtainable any other way might be obtained and thereby help in the "preventive psychiatry" aspects of team management by facilitating diagnosis and directing attention to potential difficulties. Second, a psychological test might be a useful corroboration of the validity of the subjective ratings, supporting the judgment derived from interviews. The subjective quality of the psychological tests nullified this latter hope. We spent a good part of 5 years in a fruitless attempt to develop a scale that would provide an objective basis for comparison of individuals, based on the psychological test used. However, the test was an independent subjective finding, and "could be used for comparison."

In deciding which test to use, we rejected some as too complex, others as too narrowly descriptive of a single factor, and others as too difficult to score or interpret except by their inventors. In general, the Rorschach and the Thematic Apperception tests seemed most widely used and possessed of a body of literature that would be helpful in orientation toward our own problems. The Rorschach seemed to suffer from the complexity of application and of analysis we were trying to avoid, so we settled on the Thematic Apperception Test (TAT).[2]

At first glance, the TAT is bright with promise for our purposes. In this test, a series of photographs is offered the person tested and his narration of the story each picture brings to mind is recorded. The psychologist then interprets the story on the basis of the appearance of certain figures, emotional attitudes, nature of the story line, fluency, and other factors. A similar test adapted for children is called The Children's Apperception Test (CAT).[3]

The Tomkinses in their book offer a guide to content analysis that seems simple enough so that a scale could be constructed fairly easily. The content was precisely in line with our interests. For example, the test specifically reports on the extent of influence and interaction of parents and children. The "technique involves an examination of the protocol with a frequency of introduction of parental figures, *where the picture contains none* . . . If older adults in the picture are omitted in the elaboration of a story it may signify either the parent or parental surrogates have ceased to be important or that the individual denies their existence. The degree of parental influence is to some extent a function of the scope of such parental impact and regions outside the family." [4]

Also, the story line reveals basic traits that are important in assessing the family relationship. The TAT was directed at exploring the areas of personality expression and development in relation to the family, that was a part of our own Demonstration design. However, a warning note is sounded. "The use of the TAT as a diagnostic instrument is limited by the uncertainty of inferences based upon this procedure . . . Typically we find a contrast between what the patient is willing or able to tell and his covered or unconscious anti-social wishes. These are generally sexual or aggressive wishes which occasion the individual anxiety. But there are many instances in which the suppressed or repressed wishes are not anti-social." [5]

We chose to overlook this because we were not in need of a precise diagnostic tool; we were looking for auxiliary tools. However, the weakness of the test lies just in this inability to make hard and fast classifications based on appearance or nonappearance of symbolic material in the stories. It is almost impossible to develop a scale that compares individuals when one must balance expressed against unexpressed wishes and make judgments of the cause or underlying motivation of equivalent expressed material.[6]

The Cornell Medical Index

The Cornell Medical Index (CMI) has been laboriously standardized over the years and provides useful and definite comparisons. Briefly, in this test, "yes" or "no" answers are required to a set of 195 questions about symptoms and signs of illness, the last 50 of which are particularly aimed at eliciting symptoms in the emotional area. "The presumptive evidence on the CMI of the patient having an emotional disturbance is: (1) 30 or more yes responses, (2) 3 or more questions answered both yes and no, (3) omitted answers for 6 or more questions, (4) 3 or more remarks or changes in the questions." [7] Of course, the whole of the questionnaire does not apply to these uncertain areas of personality and

53

emotional attitude, so it is unfair to compare its interpretation and use with that of the more complex projective techniques in personality testing.[8] We found this test easily given, generally acceptable, and within the limits of its applicability very useful. It would be most agreeable to have a similar simple, uniformly applicable and comparable test for personality.

Intelligence Testing

Although we used both the Bellevue-Wechsler and the Stanford-Binet intelligence tests, we did not use them routinely. They were employed only under special circumstances and always in combination with projective tests. The results were interpreted by someone who knew the child and whose judgment would be colored by this knowledge. Intelligence tests are so loaded with cultural overtones, and so dependent upon the mood of the subject and interaction between tester and subject — let alone the mood of the tester — that it is dangerous and unscientific to allow the test results alone to be decisive. After testing the reliability and validity of the Stanford-Binet and other intelligence tests among schoolchildren, the Clarkes made a number of points against their routine or unmodified use. They showed that the children's performance varies from one test to another; if only one type of test is given, a different I.Q. may be obtained from what another would yield. Even the same test given at different times may vary widely in score. Further, since the standard deviation of the Binet Test is roughly 12 points, a child who has an I.Q. score of 70 may test subnormal on one occasion and reasonably average on another, varying between 58 and 82. The Clarkes conclude: "It is clear that in the general population the concept of a rigidly constant I.Q. is contradicted by the facts; I.Q. constancy over long periods of time during years of mental growth is the exception rather than the rule."[9] Finally, even though it may measure the level of functioning, an I.Q. test doesn't necessarily measure intellectual capacity or potential. With a history of a bad or a good home mentally subnormal children show tremendously different potential. It is not unlikely that a large proportion of "feebleminded" children grow up into essentially normal adults. If used at all, an I.Q. test must be used with caution, and with other information about a child before any conclusion is reached.

Nutrition Information

Since gross dietary deficiency is rare in the United States, our nutrition form was directed at obtaining a general picture of eating habits. If defective eating habits were detected, improvement or modification could be sought. Since our information was usually obtained from the mother, the first question is, how accurate is the information given by the mother concerning food served to the family? Reed and Burke, studying this very problem in a health study at Harvard, conclude that the interview method is a reliable instrument for getting such information about dietary habits in the family.[10] It was anticipated that obesity would be the major health problem related to nutrition. Consequently we devoted a fair amount of time to defining obesity. We settled on the Metropolitan Life Insurance Height-Weight Tables, judging as obesity 20 percent or more over these ideal weights. This is unsatisfactory as there is no agreement on "ideal" weight (the tables are derived from averages) or adjustment for age, but, since a simple grid form is as yet not available for adults (like the Wetzel grid used for children), we settled for the Metropolitan tables. While obesity cannot be due entirely to exogenous factors, or even related in linear fashion to dietary intake, information about dietary intake and eating habits gave us a base from which we could move to correct obesity where found.[11]

We were also concerned about the possibility of borderline deficiency — the situation in which no overt illness is visible, but where the reserve is defective because of deficiencies in intake or metabolism. This is related to the concept of lifetime nutrition balance publicized by the American Medical Association Council on Foods and Nutrition.[12] The importance of maintaining an adequate reserve for meeting special needs at particular phases of development is logical. Adolescence and pregnancy make unusual demands on the body, aging another type of special need. During interval phases this reserve must be built up. These statements are not entirely speculative concepts. In other countries, where social crises have introduced periods of dietary inadequacy, later improvement of the diet has made a significant difference in the stillbirth rate, in the nutrition of the child, in the neo-natal mortality rate. We have vivid evidence of the effects of wartime star-

55

vation in Holland, and the effect of the long German siege on the people of Leningrad. With this in mind, it seemed desirable to make note of nutritional status and attempt to relate health improvement to nutritional improvement.

Housing Information

"There actually is limited scientific evidence to support the broad belief that there is in fact an interdependent relationship between housing quality and health. There have been creditable studies that have shown that people who live in good housing, are, in the main, healthier than those who live in sub-standard dwellings. But again there is no really solid evidence of the degree to which housing per se is related to the status of community health. Poor housing is generally associated with poor health. Both are associated with low income, poor nutrition, crowding, and lack of education. This socio-economic complex makes it especially difficult to measure precisely neighborhood-wide (let alone community-wide) relationships between housing and health." [13]

In spite of this clear statement from Pond, we developed a housing form and tried to measure correlations between housing and health. We did this for many reasons: because home accidents are a growing problem; because the likelihood of a broader range of medical services being provided in the home (as in Home Care, particularly in chronic disease) is increasing; and because there is widespread suspicion of the implication of poor housing in poor health.[14]

Since the suspicion remains, although evidence is lacking, it seems reasonable to assume that cramped space, poor lighting, physical hazards, lack of privacy, inadequate toilet facilities, insufficient playgrounds, and so on, must have some deleterious effects, and so we maintained housing data for comparison of families, and scored them on it.[15]

Occupational Adjustment and Related Information

Work is such an important part of a man's life and occupies so much of his waking time, that serious attention has to be paid to it and its effects on a man, as well as to the effects of a man's personality, needs, and frustrations on his work.

Naturally, employers and employees do not see eye to eye about the problems of the job, the adjustments, or even the nature of the psychological and social factors influencing the job and the worker's adjustment to it. We did not gain direct insights into the job relationships, but we were able to draw some important inferences. For example, the attitude of many men and women toward their jobs and the kind of jobs they held helped us to understand their total personality a little better. Disappointment or unhappiness in a job situation a generation ago would have pointed to a defect in the worker himself. Today, social psychological emphasis falls on the job rather than the worker.[16] But the work situation cannot be considered the sole determinant. A man comes to his job already sensitized. Personal conflicts and stressful home situations may also be transferred to the job, exaggerating problems and difficulties there. Furthermore the conditioning that has produced a personality type and home attitudes will undoubtedly react in this way to comparable situations on the job.[17] None of this is intended to minimize the impact of *lack* of work, or inadequate wages or insufficient job protection. It should be plain from this that there is interaction of job and worker.

Another aspect of work and the insights it gives is the so-called "security employment" — civil service — and people who select such jobs, with the reasons for selection. Today, as union contracts protect more and more workers against capricious loss of jobs and welfare funds provide pensions and other benefits, the civil service doesn't have as much of the unique security connotation it once had. But this career was selected by some, not by others.[18]

Health care *on the job* ought to have been a part of health care of the family in our Demonstration. It was not possible. We needed information about the job in order to give an additional dimension ("the working personality") to the information obtained from the interview and observations of the families; but such information was almost unobtainable. Reluctantly, we discarded the idea of having the nurse visit the plant or working place, interview the worker on the job, talk with the foreman, the employer (or city official responsible), and union stewards and officials. Since we were concerned with a small number of people, questions at their place of employment were bound to single them out, create some misunderstandings, and perhaps

57

even result in injustices to the worker. Even mentioning the idea tentatively to a number of families almost resulted in panic, and we had to give it up. Future family studies *must* include such working life information.

The measurements of occupational adjustment in the study are therefore inadequate, but helpful. They represent observations by the team of some things in a limited area (the number of job changes and expressed satisfaction or dissatisfaction).

School Health Information

We obtained much more information about the children from their schools than we did about their parents from the job setting. School visits were made — in the beginning by the Demonstration nurse or social worker, and later routinely by the nurse so that information about the child came from teachers and occasionally school nurses and principals.[19] This rating should be given greater proportional weight than the occupational adjustment rating of adults.

The argument made with regard to interaction of job and worker is equally applicable to child and school. "Attitudes engendered in the home are transported to the schoolroom where the child is reacting to his teacher and schoolmates in large measure as he does to his parents and siblings."[20] On the other hand, the teacher is bringing her problems into the schoolroom, and the size of the class, equipment, school structure, and quality all play their part in the child's success in his "work." The evaluation was intended to reflect all these factors.

- V -

THE ROLES OF THE TEAM MEMBERS

I believe that our Greater Medical Profession will run better if we go as far as is reasonably possible towards granting full professional status to every kind of trained person in it.

— T. F. Fox, "The Greater Medical Profession"

In considering the methods that might be used to carry out Demonstration objectives, the idea of a team operation seemed natural. One professional person may suffer from limitations of knowledge or experience or area of service; a team of professionals wipes out these limitations. As we looked at the objectives of the Demonstration, it was clear that a doctor, nurse, and social worker could together fulfill the description of the family doctor who was to be the center of the program. Gaps in present-day practice were bridged through the introduction of social-welfare concepts by making social work available, and the need for health education services overcome by making a public health nurse available.

One way of arranging this could have been through interagency cooperation, in which doctor, social worker, and nurse would work together while retaining his separate attachment to his agency. It seemed more fruitful to detach workers from their agencies and set up a closely knit team in which the workers would cooperate rather than the agencies. This method of approaching joint action is uncommon and somewhat hazardous. All the tendencies of professional development would appear to be against such isolated interprofessional team operations. The

59

block to team activity is seen in the varying backgrounds, lack of supervision (technical), tendency to speak different technical languages, personal problems of the participants (status), and lack of strictly defined leadership.[1] Caudill writes, "Without a substantial body of shared knowledge, the group becomes a collection of experts — each person conceived to be the supreme authority in his field, so far as the work of the group is concerned. In the stress of argument, when the expert's discipline is challenged, he tends to retreat to a highly conservative theoretical position which often serves to revive outmoded, irrelevant problems and issues. Concomitant with the foregoing is the factor of the status positions of the various members outside of the group, in terms of their professional or academic standing and community prestige."[2]

Just prior to the organization of the Family Health Maintenance Demonstration, Montefiore Hospital had had an enlightening experience in the development of a medical-care team in the Home Care Program.[3] This very positive experience persuaded us that a team operation of this kind was not only possible but attainable, and not nearly so difficult to put together as already suggested. As a matter of fact, the doctor, nurse, and social worker on the Home Care team found their own opportunities for service broadened by the intimate daily associations, and found no cause for friction in the operation. Our experience bears out that of Eaton who, in a thoughtful review of the background of difficulty in interdisciplinary team operations concludes that it is the democratic structure that is essential to good group functioning.[4] If individual roles are clearly delineated, if there is knowledge and acceptance of each other's professional role, conflict can be avoided. This is aided largely by arranging for routine communication in the form of scheduled conferences, so that flow of information is facilitated. Avoidance of conflict and facilitation of information were the most helpful elements in maintaining the team structure.

In our own team, for example, while the doctor might concern himself with medical problems, the nurse with health practices, and the social worker with family relationships, it became obvious that such things as bad nutritional habits — matters lying in the nurse's area — led to problems for the doctor and the social worker. Joint evaluation of problems and decisions were necessary. In the Home Care Program, decisions to meet the needs of seriously sick people were joint socio-medical decisions. This was of benefit both to the patient and particularly to the doctor, who found that he frequently altered what would have been his "scientific" decision when he became aware, through the nurse and social worker, of other factors affecting the patient and family. It is as if teamwork afforded the doctor stereoscopic vision. Conversely, medical consultation was of great help to the social worker and so to the patient, since emotional problems or family difficulties very often are bound up with medical needs. The same applied in the nurse's relationship to the team. Home Care thus offered an excellent point of departure and successful model for team operation in the Family Health Maintenance Demonstration.

The qualifications of the workers in the Family Health Maintenance team were consonant with our conception of its function. The doctor had to be well trained in medicine, psychiatrically oriented, and willing to work as a member of a team. The public health nurse had to have a background in educational nursing as well as bedside care; and the medical social worker had to have an interest in and some experience with psychiatric social work. Professional competence was only one facet, for ability to work as members of a team was an equally important qualification. Most important was recognition and acceptance by the team members of these factors. By the democratic nature of the operation, decisions were to be reached by consensus.

FUNCTIONING OF TEAM MEMBERS

The three members of the health team were to complement each other in obtaining information. Each was to evaluate the patient in terms of his own professional responsibility, but they would have weekly meetings to discuss the families and to deal with problems as they arose. The team member's assigned professional role was important in determining the position he took and the weight given to his decision, but all three shared in the decisions.

61

In addition, the team members held weekly meetings, individually and as a group, with the psychiatric consultant. The object of these meetings was not only to get general views and psychiatric orientation toward their work, but sometimes to seek specific help for specific problems in specific families. The psychiatrist was expected to see the problems through the eyes of the team. The team, in turn, filtered his ideas through themselves to the family. The use of the psychiatrist's insights gave an added tool in dealing with the families and strengthened the team identity.

The team therefore had the research roles of observation (noting the information according to schedules) and evaluation. It had service roles: preventive, in attempting to shore up the family against future disease or disaster; and therapeutic, in dealing with situations that had already broken down. There was also a consultative role with respect to each other which is the unique contribution of the team structure, and basically valuable to any team function.

THE DOCTOR'S JOB

As a rule, the doctor's first contact with the family took place at the initial interview to obtain a history and make a physical examination. The components of this history and examination are noted in the Appendix.

He gave the families the medical care they needed when sick, at home or in the office or hospital. If another physician's skills were required he called in the group specialists as consultants. Preventive services such as injections and periodic examinations were his responsibility.

After the information on the individual was completed, the doctor filled in the evaluation schedule on the physical condition and on whatever other area he had information or could pass judgment. Although he filled in a score and commented about physical health in all cases, he did not necessarily complete the same evaluation categories for all the subjects.

At the team conference, the doctor brought his special knowledge and background to bear on the information presented by the nurse and social worker to round out the picture of the family. His presentation of the preventive and therapeutic aspects that needed to be followed up provided the basis for the "health schedule" that the team would present to the family.

The family conference was usually the doctor's show. Although the team had been organized on, and briefed to accept, a democratic structure (no one was "boss") suitable and useful for conferences, families continued to look to the doctor for leadership. As a consequence, in presenting the findings and developing the "health schedule" for the family, the doctor took the lead and played the dominant role while the nurse and social worker played subordinate roles.

The doctor carried on his activities as an individual physician, but he was also a member of a health team. He met regularly with the others to discuss families, assess new conditions and problems, and help work out courses of action. On a weekly basis, he met with the consultant psychiatrist for general discussion and for advice on specific family problems.

Of the various types of small group meetings planned the doctor had selected teenagers as his particular interest. So over a period of years he held group meetings with teen-age boys and girls, working with the health education consultant in the organization and structure of the meetings and presenting his experiences to the other team members for discussion.

In addition the doctor shared with other team members responsibility for the general educational group meetings when they were held, discussing medical topics on occasion, and he was available to answer questions from the group and participate in the general aspects of the meetings.

As a physician, the health-team doctor was a staff member of the Montefiore Hospital and carried on service activities there, in the wards and clinics as a staff physician, and in the various medical conferences. His personal interest and training in cardiovascular physiology and disease enabled him to become a member of the cardiac team, evaluating patients for cardiac surgery, assisting in the operating room during cardiac surgery, and performing cardiac catheterizations. It should be emphasized that playing the role of the family doctor, partaking of special training in family problems, and applying himself to family practice, did not bar him from continuing to work in this highly complex specialized field of modern medicine.

Other Medical Consultants

The internist had to work out a reasonably satisfactory arrangement whereby he was the family advisor and physician to the family as a whole, while the pediatrician was the physician to the children under 13 years of age. In a sense the pediatrician was a consultant, lending his special skills to care for those patients who were his obligation and advising the internist on matters relating to the family in which he had more knowledge, but he did take responsibility for the care of the children.

The other physicians in the Medical Group with whom the health-team internist was associated were more easily recognizable as consultants. Within the framework of group practice, an obstetrician, orthopedist, or surgeon has a definite function. It was expected that the specialists would see patients only on referral and consult the internist ("family doctor") before taking over responsibility, as well as report regularly in the common record when the patient was seen. The specialists were extensions of the health team. They did not challenge the team's responsibility for family care, but added specialized knowledge and skill. They were consultants covering areas outside family practice and internal medicine.

The complexity of modern medical knowledge invites specialization which in turn magnifies technical skill. There is danger of the technician's becoming the prototype of the professional practitioner. The team approach and the use of consultants was a conscious effort to overcome the technician orientation and emphasis in family practice.

THE SOCIAL WORKER'S JOB

The new profession of medical social work emerged at the turn of the century from two sources: the almoner movement in England aimed at direct service to patients; and medical social work in the United States developed in response to the doctor's own felt need for more information about and more access to families.[5] Social work emerged as the "helping profession," helping patients directly and helping doctors to help patients. But over the years the autonomy of the profession has been fostered and the emphasis shifted so that helping the doctor has become a lesser (if any) part of the role of the medical social worker, and direct patient service the major role.[6]

We were anxious to combine the conceptions and re-emphasize the value of helping the doctor by attaching social work to daily medical practice. In this way we could expect to enhance the service value of both professions.[7] There was no intent to diminish the importance of medical social work, reduce the status of the medical social worker, or intrude the physician into social-work functions. If anything, our conception of the role of the social worker in the health team was an augmentation of role, not a contraction.[8] We asked the social worker to see herself as both a family case worker and a team member. We thought of her as a professional worker who had diagnostic and therapeutic skills which might prove useful in assisting other professional workers to do their own jobs as well as carry out a job of her own. In helping others and in gaining help from them it was thought necessary for the social worker to be part of a medical-care team, to meet with team members regularly, visit and interview families in the same setting the other team members did, and share her skills with them.

Content of the Job

One of the team members would interview the family to arrange acceptance of the program. Part of the social worker's job was to share in this responsibility. Once accepted, family members were interviewed by the social worker as a part of the base-line examination.

The Interview. The purpose of the initial interview was to obtain information from the individual about his understanding of himself in relation to his job, wife, and children and to help mark out areas of tension and dissatisfaction as well as goals, satisfactions, and interests. The interview was used somewhat as a diagnostic tool, to distinguish healthy from unhealthy elements and to determine where tension and strain exist.[9] Of course all the vital information couldn't be brought out in one interview, even if it lasted two to three hours, as some did. One can, in an initial interview, however, line up certain areas for further investigation and establish some patterns of work relations and family interaction.

65

The Demonstration interview did not differ as much in content from most family-agency intake interviews (the questions were similar) as it did in context. Those interviewed had not come specifically for help, as clients interviewed by social workers in agencies or professional offices do. Only a small number of people in the study families had consulted a psychiatrist or social agency in the past, and less than 10 percent were known to any other agency prior to our contact with them.[10] It was expected that their reactions to the interview would differ from those of agency applicants.

The fact of noninvolvement, that the social work interview was done at the request of the Demonstration rather than the patient, had great significance. First, suspicion had to be allayed that the exploration was deliberate (that is, that they were selected for investigation because we "knew something" or "had something on them"). Secondly, a balance had to be struck between arousing too much anxiety by too pointed or probing questions and getting enough information to leave the way open for study and treatment. Resistance might be evoked at some points because of unguarded revelation and fear of the social worker's opinion of the revelation. These factors are implicit in any direct interview that goes deeply into personality, feelings, and motivation. But there is a difference in dealing with these factors when the patient has come for help, as against our own situation in which the person was interviewed as part of a routine examination.

The interview schedule appended reflects the detailed information sought. In general, education and work history, religious affiliation and importance of religion, social and leisure-time activities were relatively easy to elicit. Other information was obtained with more difficulty.

Services. Routine school visits were made by the nurse. Originally it had been intended that the nurse and social worker would divide school visits between them, but by common consent, the nurse was charged wholly with this very early.

The social worker did make some school visits to fill in the details of impressions about a child. If she had a particular case for which she felt a follow-up would be useful, she made the visit and reported it from her point of view, either in addition to or instead of the nurse's visit.

The social worker then prepared a diagnostic statement, a formulation of observations and impressions of the personalities of the family members — what they knew about themselves, and how aware they were of stresses and strains within the family structure.[11] Her evaluation of the family and suggestions as to what might have to be done to help was presented to the team conference, discussed, and became part of the "health schedule" presented to the family.

The social worker completed the evaluation form on which the evidence of movement and family scoring is based. She did casework with selected patients who recognized the need and attended individual case conferences. She carried on group sessions with children who were having difficulty in school. (These corresponded to supervised play sessions but had a therapeutic aspect in addition.) With the physician and the nurse the social worker shared responsibility for the general educational meetings and health-education policies carried on by the Demonstration.

The social worker participated in the formal team activities — the family conferences and the psychiatric seminar discussions and consultative sessions — as well as in the informal relationships of practice and the exchange of information, casual advice, and opinions. At the same time she carried on extra-program activities in her own field — attending meetings and seminars in the area of her interest as a social worker and retaining contact with her professional colleagues.[12]

THE JOB OF THE PUBLIC HEALTH NURSE

The introduction of the public health nurse into the Family Health Maintenance Demonstration was the extension of a natural process of development in the field. From its inception public health nursing conceived of the nurse as an educator[13] in the face of overwhelming social problems and as a companion of the physician in helping to mitigate the effects of illness. This was framed in the nursing character. It is important to recognize that prevention, carried on through education, was an early part of the nurse's role.

Since the task of the Demonstration was to seek out sources of defect and disability in family life and their interrelation with illness, we felt that the public health nurse should play a large part in the team operation. Not only did she have to be involved in the day-to-day care of the family, but she could play a significant role in the prevention of physical and emotional illness. Experience confirmed the confidence placed in the nurse. She was a most desirable person to have on a medical-care team because of her medical knowledge and limited medical training, her acceptability to the patient, her preventive and educational role, and her integral connections with the other professions. By bringing the team a knowledge of home and family situations that the other workers lacked, she helped them to do their job better.

The Content of the Job

As did the social worker, the nurse made contact with families invited to participate in the Demonstration. She outlined the background, objectives, and goals of the program, explained the procedures necessary, and encouraged the family to consider these factors. Once a family had agreed to participate, the nurse arranged appointments and encouraged the family to complete the baseline interviews and examinations. As often as possible she would assist, or at least be present, when the doctor examined the family members. She assisted the family in filling out the Cornell Medical Index. She interpreted the doctor's recommendations and the laboratory findings and arranged for further examination or study if necessary. In many ways she acted as a catalyst and expediter of the initial processes of introduction of the family into the Demonstration.

The nurse carried out a home interview, generally with the mother of the household, to obtain information about the nutrition of the family. In this way she could discover, not only general eating habits and patterns in the family (from the typical weekly series of menus), but specific details (that day's menu) and the food idiosyncrasies of various family members. Another part of her interview included information about sleeping habits, rest and recreation, leisure and work or school activities. From the statements she compiled a record that she used in later evaluations and shared the information with the other team members. The various forms used in collecting the data are part of the Appendix.

As a part of, and yet separate from the rest of the interview, the nurse completed a housing form which yielded information on the physical condition of the housing as well as psychological factors such as crowding. The housing inquiry assumed major importance, for in her concern for home management, nutrition problems, child-rearing, and sleeping and living arrangements, the nurse found housing a formidable element in the design of family health.[14]

The nurse regularly visited the schools, obtaining information from teachers, and principals, and occasionally from school nurses, about the child or family concerned.

After assessing the information and observations, the nurse completed the Evaluation Form.

In carrying out team activities, she met regularly with the doctor and social worker, attended team and family conferences, and participated in discussions with the psychiatric consultant. She was of help to the team through the evaluation of family environmental and health needs, and in team planning with the families to meet these needs.

As part of the Demonstration activities she attended group meetings of Demonstration families and carried on small discussion groups for parents of school-age children, pregnant women, and mothers of preschool children. She also ran a group session for overweight family members.

As part of the preventive role, the nurse made periodic home visits, helped with budgets and menus, advised on family problems, and made herself available for such consultations in the home or office as might be desired or requested. She gave talks, distributed literature, recommended books, and sometimes demonstrated washing a baby or cooking a meal. She supervised corrective exercises and aided with planning family budgets and food purchases. This health counseling and teaching function was the bulk of her activity.

As part of her therapeutic role, the nurse was present in the doctor's office as often as possible to assist him and speak with patients after his visit to interpret and assist in carrying out the doctor's orders. She visited the home when there was sickness and gave treatments or passed along information to the doctor. This part of her job gave rise to some dissatisfaction because she felt there was not time to do this and carry on her manifold educational activities as well.

The health team had to have a connection with two different camps. One of these provided the consultation services of the medical group, all the medical specialties used today in diagnosing and treating disease. Since the family doctor had restricted his qualifications to family practice and adult medicine, specialists in the other fields of medical practice — such as obstetrics and gynecology, orthopedics, surgery, dermatology, allergy, otology, and ophthalmology — were necessary. Skillful representatives of these specialties were provided as part of the Montefiore Medical Group structure. These specialists saw patients referred by the health team, and their notes and recommendations would be considered by the team or acted upon by the physician.

The other camp was comprised of a group of specialists whose skills helped the team to understand and deal with the socioeconomic and psychological aspects of family life and to assist in the preventive activities that were intended to be the cornerstone of team activity. A health educator, psychiatrist, psychologist, and social scientist were included in this category of consultants. Their special skills were used to outline areas of difficulty, evaluate situations, and recommend courses of action with regard to family problems. In addition the consultants advised the team members carrying out plans or programs. They were guides and advisors to the team as the team itself was to be guide and advisor to the families. The consultants would not give service to families — this would remain the prerogative of the team — but would give service to the *team*. This decision to separate them from their ordinary client relationship had an important influence on the way the consultants saw themselves in the Demonstration. In addition, the emphasis on prevention served to modify the consultants' conception of their own role.

The Health Educator

A health educator was employed, on a part-time basis, to implement the preventive medicine function of the Family Health Maintenance Demonstration. His duties were:

70

To stimulate the interest and involvement of the team members in educational efforts;

To suggest or demonstrate to team members appropriate educational methods;

To present for consideration to the team basic goals and current assumptions of health education.

By the very nature of the Demonstration the health educator was charged with a responsibility that transcended custom in his field, even as the Demonstration involved team members themselves in activities that went beyond traditional considerations of their roles.

The health educator was to apply his special skills and knowledge of individual and group motivation to gain acceptance among patients for modification of health practices. He would offer the team insights as to what might be useful in helping people to recognize their problems, so that the team might give the patients specific medical information in ways that would be acceptable to them. It meant organizing, or helping the team to organize, small group meetings which the team members were to conduct.[15]

At first the health educator himself demonstrated how such small group meetings could be run. Then similar groups were organized for the team members to take as their individual responsibility. The health educator provided lists of pamphlets and reading material and these were made available for distribution to patients and set up a reading list of books for team and patients to find information not available in pamphlets. He selected films to be shown at general meetings and at the small group meetings with content relevant to helping people to visualize better the problems they had come together to discuss. At general meetings with the team he discussed educational methods and the functions of health education and suggested desirable topics for future consideration.[16]

The Psychologist

The psychologist was a working consultant in a somewhat different sense from the other consultants. The largest part of his role lay in administering tests and offering interpretations of these tests to be used by the team members. Originally it had been in-

71

tended that a specially designed interpretive scheme would be devised to give the TAT a specific application to Demonstration evaluations. This turned out to be impractical, although a great deal of time and effort was expended in this direction. Research planning remained an element of the psychologist's contribution, but diagnostic testing was the important aspect of his role. By narrowing the range of his activity, we may have filtered out some important service and knowledge that a psychologist has to offer. However, this was a deliberate restriction. In addition to routine testing, the psychologist did intensive diagnostic testing on family members with special problems referred by the working team: such problems as reading or speech difficulties in children and chronic psychosomatic disorders in adults might be tested.

The Thematic Apperception Test was selected as the projective test most likely to permit the indirect expression of beliefs, values, and expectancies which govern behavior but which are not in the awareness of the individual. Despite our inability to develop an objective score on these factors of interest, certain observations could be made and impressions gathered from the testing. In a large number of individuals, similar patterns of response were evident. Some of these trends were: ubiquitous presence of anxiety and tension as sources of unhappiness and harassment in the daily lives of both adults and children; manifest disturbance in important aspects of life functioning, in work, sexuality, and social relationships; inability of married adults to emancipate themselves from the direct control which their parents continued to exercise over their lives.[17]

Two other points are noteworthy, keeping in mind that these are *impressions*. First is the general congruence of team impression and psychological interpretation. Secondly, 3 to 4 years after taking a TAT, those who took the final test noted that the pictures "looked familiar." There is a hint in this that the TAT may not be useful in follow-up studies because of the memory factor.

The Psychiatrist

As part of the prepaid Health Insurance Plan service, the Montefiore Medical Group had a psychiatrist available for consultation and referral for the purpose of establishing a psychiatric diagnosis or referring patients for psychiatric treatment. However, we felt that the team needed more in the way of psychiatric orientation. Since the team was to do more in the way of psychiatric service than the average physician in the Group did, we had to take into consideration psychiatric factors that were ordinarily either overlooked or ignored in practice even by competent internists. An effort had to be made to permeate the health team with psychiatric concepts so that it could deal with a good bit of what might ordinarily be considered psychiatric problems without referring the patient to a psychiatrist or to a psychiatric clinic.

This is not a new development, nor is the idea unique to the Demonstration. The conception of a larger role for nonpsychiatric professional people in dealing with psychiatric problems has occurred to educators and to psychiatrists themselves.[18] The reasoning stems partly from purely statistical considerations, that it would be impossible for all those who need psychiatric service to be treated by psychiatrists. Not only are there too few psychiatrists to deal with all the problems that arise but it is questionable whether it would be desirable for every person who has a neurotic complaint, an emotional disturbance, or a social problem to be referred to a psychiatrist for short- or long-term care. It seems more desirable for most problems to be handled at a level that would correspond with the patient's understanding of his need and where he *customarily obtains medical service.* The health team, to serve a useful function in giving the family advice and guidance, was designed to extend itself to do more in the way of emotional counseling and looking after minor (or relatively minor) neurotic disturbance than the average physician does now.[19]

A psychiatrist consultant to the team was seen as a consultant who would broaden the knowledge of the health team with regard to psychiatric care and problems; give them some insights into the generality of psychiatric problems that patients might bring; be available for regular consultation to discuss general problems; and advise on specific cases. It was not considered desirable for the psychiatrist to deal with the patients himself. If he became involved in therapy he would be an additional person dealing with the family, and because of the team focus this was undesirable. Then, if severe cases of psycho-neurosis or psychosis that ought to be in psychiatric treatment were taken care of within the Demonstration, within a short time the psychiatrist would be involved in patient care to such a degree that he would not have time to be a consultant. If he were to remain available for consultation and education of the team, enabling them to deal more effectively with what nonpsychiatrists can handle, the psychiatrist could not deal with patients himself.

Specifically, the psychiatrist offered direct educational service and held regularly scheduled conferences with team members — both individually and as a group. The different levels of knowledge of the members about psychiatry meant that an important function of the psychiatrist consultant was to assist in the development of each team member's knowledge about psychiatry so as to allow him to play his assigned role adequately. Naturally, no one would be expected to be as expert in any consultant area as the consultants themselves. The object was not to make psychiatrists out of team members, but to develop psychiatrically oriented team members. Psychiatry was to help them to do their own job better, not to do a different job. To the physician, a great contribution that psychiatry made to his job performance was to impress upon him the necessity for listening. Not only did he get to hear things about patients, but the opportunity to talk was received with gratitude by patients and may even have been therapeutic in itself.[20] Naturally, the social worker with her background of psychoanalytic training and casework experience, brought a much more sophisticated approach and presentation of problems to the psychiatrist.

The Social Scientist

Of the many roles that a social scientist could play in connection with the operation of the Family Health Maintenance Demonstration, two are outstanding: he could remain outside the group operation, observing and reporting as an outsider; or he could enter into the team operation as the other consultants did, sharing his knowledge with the team and advising on problems as they arose. We tried to get some of both into the Demonstration. The difficulty is that a social scientist observing and reporting on the *team operation* to the team will very rapidly limit his own usefulness. As he begins to be seen as a critic, the team operation may become so modified in his presence as to interfere with continued successful performance. So in the beginning the outsider's role, interpreted as research activity, was the larger role. At no time did the social scientist play a consultant's role to the degree that the psychiatrist or health educator did. However, over the years, as bits of research information were circulated among team members, questions and discussion followed, and so the imprint of the findings was left on the team members and presumably on the program, but no direct channel of consultation was developed.

The first consultant social scientist[21] devoted a good deal of time to establishing the sociological characteristics of the families, and most of the planning and the tables as they were influenced by sociological concepts are her work. She also was interested in the attitude of families toward the project and worked in tandem with the health educator in the development of the programs for group meetings. Observations of the team in operation and family attitudes were carried on too briefly for effective reporting, but she offered some helpful impressions. She pointed out the cultural factors that influenced our study families, the varying socio-economic factors, religious and ethnic background, and other sources of family tension. She gave team members insights about contradictory cultural goals (emphasis on academic achievement on the one hand, emphasis on financial success on the other) that modified personality as seen in the interviews. And she offered the team members themselves observations on their own relations to relation to patients on the one hand and to the consultants on the other.

Dr. Eliot Freidson, who took over as consultant in 1955, chose a research role entirely and plunged into very productive studies, ideas which continue to generate fresh studies. He set out to develop a research program that would essentially explore the relationship between patient behavior and the organization of health services. This exploration involved study of the interaction of the interprofessional Family Health Maintenance Demonstration teams, patients' conceptions of medical care and of the roles of the team members who supplied them with care, and the bearing of the organization of care on patient attitudes and the utilization patterns.

At first he was interested in looking at interprofessional team performances. He recorded team conferences on particular families and then team conferences with families. From his observations, he drew conclusions about the nature of the interaction of the team members with each other and with patients as well as the reactions of patients to the kind of care given and the kind of role played by different team members. Then he studied patient attitudes toward solo practice, toward the Montefiore Medical Group, and toward the Family Health Maintenance Demonstration to discover how the patients' conception of medical care was fulfilled by each medical care system. Later, he focused upon instances in which patients did not do what we expected of them, particularly instances of resistance to referral to the social worker and instances in which patients used solo practitioners in lieu of the Family Health Maintenance Demonstration or Montefiore Medical Group services.[22] I would emphasize that the presence of a social scientist, broadly engaged in research and consultation in connection with the Demonstration, was in itself helpful. By attending conferences and informal discussions the social scientist was able to call attention to sociological factors that might otherwise have been ignored or overlooked. For example, a great deal has been written about the influence of cultural factors and medical care in nutrition, but always in terms of "foreign" cultures, so that we tend to believe that these are problems for the Spanish-Americans in Colorado or immigrants in New York City. But class and culture interact among us all, and misunderstanding might develop between doctor and patient over the definition of what constitutes illness — with a resulting friction and failure to accept treatment.[23]

What the doctor is, rather than what he thinks he is or would like to be, may be broached through the social scientist's exploration. If a "Family Health Project" (or any organization of medical service) doesn't jibe with the doctor's conception of what he ought to be doing, a viable program will not ensue. Some studies, available and in progress, indicate what doctors are like, why people select medicine as a career, what the elements of a career line are, and what attitudes doctors have toward medical practice, as well as doctors' views about working in an organization as opposed to solo practice.[24] Much work still remains to be done to allow us to see doctors in full dimension and in relation to the manifold problems of practice, so that the social scientists may aid in orienting us toward this important problem of organizing a new type of medical service — the health team.[25]

In summary, the health team was organized to provide both preventive and therapeutic medical care to patients along lines that corresponded with the expectations of patients and the modern trends in the direction of professional performance. A specialized physician — an internist — joined forces with a public health nurse and a social worker to form this team. Consultant specialists in medicine, psychiatry, psychology, social science, and health education assisted the team in discharging their functions. The varieties of activity in advice and guidance, health promotion, and preventive medicine, as well as medical care, were worked out by the team members in concert and their individual professional skills informed each other to augment the team's activity.

PART TWO

RESULTS OF THE FAMILY HEALTH

MAINTENANCE DEMONSTRATION

~ VI ~

REACTIONS TO HEALTH-TEAM SERVICE

We cannot think first and act afterwards. From the moment
of birth we are immersed in action, and can only fitfully guide it
by taking thought.
                                                    — A. N. Whitehead

Engaged in research and service simultaneously, the Demonstration was "immersed in action," but we tried to take thought. It was not without trepidation that we had set out on this venturesome experiment. We realized that, since medical care is only a small part of life, in attempting to influence families through this small part, we were probably taking on much more than we could hope to accomplish. In planning we became aware of many difficulties ourselves; other obstacles were made known to us by critical observers. Some of the critics were disturbed by the breadth of the research design. Some felt that we concentrated on individual physical and emotional factors at the expense of productive exploration of the environmental and social fields. Those who saw personal emotional factors as preeminent determinants of family health considered our approach superficial, one that must fail and so undermine their position. Even those who accepted the research design of the Demonstration argued for limiting the study to a narrower range of observations.

In truth, all the criticisms have some substance. We could not examine every facet of family life: what we overlooked may be more important than what we noted. Important values or influences that we failed to uncover may well exist. It is an enormous

81

task to observe and note events in the lives of so many families over a 4-year period. With our imprecise measuring tools and inadequate concepts of causation, it took great self-confidence to note events in the belief that we could derive correlations or etiological relationships from them. Considering the complexity of modern society and the limited observations at our disposal, we can be certain that our observations do not fill in the whole story of health and disease in family life.

However, the broad range of observations had value if only as a "reconnaissance in force." A few interrelations of physical and emotional illness were noted, a few patterns that may be useful in medical practice were demonstrated, and a few social aspects of medical practice became visible. As a result, the path of future Demonstrations may be easier and future research may be more sharply and seriously focused.

We had set out to see if we could: (1) establish a new medical-care structure, containing preventive *and* therapeutic elements; (2) modify professional roles to carry out this combined function; (3) influence families favorably in their physical and emotional health; (4) measure this influence; and (5) accumulate data on family life and health practices.

With regard to (1) and (2), it seems clear enough that a new medical-care structure, with somewhat altered roles for the participants, is possible and feasible.

In connection with this view of family life in relation to a modified form of medical practice, an important general principle emerged as a limiting factor in any assessment of the program. It wasn't the modern scientific aspect of the program which made it viable for patients. People do not see physical, mathematical, and chemical formulas when they envision medicine; they see the relief of pain or the cure of disease. They expect science to be a part of medicine, not vice versa. Medicine is only partly to be considered the study of disease, because it is concerned with personal and social relationships of people with or without disease. When it affects to diagnose and treat disease (or prevent it) it is in larger part a social rather than a biological science. Medical service is expected to provide something extra, something that is unlikely to be a part of the natural scientist's conception of disease treatment.[1]

Many observers have noted that there is dissatisfaction with doctors' attitudes, and that this is not restricted to one section of the country. In newspaper reports, magazine articles, and books physicians may be viewed as cold, callous, indifferent, interested only in money. These statements are usually impressions rather than personal experiences. Intake interviews by a nurse or social worker prior to participation in our own program elicited many such hostile comments. People expressed a certain suspicion of physicians, and hinted at economic motivation. They felt that visits with doctors were too abrupt and rushed, and they expressed a need for discussion and explanation that was not usually supplied. The failure of the profession to meet popular expectations is not from the lack of laboratory science. Awareness of modern "miracle" surgery, "miracle" drugs, "miracle" diagnosis is widespread, yet something seems to be missing. Apparently what is missing is responsiveness on the part of doctors to the social needs of patients. The theoretical primary nature of the efficacy of treatment should really be subordinated to the satisfaction of social need. The "felt necessity" has priority over the professionally determined one.

The prespecialization physician took cognizance of the various systems in diagnosis and treatment (an analytic role) and also put together the meaning of the diagnostic and therapeutic deductions for the entire patient (a synthetic role). He saw his patient as an individual, part of a family and society; as a physiological engine, psychological personality, and citizen. The accumulation of modern scientific knowledge which has made specialization in medical practice necessary and professionally valuable, leaves a gap. While logically group practice cements the fragments which specialization creates, there remains a loose piece. Group practice generally omits the synthetic role. And it is the synthetic role that seems most closely related to patient satisfaction. The health team would seem able to supply the element lacking in group practice, and so meet patient needs in the area of satisfaction. The Demonstration type of practice, combining the scientific element of modern practice with the location of the health team in the structure of a group practice unit, should offer a greater degree of satisfaction to patients.

PATIENT REACTIONS

Measurement of morbidity and mortality alone do not wholly measure medical-care need. I say this in full awareness of the tremendous toll of epidemic disease in other parts of the world, and of the extent of chronic illness in our own country. The health team, although a revolutionary new pattern of service, did not appreciably alter the amount of illness found or treated. The impact of the program on the health of the study families as measured by morbidity was very little different from the impact of the relatively orthodox medical-care system on the control families.[2] But if we believe that disease treatment alone is not the sole job of the doctor, that answering the felt needs of the patient is just as important, then the values inherent in patient satisfaction with the Demonstration have great meaning. It was such satisfaction that must have kept families from moving away from the Bronx so that they could continue their participation in the program. This is what kept study families in the Group while control families dropped out.

From Table 2 it can be seen that 16.9 percent of the study families dropped out during the 4 follow-up years, compared to

Table 2. Families[a] withdrawing from Montefiore Medical Group.

Year	Number		Percent	
	Study	Control	Study	Control
Follow-up:				
First	2	9	1.6	5.6
Second	6	14	4.8	8.6
Third	9	14	7.3	8.6
Fourth	4	12	3.2	7.4
Total	21	49	16.9	30.2
Annual average	5.25	12.25	4.2	7.6
After completion of FHMD:[b]				
First	11	10	8.9	6.2
Second	3	1	2.4	0.6
Total	14	11	11.3	6.8

[a] Families originally present: study, 124; control, 162.

[b] For control families, year after completing an equivalent time period to matched study family (4 years) of membership in Montefiore Medical Group.

30.2 percent in the control group. The annual average withdrawal was 5.3 families for the study group, and 12.3 of the number present at the start for the control families. But after the Family Health Maintenance Demonstration was completed, the situation was reversed and study families began to drop out of the Montefiore Medical Group much more rapidly. Over the 2-year period following completion of the Demonstration, 14 study families and 11 control families dropped out. The apparent greater adherence by the study families to the Medical Group disappears once they are separated from the Demonstration.

Movement out of a group medical plan like HIP is occasioned by many events quite independent of dissatisfaction. People move to the suburbs; workers or managers are transferred to other jobs. An employer who paid all or a part of the insurance may drop the policy (or the worker leaves covered employment) and the individual may not wish to continue his insurance payment because he can't or won't pay the full premium on his own. About 7 percent of subscribers leave the group each year for all these reasons. On this basis, we would expect that 10 families would have left the Family Health Maintenance Demonstration each year of service, or a total of 40 families. More than the expected number of control families left (49), but far less than the expected number of study families left (21).

Furthermore, of the 21 families who did leave the Demonstration, only 3 left for overt reasons of dissatisfaction. For the others, better jobs or better housing forced a separation, and 18 families moved for these reasons. But it is an inescapable fact that a number of families remained in the Montefiore Medical Group, paid their own insurance premiums (an added burden), or held off from moving into new housing only because they wanted to remain as participants in this novel medical-care scheme. Family after family indicated in an attitude survey that the Demonstration met their needs for, or satisfied their conception of, family practice. The concrete fact that some families remained, only to move out as soon as the Demonstration was completed, supports the attitude survey strongly.

This fulfillment of a felt need for a special kind of family practice seems to have been what kept them attached to the idea of the Demonstration. There were undoubtedly families who felt that the team had no business prying into their emotional lives and would have none of our advice and guidance with respect to child-rearing practices or marital relations. There were families that may have become impatient with the elaborate, time-consuming, repeated studies and interviews, and families that may have resented the addition of the nurse and social worker and wouldn't use their services.

Despite the fact that some families may have tried to insulate their emotional lives and seal off from view the underlying unconscious events that motivated them, and despite the fact that with regard to physical disease they may have been only slightly better off than the people in the control group, they still felt a loyalty and attachment to the program. It is not an unlikely assumption that they looked upon the Demonstration as the fulfillment of their conception of a medical-care system.

Other evidence of satisfaction came out clearly in the conference held by the social scientist in which he asked a sample of families to specify both what they liked and what they didn't like about the Demonstration. Except for the fact that people paid money to remain and stayed under difficulties, one might accept the lack of negative comment as tactful. But there was *no* negative comment. When Dr. Freidson asked, "What was 'extra' in Family Health?," the answer given by one of the patients is typical. "Well, to me it was more personal. It's more as if he were your own family doctor on the outside." Another said, "I had a family doctor for years, before HIP . . . since I was about 12 . . . I always felt free to call on him . . . he always had time . . . when I went into HIP I lost that feeling at the beginning . . . When I went into Family Health, I got that same feeling that I had with my family doctor originally. And *they* [italics added] would call up occasionally — call up on the phone and asked me how [the child] was doing or was there anything that bothered me." [3]

They refers to the health team, not just to the physician, as the source of satisfaction. Unquestionably the added attention derived from the research character of the Demonstration was important in developing the family's feeling about the interest and the concern of the team members. This "special" quality also made the family more accepting of the whole Montefiore Medical Group environment. Actually, of course, the Demonstration was located in the same building; the doctor was part of the same Group structure; the nurses, attendants, and telephone operators were Group personnel. The patient's feeling that something was different and better about the Demonstration approach derived from the relationship of the program to him rather than from anything physically different in the circumstances.

Another bit of evidence in the same direction stems from the reaction of patients and doctors to the situation which arose when study families returned to the Medical Group after 4 years in the Demonstration. Doctors who saw ex-Demonstration patients often complained that they were too "demanding." How much of this was due to the patients' actual demands arising from their testing the new situation and how much from change in patients' expectations is not certain, but for a period of time friction between patients and doctors resulted. During the first year after they had left the Demonstration, patients came back from time to time to talk with the nurse or social worker or clerk, complaining that they missed the Demonstration and wanted to come "home" to people who were "interested in them" and be cared for as before. Some families changed from doctor to doctor, indicating their dissatisfaction with the Group service after the Demonstration service.

This tendency can be seen in Table 3 where it is shown that, during the first year after completion of the Family Health Maintenance Demonstration, 13 of the 98 study families who completed the Demonstration and remained at least 6 months there-

Table 3. Families[a] changing to new family physician during first year after completion of FHMD.

	Number		Percent	
Number of changes	Study	Control	Study	Control
0	85	101	86.7	91.8
1 or more	13[b]	9	13.3	8.2

[a] Study families who completed FHMD and control families completing an equivalent time of membership in the Montefiore Medical Group, who remained members of the Montefiore Medical Group for at least 6 months afterward. (Five study families and 3 control families withdrew in less than 5 months.)

[b] Three families changed twice.

after changed from one doctor to another. (Three changed to still another doctor during that year.) Of the 110 control families, only 9 made a change of family doctor.

A corollary to the satisfaction of patients was the satisfaction of the professional people working in the program, an indication that they were exercising their professional roles in an acceptable and agreeable way.

The Doctor

One of the doctor's satisfactions was the greater amount of time he had available to spend with patients. The Family Health Maintenance Demonstration physician was able to devote more time to his individual patients than family physicians in the Group because he had a smaller number of patients. However, since the Demonstration internist was charged with conferences, research activities, and other work in connection with the Demonstration, he did not have quite 5 times as much time available for the $\frac{1}{5}$ the number of patients he cared for (280 patients as compared to 1500 for a full-time Group family internist). On the basis of 1.6 visits per year (control families utilization rate) for 280 people, the expected number of family physician services per year would be 448. In the Demonstration, there were 1134 services, many more than expected. However, the doctor would still have much more time available for his patients since his hours as a full-time physician would be the same as those of the family doctor for the control families. This gain in time available plus more frequent visiting was one of the sources of satisfaction to the patients. ("He didn't have too many patients. He took time with you. He had time to give you.")

The family physician in the Demonstration also used this time to advantage. He made more diagnoses and found more cases of illness and he exerted a sparing influence on referrals, as can be seen in Table 27.[4] The increase in family-physician time was offset to some degree by the lessened percentage of specialist services used by the Demonstration families. The burden of added service imposed by an open system fell upon the family doctor and was not passed along to specialists. Even in his case, the burden diminished so that over the 4-year period family-doctor visits did decline and in the last year were down to twice the rate in the study as in the control groups.[5] By spending an average of 10 minutes more per visit, and seeing patients more frequently, the Demonstration physician was able to discharge his role more satisfactorily to the patient and more effectively. The family physician was obviously taking more responsibility, reducing referrals that might otherwise be made out of concession to patient demands or pressure of his own work.[6]

There were other reasons why the doctor enjoyed team participation. Not only did he have access to a full range of medical specialists whom he could use while exercising his professional role of family advisor, but he could use the skills of a public health nurse in routine daily practice. She could relieve him of many of the burdens of supervision in cases of illness. He could give her instructions about care in the home and ask her to help with advice, so that families got the extended range of the doctor's service through a professionally trained "assistant." In return he received information from the nurse about what went on in the family while the medical care was being carried out. He had a useful and gratifying professional channel of communication with the family which most physicians lack.

Further, he had access to the services of a social worker whose attitudes toward emotional illness and whose insight into families and their emotional health could help him in dealing both with patients with physical illness and with patients whose presenting symptoms of physical illness were either a mask for, or a complication of, emotional illness. He had the same sort of extended observation into the emotional lives of the patients through the social worker that he had into the physical life and environment through the public health nurse.

This is not to say that every doctor would find a team role congenial. The tradition of medical practice, with its emphasis on the solitary nature of responsibility and independent decisions regarding diagnosis and treatment, probably influences a certain type of person to enter the profession. Perhaps some doctors would grow restive under the necessity of team conferences and sharing decisions. I submit only that there were compensations for a conscientious physician in such a setting — that he could devote more of himself, obtain more information, and have more help to do a good job of patient care.

The Nurse

The public health nurse found in the health team a niche that represented the fruition of modern nursing aims. By and large, in agency practice the public health nurse must carry on within a framework that precludes initiative. She is under a doctor's instructions and, although her functions of health education and mother and child care offer some leeway, she is limited by those instructions. The doctor must diagnose and prescribe before the nurse is allowed to use her skills of health education and health supervision. In modern settings lines of communication with the practicing physician are tenuous at best and independent action limited. Yet the satisfactions of nursing are to be enjoyed principally where the nurse is able to proceed flexibly and freely in her field.[7] The daily contacts of doctor and nurse, scheduled team conference, and access to patients in advance of nursing problems, actually spelled out such flexible conditions.

The public health nurse found satisfaction in a daily team role. In the ordinary scheme of medical care, the public health nurse and the social worker are rarely engaged in medical service as a continuing process. An occasion of illness or dramatic need calls forth the nurse's service. The need met, or the occasion over, further contact with the patient ceases. In the Demonstration continuity of supervision was a routine matter.

Furthermore, the public health nurse working with an agency carries out agency objectives primarily with specific patients (or specific illnesses if she is specialized). In the Demonstration the public health nurse offered continuity of service in a family context. Just as we think it desirable that American medicine be structured so that there be a family physician, the Demonstration team was structured to provide a family nurse. She was in immediate contact with each family as it joined the program, and was given an opportunity to deal with family members, without a disease focus, before a problem existed that they were aware of or for which they might seek help.

In this connection she could emphasize another important aspect of modern public health nursing. She had a preventive role as the one who could recognize the need for and make available to families the opportunities and resources for forestalling illness. It was in these facets of her role — daily practice, family practice, and preventive practice — that the nurse found increased professional satisfactions.

The Social Worker

The social worker, her own field illuminated by medical information provided by the doctor and the observations of the nurse, was able to broaden her activities. She was party to diagnosis and difficulties much earlier than is common in agency case work, and so became aware of larger areas of need and service. In addition she could take advantage of the opportunity to contribute to the practice of other team members.[8]

Doctor, nurse, social worker — each seemed to find reward in the team process over and above the fulfillment of his own role. The sum of the experience, like that of patient satisfaction, points to the acceptability of health-team operation in daily medical practice.

THE PATIENTS VIEW THE TEAM

What was provided by the team and what was accepted by the patient was regarded differently by the participants. It is amusing now to look back on how carefully we tried to structure the team "democratically," so as to shore up the status of the paramedical people and put them on an equal footing with the doctor. We took great pains to establish a team "having no captain." Theoretically all were equal in decision-making, deferring to each other's superior judgment in specific areas, respecting each other's skills, and arriving at decisions by common consent. It is amusing because *we* decided the team should operate this way. The patients decided otherwise.

The Doctor

In Emerson's sense that an institution is the lengthened shadow of a man, medicine (the healing art) is the lengthened shadow of the doctor. Patient definition of "medical care" ranged very widely, but for problems touching on important illness or aberrant behavior the doctor was considered the logical person to

91

consult first. If the doctor was not available, the nurse was the next most desirable consultant. Of course, some families defined "medical care" differently — children's behavior in school was not generally accepted as a medical problem. In Freidson's study of patient selection of staff for various types of services, he showed that more respondents would ask the social worker first about school problems, for example, then the nurse, then the doctor. However, patients rated staff as desirable consultants in medical affairs in the following order: physician, nurse, clerk, social worker.

The view of the doctor as the key to medical practice cut across class lines. Poor or rich, well- or ill-educated, from lower or upper occupational class, patients preferred the doctor's ministrations. In the lower social scale, it is true, patients would more readily accept a nurse's diagnosis or treatment, not wanting to "bother" the doctor, but their indicated preference was for his service.

The Nurse

Differences in preference demonstrated by patients does not invalidate the idea of the health team as acceptable and useful to the majority of the participants. This acceptability simply did not extend to equal appreciation or utilization of the team personnel. Utilization reflects both appreciation of role and actual need. Regardless of class, although utilization varied, the preference did not. The relationship with the nurse was felt to be the most comfortable one, compared with both the doctor[9] and social worker.

Table 4 shows that a larger proportion of study-family members used the services of the family physician or pediatrician during their 4 years in the Family Health Maintenance Demonstration than they did the services of the public health nurse or the social worker. The services of the social worker were used by the smallest proportion. Some 66 percent of the study-family members used the services of the family physician or pediatrician during their first year of participation. Although this proportion dropped steadily as time progressed, and was 53 percent by the fourth year, the weighted 4-year average was 58.7 percent, nearly three-fifths of the total number of study-family members.

Table 4. Percent of study-family members using services of professional staff, by staff member used and follow-up year.[a]

Staff member	Weighted 4-year average of percents in each year[b]	Follow-up year			
		First	Second	Third	Fourth
Family physician or pediatrician	58.7	66.2	59.1	56.1	52.9
Public health nurse	41.1	72.5	38.8	29.3	21.6
Social worker	22.8	33.7	25.0	19.1	12.4

[a] A study-family member is here defined as using the services of a professional staff member in a specific follow-up year only when he used 3 or more services by that staff member during the follow-up year.

[b] Weighted by the number of study-family members in each year, as follows: first, 523; second, 513; third, 508; and fourth, 476.

Public health nursing services dropped more sharply (73 to 26 percent) with an average of 41 percent of families using them; and use of the social worker was consistently in the smallest proportion, dropping from 34 to 12 percent and averaging 23 percent of the families. The same pattern was evident for each family member, each year of study.

While the doctor held the same position of esteem in patients' eyes that he held in solo practice, the nurse achieved the medical-care status of a substitute or surrogate for the doctor in his absence or by his designation. This is not unexpected and fits well with the characteristics of public health nurses.[10] Nurses seem to identify more with patients (and patients with them) either because of the personality attributes that caused them to select nursing, or because of class similarity to their patients. They are psychologically prepared and obviously willing to do the "dirty" work of bedside care and be cheerful and helpful in the face of difficult, unpleasant — in the presence of infectious disease, actually dangerous — work. The recognition of this by patients causes them to see the public health nurse as a "doing" person, and so a "good" person. She was liked by the families; they could respond to her. In return, the nurse tended to be more favorably inclined toward the families and more optimistic; she took a more sanguine view of their defects. This is reflected noticeably in the final evaluation wherein areas marked by the nurse the study families showed positive growth.

93

A patient remarked, "Miss A was very nice and gave me many helpful hints. She came here in the morning, showed me how to bathe the baby and any problems that I had, I mean I felt no hesitation in calling on her and believe me, I had a few . . . it was never too much trouble for her — on the phone or if I happened to stop in at Family Health. She came here quite a few times to see how the baby was doing and helped out with the feeding schedule, to make it easier for me."

Accepted by the families as having a medical role to play, the nurse was so consulted, with or without the presence of significant illness. Even in the problems of child-rearing, where the social worker had equal interest and could have been equally helpful, it was to the nurse that the families turned. Unlike social work, there were no pejorative connotations attached to public health nursing and the nurse's job was not seen in a psychiatric context. The nurse could criticize the sleeping arrangements in a family, for example, without this implying a psychiatric diagnosis. Her greater acceptability tended to displace the doctor somewhat, too, in the role of advisor and educator. Not only the current picture of the doctor as scientist and specialist, but the common understanding of the function of the nurse fostered this. While American medicine does not tolerate a "secondary practitioner" in theory, in reality the public health nurse in some ways discharges this role.[11]

Evidence of attachment to the nurse, both in her own capacity and in her capacity as team representative, was seen early and all through the program. It was even evident in patients after they had left the Demonstration. A number of people had no hesitation in coming back, although they were no longer on the program, to ask the nurse for guidance and help in critical family situations. In one case, a pregnant woman whose father was dying of some obscure malady found herself unable to cope with mounting misfortune. Her husband's new business venture began to fail; he himself developed pneumonia and was convalescent a long time. She found herself breaking into tears over little things and avoiding contacts with neighbors. Remembering only the discomfort and dread when her first baby had been born, she was afraid to go to the hospital to have this baby. She was deluged with fears. Her family doctor advised psychiatric care, which she

94

refused. Although she had been separated from the Demonstration for over a year, she felt impelled to return and talk with the nurse. The nurse talked with her, arranged to see her again at home, and spent several hours with her on different occasions. Advised by the nurse to take the doctor's advice and seek psychiatric care, the woman went. In a few months she had recovered sufficiently to cope with her problems, none of which remitted. Her gratitude was directed, not to her family physician nor to the psychiatrist, but to the nurse.

In Freidson's tables (one of which — Table 5 — is reproduced here), the responses of the study-family members to specific ques-

Table 5. Choice between staff workers (percent) by Warner occupational scale, administered Winter 1957 to study families.

Question: "If it were necessary to choose between having the services of a public health nurse . . . and the services of a social worker . . . how would you choose? Make your choice on the basis of your own needs and past experience."

	Warner occupational scale class		
Answer	1 & 2 (highest)	3 & 4	5 & 6 (lowest)
If I couldn't have both, would prefer having a social worker	37	26	17
If I couldn't have both, would prefer having a public health nurse	46	62	67
Makes no difference which one	17	12	16
Number of respondents	59	71	81

Source: Freidson, "Patients' Views of Medical Practice."

tions of preference among staff members elicited unequivocal selection of the nurse. The questions were of this type: "To whom have you made the greatest number of office visits for which you made an advance appointment?" "Whom have you called (most) on the phone for one thing or another?" "With whom have you had the greatest number of informal chats?" Overwhelmingly, the lower-class[12] respondents preferred the public health nurse for service. The other classes did not display such marked response, but the evidence of the nurse's general acceptability is clear.

Well liked and understood, her role clearly defined, close to the social class of those she served, the public health nurse had a secure and pleasant place in the program — to her taste, and to the patients' as well. In addition, as a colleague who accepted instruction from the doctor and carried out his instructions, saving him steps and trouble, responding to his unvoiced unwillingness to do the things she did, the nurse had the doctor's respect and gratitude as well.

The Social Worker

For the social worker life was not so easy. From the analysis of preferences, patients placed social workers below doctors and nurses in the order of desirability for dealing with medical problems. In every sense that nursing is understood and accepted, social work may not yet be.

Social-work norms in the United States are middle-class norms,[13] and the training requirements (at least 2 years after college and a Master's degree) tend to reinforce middle-class attitudes and standards. Problems filtered through class bias usually result in unacceptable solutions to those of different class.[14] Resistance to social work may also derive from previous experiences. Family members may have had experience with social work that had struck a jarring note.[15]

By contrast with the nurse stereotype which is admired, the social-worker stereotype seemed to have been mistrusted and misunderstood by Demonstration families, particularly by those low on the occupational scale. But even for those higher on the scale, who may not have had unpleasant previous experiences to discolor their picture of social work, an alternate reason for dislike may be found in social-work identification with psychiatry, and thereby with mental illness. Social-work intervention in a case, even suggested interview with a social worker, struck an ominous note. So social work was generally not considered by the patients to be part of *health* services.[16] Associated with the idea of mental illness and welfare, the social worker's job was sharply separated from activities to be tolerated on behalf of an active person in good physical health. To convince the families of the need for the social worker implied acknowledgment of a disturbed family situation. Few families in our culture care to accept a diagnosis of psychiatric disorder, so long as there remains a difference in people's minds between psychiatric and physical illness. They would be reluctant to come in as presumably normal, functioning families without any problems and without any difficulties, and have the social worker say to them, "there are some weak areas that have to be worked with," which translates to them in effect as "your family suffers from mental illness."

In the light of this, it is not surprising that the social worker responded to the patients differently from the nurse. Where the nurse was optimistic in the evaluations, the social worker was pessimistic. In evaluation scores, the social worker marked lower in areas marked by both on the same individual. The nurse marked more people "excellent" than the social worker did. In the initial evaluation the number of "excellents" in the public health nurse's evaluation of personal adjustment had exceeded the social worker's by about one-third; by the final evaluation this number had risen to nearly two-thirds.

Table 6 shows that the degree of correspondence[17] in their

Table 6. Degree of correspondence of ratings of study-family members between the social worker and the public health nurse.

Area of evaluation	Initial evaluation		Final evaluation	
	Number of subjects	Coefficient of correlation[a]	Number of subjects	Coefficient of correlation[a]
Personal adjustment	422	+0.66	465	+0.49
Family relationship:				
Husband and wife	102	.68	106	.30
Father and children	198	.61	251	.41
Mother and children	203	.69	262	.37
Recreational adjustment	458	.51	447	.45
Occupational adjustment of father	117	.58	119	.36
Educational achievement of children	117	.67	190	.62

[a] While the data do not conform to usual requisites for the coefficient of correlation, nevertheless the coefficient does give a rapid idea of the degree of correspondence.

evaluations of the same individual declined with the passage of time, that is, from their initial to their final evaluation of each member of the study families. Decline was evident in each area of evaluation, and in some areas the decline was quite sharp. For example, on personal adjustment evaluated for 422 individuals the correlation coefficient (used here to measure the degree of correspondence between the social worker and the public health nurse), dropped from +0.66 for their initial evaluations to +0.49 for their final evaluations. Agreement between these professional staff members on their evaluation of the family relationship of the spouses and of parents with children dropped also.[18]

This is a consistent pattern and actually a test of internal consistency of these subjective evaluations. In evaluations of the same individual, the public health nurse changed her grade from the initial to the final rating in the direction of improvement, while the social worker changed her grade in the direction of deterioration. Thus, in the social worker's evaluation of the personal adjustment of the individuals in the study families, 14.1 percent were judged to have worsened. For the spouses the corresponding percentage deemed by the social worker to have deteriorated was 23.9 percent; for father and children it was 32.1 percent; and for mother and children it was 17.1 percent. Only in her evaluation of the occupational adjustment of the father did the social worker detect improvement.

The situation was completely reversed in the evaluations by the public health nurse. She detected improvement between the initial and final evaluation in nutrition for 22.0 percent of the individuals in the study families; for housing in 32.3 percent; for sleep and rest in 25.9 percent; and for educational achievement of the children in 17.8 percent. Only in her evaluation of recreational adjustment did she detect a deterioration between initial and final rating, and that for 18.5 percent of the individuals.[19]

Some weight ought to be given to the fact that the training of the social worker, like that of the physician, is problem (or disease) oriented. The social worker doesn't expect wellness. She looks at people diagnostically, from the standpoint of what is wrong, on the basic assumption that there always is something wrong. With familiarity and with the opportunity over a 4-year period to elicit more symptoms and to find more problems, the social worker is very likely to discover in the end that the patient was endowed with considerably more in the way of difficulty and defect than she found in the beginning. In the end, it would not be expected that the patients could be thought improved.[20]

The difficulties in integrating a social worker into the health team were greater than those in the integration of doctor and nurse and do not seem amenable to easy, swift solution. For example, social-worker interviewing was carried out in the office, and only rarely would a family member be interviewed at home. The social worker found the home environment constrictive because of the lack of privacy, less productive and of lesser value than the office interview. Although home visiting had been visualized, the social workers resisted. They felt that a home visit should have a purpose, that visiting merely to be in the home not only was of little value but actually was detrimental to the purpose of the interview. Obtaining expression of extremely personal and private feelings in the home environment was said to be much more difficult than in the office setting where confidences of this sort are expected to be extracted. Therefore, home visiting by social workers was the exception rather than the rule.

While administrative obstacles may have played a part through faulty assignment of cases, characteristics of the individual workers, and the professional conceptions of "proper" roles, the greatest obstacles lay in an area least easily dealt with — the patient's conceptions of professional roles and the place of these roles in their daily health problems.

If these obstacles can be overcome, the social worker could expect to derive satisfactions from enrichment of therapeutic role by the added illumination and support offered by daily contacts with nurse and physician.

OBSTACLES TO PROFESSIONAL SATISFACTION

The Doctor

It became evident early that to be a family adviser one should have responsibility for the entire family. The families themselves in discussion with team members mentioned a degree of confusion as to where to turn for advice. The team members found themselves in a situation from time to time in which both pediatrician and internist were involved, perplexing the parents and the team members as to which source of advice should be consulted — or perhaps whether it shouldn't be both. The doctor, well trained as an internist, found difficulty in being a family adviser of a generic type because a part of the family (children under 13) were not under his direct care, and were looked after

99

by a pediatrician. We did arrange for pediatrician and internist to confer, and arbitrarily assigned to the internist the role of family adviser. Yet, it was hard for the internist to be such a family guide without being a pediatrician. Unfortunately, there is as yet no specialty that encompasses this kind of family practice. Desirable as it may be, it is difficult to see how such a specialty could be developed in the near future.[21]

The Public Health Nurse

An obstacle to full satisfaction for the public health nurse was the cleavage between her role as a family visitor and adviser and her role as physician's assistant. It was thought desirable that the public health nurse should work in the office with the doctor when he was seeing patients, but family visiting conflicted with office hours. When an office nurse was provided to work with the doctor on occasion, matters were brought up in the doctor's office that would have to be transmitted at second hand to the public health nurse. This was a real disadvantage. It is not impossible to visualize a group of teams working together in some future family-oriented group practice, where nursing obligations for teaching, visiting, and office work can be divided among the nurse members of the team and dispose of this obstacle.

The Social Worker

The difficulties with regard to patient attitudes, and a divergence in professional conception of role from the one assigned in the Demonstration, have already been discussed as complications of the social worker's task, inhibiting satisfaction. The conception of role derives from standard patterns of professional responsibility. Visiting schools and homes, for example, was a responsibility which nurses discharged without complaint. Visiting away from the office was a reluctant duty for social workers. Reconciliation to a family practice concept, in the doctor's or nurse's sense, was difficult.

Chapter X provides a detailed assessment of the health team. Here, reaction to team service can be summed up briefly. The patients and staff liked it: the patients particularly because the team represented a model of medical care and guidance they had always longed for; and the staff because it permitted ideal fulfillment of professional roles. There were some difficulties, but these represent problems in adjustment rather than basic defects of organization. Even differences in conception of professional role can be utilized to modify future team operations and do not present real obstacles. The team is a feasible health-service form, and in acceptability to patients is superior to group practice while equal to it in modern scientific terms.

101

~VII~

CHANGES IN THE HEALTH OF
DEMONSTRATION FAMILIES

Citius emergit veritas ex errore quam ex confusione.

— Francis Bacon

As one of the major objectives of the program, we had added a series of health promotional activities to a comprehensive medical service in an effort to prevent emotional difficulties and family breakdown, and thereby improve family health. The health team seemed to be viable, but did it improve health? Did it prevent disease and family disorganization? Did it modify behavior so as to prevent emotional difficulties in the family members and hold together threatened family structure?

Although it was difficult to measure the health of the participants and define the effect of the program on health because of the subjectivity of recording, ambiguities of diagnosis, and brevity of the Demonstration, interesting clues pointed up the value of this kind of health supervision.

THE EVALUATIONS

In order to assess changes in the physical health and adjustment of the study families, tests were given both at the initiation and conclusion of their participation in the Family Health Maintenance Demonstration. Final evaluations for control families were carried out at approximately the same time that the corresponding study families terminated their participation. Table 7 sum-

Table 7. Number of evaluations by area and by staff members making the evaluation.[a]

Staff member	Evaluation	Study families[b]	Control families[c]
Physician	Family medical history	507	324
	Physical condition	483	332
Public health nurse	Nutrition	440	325
	Sleep and rest	466	328
	Educational achievement of children	135	141
	Recreational adjustment	459	326
	Housing	465	329
Social worker	Personal adjustment	447	317
	Family relationships of —		
	Spouses	219	144
	Children and father	218	169
	Children and mother	225	173
	Occupational adjustment of father	107	70

[a] Except in family relationships, all evaluations are of individual family members.

[b] Includes only those members for whom rating was made at both initial and final evaluations.

[c] Includes only those members for whom rating was made.

marizes the areas of evaluation, the staff member making the evaluation, and the number of these evaluations, for both.

While it was expected that all the team members would register evaluations in all areas, in some areas such duplication was unnecessary or impossible. The physician evaluated on matters directly relevant to physical health — family medical history and physical condition. The public health nurse evaluated on matters that were assigned to her area of competence — nutrition, sleep and rest, housing. The social workers evaluated primarily on personal adjustment and the various family relationships. However, there was some overlapping; consequently, it was possible to compare markings of nurses and social workers — in the areas of personal adjustment, for example.

The number of families evaluated was not the same for the study as for the control group. Evaluations made for the study families always exceeded the number made for the control families. This is not surprising in that the study families had closer contacts with the health team, and more incentive to cooperate. Furthermore, the number of evaluations made by the staff varied by area of evaluation. For example, the physician made 507 evaluations of family history in the initial evaluations of study families, but only 483 evaluations of physical condition. In the control families the comparable figures were 324 and 332, respectively. These differences stem from the fact that the evaluations had to be done piecemeal, each at a different time. No individual or family could spend, on one occasion, the hours required for doing all the evaluations. Among the study families, the family history would surely be known. Yet one or two would escape the final physical examination. Among the controls, some histories as well as physical examinations would be missed. Although only 70 control families were complete, there were others who had some part of the evaluation done; and of the 40 incomplete, they were not untouched. The total available number to be evaluated at different times is noted in Table 8.

Table 8. History of participation.

Families	Study		Control	
Total invited	159		162	
Agreed to participate	124		—	
Terminated before initial evaluation	0		12	
Available for initial evaluation[a]	124		150	
Complete		124		132
Not complete		0		18
Terminated before final evaluation	21		40	
Available for final evaluation	103		110	
Complete		103		70
Not complete		0		40

[a] For Controls, "Initial Evaluation" refers to mail questionnaires only.

Finally, the number of evaluations was necessarily different where it concerned a different base — for example, the family as a whole, children, fathers, family relationship. In the initial evaluations of study families, the 507 evaluations of family medical history exceeded the 135 made of educational achievement of the children, 219 of family relationships between the spouses, and 107 of the occupational adjustment of the father.

Turning to the content of the evaluation, it may be recalled that each area for evaluation was rated excellent, good, fair, or poor, depending upon staff judgments and scores on the Cornell Medical Index and other tests. To permit clearer exposition and understanding of the results of these ratings, however, each was arbitrarily assigned the following weight: excellent, 4; good, 3; fair, 2; and poor, 1. On the basis of these weights, a mean for the entire group of patients could be computed. If exactly the same proportion of patients was rated 4, that was rated 3, 2, or 1, the average thus computed would equal 2.5. The maximum mean that could be obtained by any group by this procedure is 4.0 (all "excellent" ratings) and the minimum is 1.0 (all "poor" ratings).

EVIDENCE OF IMPROVEMENT IN FAMILY HEALTH

The evidence of benefit to the participants in a measurable way is unequivocal in some important areas, disappointingly indecisive in other areas. In the areas evaluated by the physician — family medical history and physical condition — members of the study families improved between their initial and final evaluations. For family medical history the improvement was negligible, from a weighted mean of 2.4 to 2.5, but for physical condition the improvement was much greater, from 2.7 to 3.1 (see Table 9).

The slight improvement in family medical history consisted of changes from initial evaluations in which 3.4 percent rated "ex-

Table 9. Averages[a] of evaluation ratings by area and staff member.[b]

| Staff member | Evaluation | Study families | | | Control families |
		Initial evaluation	Final evaluation	Change	
Physician	Family medical history	2.40	2.48	0.08	2.69
	Physical condition	2.67	3.07	.40	2.97
Public health	Nutrition	3.12	3.31	.19	3.17
nurse	Sleep and rest	3.32	3.52	.20	3.55
	Educational achievement of children	3.50	3.66	.16	3.75
	Recreational adjustment	3.51	3.48	(−) .03	3.56
	Housing	2.69	3.25	.56	2.72
Social worker	Personal adjustment	2.91	2.66	(−) .25	2.82
	Family relationship of				
	Husband and wife	3.02	2.67	(−) .35	2.92
	Father and children	3.20	2.79	(−) .41	3.09
	Mother and children	2.96	2.61	(−) .35	3.02
	Occupational adjustment of father	3.26	3.42	.16	3.57

[a] Weights: excellent, 4; good, 3; fair, 2; poor, 1.
[b] Except in family relationships, all evaluations are of individual family members.

105

cellent," to final evaluations in which 3.7 percent rated "excellent," and in "good" ratings, from 44.8 to 51.1 percent of all study-family members. There were corresponding declines in the proportions rated "fair" and "poor," 39.8 to 35.1 percent and 12.0 to 10.1 percent, respectively.

The substantial improvement in physical condition consisted mainly in the large shift in the proportion rated "good" — from 36.6 percent of members of study families in their initial evaluations to 68.2 percent in their final evaluations (the corresponding change in the proportion of "excellent" ratings was only from 16.4 to 20.3 percent). Balancing the large upward shift in "good" ratings was the large downward shift in "fair" ratings, 44.1 to 9.7 percent. Again, the decline in "poor" ratings was minor, 2.9 to 1.8 percent.

In the area of family medical history, both initial and final evaluations of the study-family members resulted in means slightly below that which would have been obtained — 2.5 — if the ratings had been distributed in 4 exactly equal proportions. However, the control families did much better — their mean was 2.7. The difference between them and the study families consisted in their higher proportion of "excellent" ratings, 12.3 percent, and correspondingly lower proportions of "fair" and "poor" ratings. (It was easier to get more family history material in the study families. This may explain the quantitative difference from controls.)

In the area of physical condition, the mean scores in both initial and final evaluations of study-family members were above 2.5. The means of the controls, 3.0, fell between initial and final means of the study-family scores. As Table 10 shows, the percentage distribution of scores for physical condition was quite different for the control-family members. The higher proportion of ratings of "excellent" may be interpreted as evidence of better physical condition of controls to begin with — which is doubtful — or a differing experience with the families on the part of the health team — which is more likely. The greater case finding in the study group unquestionably contributed to the final evaluation, and diminished the number of "excellents." But, still, taking "excellent" and "good" together the study families exceeded the control families in these combined categories by a sizable amount (88.5 to

Table 10. Distribution (percent) of evaluation ratings of individual family members in areas evaluated by the physician.

Area	Study families		Control families
	Initial	Final	
Family medical history:			
Excellent	3.4	3.7	12.3
Good	44.8	51.1	51.0
Fair	39.8	35.1	29.9
Poor	12.0	10.1	6.8
Physical condition:			
Excellent	16.4	20.3	24.2
Good	36.6	68.2	51.4
Fair	44.1	9.7	22.0
Poor	2.9	1.8	2.4

75.6 percent). On the basis of these data, the Family Health Maintenance Demonstration was apparently successful in improving the physical health of the study-family members.

At the same time, all the change in all the families was not in an upward direction, toward improvement. Keep in mind that 35 percent of all those evaluated did not change at all (see Table 11), and that there was no discernible pattern in the improvement

Table 11. Change from initial to final evaluation in study families.

Member of family	Change in physical condition (percent)		
	Improved	No change	Deteriorated
Father	55.9	37.3	6.8
Mother	47.1	48.7	4.2
Child	47.2	27.8	25.0
Total	49.3	35.2	15.5

or lack of it. Of those originally marked "excellent," 22.4 percent deteriorated. Of those originally graded "fair," 52 percent improved. Only in a general way, taking the study families as a whole, can it be said that improvement was shown. Nor is the improvement or deterioration uniform among mothers, fathers, and children (see Table 12). Nevertheless, the trend is clear.

In the ratings of the public health nurse, even initially the averages were considerably above 2.5. This no doubt reflects the

Table 12. Distribution of evaluation ratings in areas evaluated by the physician.

Evaluation	Member of family	Evaluation of physical condition (percent)			
		Excellent	Good	Fair	Poor
Initial (study families)	Father	5.1	44.9	47.5	2.5
	Mother	2.5	42.3	47.1	7.6
	Child	29.0	28.2	42.0	0.8
	Total	16.8	35.8	44.6	2.9
Final (study families)	Father	20.3	70.3	6.8	2.5
	Mother	7.6	75.6	13.4	3.4
	Child	24.2	65.1	9.9	0.8
	Total	19.2	68.9	10.0	1.8
Control families	Father	29.2	51.4	19.4	0
	Mother	23.7	46.0	23.7	6.6
	Child	22.4	53.6	22.4	1.6
	Total	24.2	51.4	21.0	2.4

relatively high standard of living of our families. Nevertheless, and despite this initially high level, improvement was indicated in 4 of the 5 areas in which the nurses made their evaluations. In one — housing — the degree of improvement was substantial.

The average of study-family members for nutrition rose from 3.1 to 3.3. For sleep and rest it was from 3.3 to 3.5; and for educational achievement of the children from 3.5 to 3.7. The comparable rise in housing was truly impressive, from 2.7 to 3.3. Only in recreational adjustment was there no real change — as the averages of ratings for members of the study families stayed at about 3.5.

This increase in the study-family members' average for housing from initial to final evaluation was all the more significant because apparently no such change took place for members of the control families. Their average, 2.7, was very much like that for the initial evaluation of the study-family members. For nutrition also, although the increase in the average of the study-family members was not impressive, it did succeed in bringing their average scores above that of the controls.

Finally, of the 5 areas evaluated by the social worker, the averages of the ratings of study-family members declined from initial to final evaluation in 4 of these. For personal adjustment, the drop

108

in average rating was 2.9 to 2.7. The controls averaged 2.8. Similarly, for those areas of evaluation representing family relationships, each dropped from initial to final evaluation in the study families, and in this instance the differences were larger. In each of these the averages in the initial evaluations of the study families were fairly close to the corresponding averages for the controls in their final evaluations. Among all the areas evaluated by the social worker only in the case of occupational adjustment of the father was there a small increase in the average rating between initial and final evaluation of the study families. It rose from 3.3 to 3.4, but the average rating for the controls was even higher, 3.6.

THE MEANING OF THE DIFFERENCES

These findings require some elucidation. There is evidence that the study families were physically healthier at the end of the program than they were in the beginning, and that at the end of the program slightly more of them were judged healthy than were the control families. Improved nutrition would be expected to go hand in hand with improvement of physical health generally, and nutrition is improved in the study families. Other areas, such as sleep and rest or educational achievement of the children, reflect no greater improvement among study families than among controls, and the difference in recreational adjustment is insignificant and unimportant. But in housing there is an interesting implication in the improvement.

Nutrition is closely tied to health in many different ways, and the improvement evident is welcome. If health and nutrition didn't go up or down together, that would be puzzling and difficult. But the large and significant improvement in housing among study families, not reflected in the control families, is grounds for suspecting that we did succeed in getting the families to improve their housing, either through moving to new quarters or readjusting their living arrangements.[1] Enthusiastic acceptance of the significance of this finding is dampened somewhat by the knowledge that a few families with poor housing do not appear in the final evaluation, and so overemphasize the apparent improvement (see Table 24).

No wholly satisfactory explanation can be made for the absence of evidence of improvement in the emotional area, and actual evidence of deterioration vis-à-vis the control families. It is possible the Demonstration affected the emotional health of study families adversely, or it may be that in 4 years of close communication more evidence of family difficulties became available than could be brought out in a single final interview with the control families. Again, our criteria may have been off the mark, our measurements crude or inaccurate (certainly the 4-step scale of marking is too coarse to be satisfactory), or we ourselves not up to the job.[2]

CORRELATES OF IMPROVED HEALTH

Having seen the degree of improvement that could be measured, we may explore the characteristics of the families or persons judged by our staff to have been improved in health over the years of observation.

One index of improvement likely to be objective is the physician's evaluation of physical health. Study-family parents whose rating on physical condition improved between the initial and final evaluations were almost identical with all study-family parents in age, but in other characteristics they differed a bit (see Table 13). The parents who displayed improvement in physical condition constituted about 1 in 6. Among the younger parents (20–34 years), it was slightly greater than among the older parents (35–54 years), but in neither age group was the proportion much different from that for all parents.

By education, however, the "improved" parents constituted somewhat higher proportions among both highest and lowest education attainment groups (20 percent of all parents in each of these groups). These educational groups were also the lowest utilizers of medical services. "Improved" parents were a much lower proportion of parents of medium educational attainment, and medium educational level is characterized by *high* utilization of services. The "improved" parents constituted a larger proportion of parents who were ranked high and low in social class (measured by occupation), who are relatively low utilizers of service, and a smaller proportion of the middle class who are relatively higher users of medical service. "Improved" parents

Table 13. Number of study-family parents[a] whose physical condition improved from initial to final evaluation according to selected characteristics.

	Fathers			Mothers		
	Improved			Improved		
Characteristic	Number	Percent	Total	Number	Percent	Total
Total	24	20.3	118	14	11.8	119
Age:						
20–34	9	23.1	39	8	12.9	62
35–54	15	19.0	79	6	10.5	57
Education						
High	11	22.4	49	6	16.7	36
Medium	5	12.5	40	5	8.8	57
Low	8	27.6	29	3	11.5	26
Social class:						
High	8	22.9	35	4	14.3	28
Medium	5	14.3	35	6	12.5	48
Low	11	22.9	48	4	9.3	43
Score on Cornell Medical Index:						
0–9	10	25.6	39	1	5.6	18
10–29	11	16.7	66	7	10.9	64
Over 29	3	23.1	13	6	16.2	37

[a] Includes only those for whom both initial and final evaluation of physical condition are known.

were least represented among those with middle range scores in the Cornell Medical Index, but this did not correlate with use of services since a high CMI score was correlated with very high utilization (see Table 39).

Interestingly, this description of improvement and its relation to the factors reviewed is a function more of the fathers' situation than of the mothers'. While in the area of age and educational attainment fathers and mothers responded similarly, the fathers contributed more heavily in percentages improved. In social class and in the CMI relationship the mothers responded differently, and it is the higher proportion of fathers responding that gives the characteristic pattern for parents in these areas. Mothers in the lowest social class contributed a very small percentage to improvement, unlike the fathers. Mothers with a low score on the CMI contributed little to improvement, again unlike the fathers, and most surprisingly in both medium and high score CMI re-

111

sponses they showed the most improvement. It is in this that the mothers show a greater inconsistency than the fathers in relation to use of services as an index of improvement.

The characteristic consonant with the data is that study-family parents (not individuals) whose rating on physical condition improved between the initial and final evaluation did differ significantly from all parents in their use of the services of the Demonstration staff members (see Table 14). "Improved" parents aver-

Table 14. Average annual use per person of services of staff members by study-family parents and by those parents whose physical condition improved from initial to final evaluation.

Staff member	Study-family parents	Parents with improved physical condition	Ratio (percent)
All physicians	6.0	5.3	88
Family physician	4.1	3.9	95
Specialist	1.9	1.4	74
Public health nurse	2.8	2.3	82
Social worker	2.9	3.3	114

aged 5.3 as their annual use of physicians' services over the entire 4-year period of participation, sensibly less than the 6.0 of all parents. And their use of physicians' services was less, regardless of type of physician used. They also averaged fewer services by the public health nurse than the annual mean for all parents. Only in the case of services by the social worker did "improved" parents average a larger number of services than the figure for all parents.

This exposition of average annual utilization over the 4 years of observation in the Family Health Maintenance Demonstration would be at best puzzling and at most damaging, if the implication were true, that improvement in physical health was associated with staying away from the doctor and nurse and consulting the social worker. But, as Table 15 shows, the picture is strikingly different when individual follow-up years are considered. During the first follow-up year, for example, parents who later improved actually averaged a larger number of physician services whether family physician or specialists, than all parents. By the fourth follow-up year, the situation was reversed and use by "improved"

112

Table 15. Average annual use per person of services of staff members during first and fourth follow-up years by study-family parents and by those parents whose physical condition improved.

Follow-up year	Staff member	All parents		Parents improved on physical condition		Ratio (percent)	
First	All physicians	7.2		8.4		117	
	Family physicians		4.9		6.2		127
	Specialists		2.3		2.2		96
	Public health nurse	4.1		3.4		83	
	Social worker	4.0		4.4		110	
Fourth	All physicians	5.4		3.7		69	
	Family physicians		3.7		2.7		73
	Specialists		1.7		1.0		59
	Public health nurse	2.0		1.7		85	
	Social worker	1.8		2.4		133	

parents was considerably lower than the comparable averages for all parents, except in the use of the social worker, a third less in family doctor services, and 50 percent less in specialist services.

One is tempted to say here that early and prompt use of services of the physician may have been responsible for the improvement of physical health.[3] Certainly the result was to reduce the use of medical services in the later stages of the Demonstration. The full sparing effect on specialists' services is quite visible in these numbers.

For use of services of the public health nurse, the ratio of average use by "improved" parents as a percentage of average use by all parents remained relatively unchanged between the first and fourth follow-up years, while the actual utilization was cut in half. During the first follow-up year "improved" parents averaged 3.4 services by the public health nurse, or only 83 percent of the comparable average of all parents. In the fourth follow-up year their average was 85 percent of the average of all parents. The ratio of average use of social-work services by "improved" parents did actually increase over the years even though average services declined by about half. Why this should be so is not clear, except that it may be speculated that improvement was associated with a better understanding of the use of medical services — less need for physician and nurse, more need for counseling. It is plain that, while use declines over the period of observation, use of physician services declines far more in "improved" families.

IMPROVEMENT AS A FUNCTION OF SYMPTOMATOLOGY

In addition to utilization, the presence or absence of symptoms might be expected to play a part in, or be related to, improvement. However, the score made by the study-family parents on the Cornell Medical Index at the initial evaluation was not very useful as a predictor of improvement of physical condition. Compared to the 16.0 percent of all study-family parents who demonstrated such improvement (see Table 13), those who scored very low on the CMI and those who scored very high were somewhat more likely to have demonstrated this improvement than were all parents. Those whose scores fell in the middle had a somewhat smaller percent of their number improving.

If we use "Personal Adjustment" rather than the physical condition for comparison, the CMI scores of study families were no more clearly related than they were for physical condition. Among 219 study-family parents for whom these data were available, 15 "deteriorated" in their scores on personal adjustment (see Table 16). Those parents whose scores on the initial CMI were

Table 16. Study-family parents[a] whose rating on personal adjustment deteriorated from initial to final evaluation by score on the Cornell Medical Index.

Initial CMI score	All parents	Parents whose rating deteriorated	
		Number	Percent of all parents
0–9	51	5	9.8
10–29	122	10	8.2
Over 29	46	0	0.0
Total	219	15	6.8

[a] Includes only parents for whom both initial and final evaluations of personal adjustment are known.

low or medium were more likely to have deteriorated than those who had a high score where none deteriorated.

It is clear that neither in improvement (as in physical health) or in deterioration (as in personal adjustment) does the Cornell Medical Index provide a helpful prediction of what will happen to a family over a period of time. Symptoms seem to increase with time — not exactly surprising — but there is no change of ratio between improved and not improved in this regard. This is not to diminish the screening value of the Cornell Medical Index at all — its use in bringing out symptomatology cannot be gainsaid — but as a predictive test in an individual case it proved ineffective.

The social worker's score on personal adjustment was also ineffective as a rougher but more immediately clinical measure of symptomatology. Table 17 indicates that the members of the

Table 17. Personal adjustment related to change in physical condition from initial to final evaluation (study-family members only).

Initial rating of personal adjustment	Change in physical condition							
	Number				Percent			
	Im-proved	No change	Deteri-orated	Total	Im-proved	No change	Deteri-orated	Total
Excellent	38	28	19	85	15.8	16.6	27.9	17.8
Good	138	98	34	270	57.3	58.0	50.0	56.5
Fair	61	41	15	117	25.3	24.2	22.1	24.5
Poor	4	2	0	6	1.6	1.2	0.0	1.2
Total	241	169	68	478	100.0	100.0	100.0	100.0

study families who improved in physical health were not represented to any greater degree among the "excellent" and "good" of the "Personal Adjustment" category, than those who did not improve. But the rating of a study-family member on the social worker's evaluation of his personal adjustment did serve as a *reverse* predictor of subsequent change (from initial to final evaluation) in the rating of the family physician or pediatrician on his physical condition. Of those rated "excellent" on personal adjustment, less than one-half improved in physical condition. Of those rated "good" or "fair," the corresponding proportion improving was somewhat over one-half. (Of those rated "poor" the numbers were too few to be significant.) In contrast, the pattern was directly opposite when persons deteriorating in physical condition were considered. The proportion deteriorating was higher among those rated "excellent" on personal adjustment than among those rated "good" or "fair."

Further, there was no correspondence between ratings on the Cornell Medical Index and other areas of evaluation (see Table 18). The extent of correspondence was measured in terms of the

115

Table 18. Degree of correspondence[a] between rating on Cornell Medical Index and some areas of evaluation[b] (study-family parents only).

Staff member	Evaluation	Coefficient of correlation	
		Father	Mother
Physician	Physical condition	0.25	0.18
Public health nurse	Nutrition	.12	.04
	Sleep and rest	.22	.25
	Recreation	.02	.03
	Housing	.08	.02
Social worker	Personal adjustment	.15	.05
	Relationship to spouse	.20	.20
	Occupational adjustment	.02	—

[a] While the data do not conform to usual requisites for the coefficient of correlation, nevertheless the coefficient does give a rapid idea of the degree of correspondence.

[b] The rating scale used for each area of evaluation was: excellent, good, fair, and poor.

correlation coefficient, all of which indicated a very low order of correlation. Apparently there is little correlation between high symptom expression and evaluation of physical illness or emotional difficulty. The Cornell Medical Index selected 50 parents as disturbed, or with emotional problems (30 or more "yeses"). Only 1 of these was also selected as poorly adjusted on the evaluation scale; 1 was selected as having poor relationship with spouse; and only 6 were selected as being in poor physical condition (one of these was the poorly adjusted fellow). This tends to contradict some accepted notions of psychosomatic medicine, and ought to be the subject of future study.

EVALUATION CORRESPONDENCE WITHIN FAMILIES

Families were not uniform in their evaluation scores. Parents who were "1" did not necessarily have children who were "1," nor did "4" parents have "4" children. Nor was this corrected by time: the children not only did not resemble the parents in the beginning, but they were not more likely to become like the parents or achieve the parents' score at the end of the program.

These trends are evident from the data of Table 19. In only 30 of the 102 study families did the social worker, in evaluating the social adjustment of family members, give an identical rating on

116

Table 19. Number of study families (out of 102) in which the social worker evaluating the personal adjustment of members gave identical ratings to parents and to their oldest child.

Evaluation	Rating	Father, mother, and child	Father and child only	Total for father and child	Mother and child only	Total for mother and child
				Family relationship		
Initial	Excellent	1	3	4	1	2
	Good	23	11	34	13	36
	Fair	6	3	9	6	12
	Poor	0	0	0	0	0
Final	Excellent	1	2	3	0	1
	Good	17	12	29	8	25
	Fair	16	2	18	11	27
	Poor	0	0	0	0	0

initial evaluation to father, mother, and oldest child. At the final evaluation this number had increased only slightly.

In addition to the families in which all 3 members were rated identically, there were some families in which only one parent was rated identically with the oldest child. When these numbers are added to the initial 30 and final 34 in which all 3 family members were given identical ratings, the number for mother and child becomes 50 and father and child 47 in the initial evaluations, and 53 and 50, respectively in the final evaluations.

Most of these identical ratings, either all 3 family members or child and either parent, were "good" ratings in the initial evaluation. This was to be expected, since well over one-half of all ratings of personal adjustment were "good" in the initial evaluation. Similarly, in the final evaluation, the proportion of identical "fair" ratings increased, as was the case with "fair" ratings for all study-family members, whether identical or not. Eliminating "good" and "fair," and considering only the "excellent" or "poor" ratings, a decline is evident from the data of Table 20. The total of "excellents" was halved, and the number of "poor" so small as not to provide sufficient ground for discussion. However, it is plain that within families there was no uniformity in this evaluation and no visible modification of this by virtue of the Demonstration.

While there is not necessarily a correlation between parent

117

Table 20. Number of study families (out of 102) in which the social worker evaluating the personal adjustment of members gave "excellent" or "poor" ratings to a parent, to the oldest child, or to both.

Evaluation	Rating	Father	Mother	Oldest child
Initial	Total number "excellent"	12	4	20
	Also having "excellent" oldest child	4	2	
	Total number "poor"	0	2	2
	Also having "poor" oldest child	0	0	
Final	Total number "excellent"	6	3	10
	Also having "excellent" oldest child	3	1	
	Total number "poor"	1	1	2
	Also having "poor" oldest child	0	0	

scores in the adjustment evaluation area and children's scores in those areas, however, the rating by the social worker on her evaluation of the relationship between spouses was strongly associated with the rating on her evaluation of the personal adjustment of their children (Table 21). Where the social worker had

Table 21. Personal adjustment of study-family children by initial evaluation of relation between spouses.

Evaluation of relation between spouses	Number of pairs of spouses	Number				Percent			
		Excellent	Good	Fair	Poor	Excellent	Good	Fair	Poor
Excellent	36	26	36	6	1	37.7	52.2	8.7	1.4
Good	57	36	64	20	0	30.0	53.3	16.7	0
Fair	31	9	38	15	3	13.8	58.5	23.1	4.6
Poor	0	0	0	0	0	0	0	0	0
Total	124	71	138	41	4	28.0	54.3	16.1	1.6

rated the relationship between spouses as "excellent," 37.7 percent of their children were also rated "excellent" in personal adjustment. Where the parents had been rated "good" or "fair," the corresponding figures for the personal adjustment of their children as "excellent" were only 30.0 and 13.8 percent. (There were no cases of spouses rated poor in their relationship.) The situation was reversed with reference to the "fair" ratings on children's personal adjustment. Only 8.7 percent of the children of "excellent" parents were rated as "fair," compared to 16.7 percent of parents rated "good" and 23.1 percent of parents rated "fair." This seems quite logical.[4]

PROBLEMS OF EVALUATING HEALTH

The Family Health Maintenance Demonstration showed that study families over a 4-year period benefited in their physical health (and nutrition), by the evaluation criteria used, as compared with control families. Emotional health, on the other hand, by our criteria, showed no improvement of study families over control families. Some of the correlates of these findings are that the improvements (and lack of them) are not related to over-all high utilization of medical services or to prevalence or absence of symptoms and difficulties. There does seem to be a clear correlation between high use of service *early*, a willingness to undertake treatment, and eventual improvement of physical health. The improvement in housing might also be a condition of willingness to undertake treatment, since the control families did not exhibit this improvement at all.

It was not easy to demonstrate changes in family health. One difficulty arose from the need for interpreting the changes that did (or did not) occur within the study families. Because of the nature of the data and observations underlying physical examinations, it may be that our most secure and objective measurement of health was contained in the physician's evaluation. Here, happily, we were able to demonstrate a change of respectable proportions. Many of the nurse's evaluations (housing, nutrition) were in areas that lent themselves to objectivity as easily, or more easily, than the physician's. So, although the nurse was optimistic compared to the social worker, we may accept the findings of modest improvement in these areas with some equanimity.

In the field of emotional health, where there is evident sharp decline between initial and final evaluation, we are faced with a choice of unpalatable interpretations. Either the measurements are of no value, or the families deteriorated under supervision. We are naturally reluctant to admit that it would be possible for families to deteriorate under Demonstration care. While we are equally reluctant to admit that the measurements are valueless, it must be obvious that the assessment of personal adjustment and family interaction are areas embodying fewer objective criteria

119

and less concrete data than do housing, nutrition, or physical condition. This would make for less certainty in interpretation. The social worker's more pessimistic attitude would not influence the results since both initial and final evaluations are equally affected. In the matter of choice of analysis of the results, perhaps it would be best to leave it that we could not demonstrate a change for the better in the emotional relationships of the study families.

A second problem of interpretation lies in the comparison between study and control families. Although we made an effort to get some information on the control families in the beginning, we did not do a thorough initial evaluation, assuming that, as matched controls, the matching process guaranteed the similarity of study and control families. We did have Cornell Medical Index material on both initial and final status, however, and in this area both study and control families are logically comparable. Table 22 demonstrates the similarity of the groups. In addition, it

Table 22. Parents' Median Cornell Medical Index score (number of "yeses").

| | Initial evaluation | | | | Final evaluation | | | |
| | Study | | Control | | Study | | Control | |
Parents	Score	No.	Score	No.	Score	No.	Score	No.
Fathers	14.2	124	14.2	122	10.7	77	13.7	70
Mothers	21.4	124	16.9	128	17.6	82	17.0	73

demonstrates the dimension of improvement. At the end of their participation in the Family Health Maintenance Demonstration, the study-family parents had improved their CMI scores markedly; the control family parents changed relatively little.

This trend was noticeable in both fathers and mothers. Among both study and control families, fathers' median CMI scores were consistently lower than those for mothers, whether at initial or final evaluation. As Table 23 indicates, in most instances the decline in median scores between initial and final evaluation for the study-family parents was the result of an increase in the proportion of parents classified in the lowest score category (0–9 "yeses"). And the proportions classified in the highest category

Table 23. Distribution of Cornell Medical Index "yeses" among study-family parents.

Parents	Number of "yeses"	Initial evaluation (percent)	Final evaluation (percent)
All parents	0–9	24.6	35.2
	10–29	54.9	51.6
	Over 29	20.5	13.2
Fathers	0–9	33.9	48.1
	10–29	55.6	44.1
	Over 29	10.5	7.8
Mothers	0–9	15.3	23.2
	10–29	54.0	58.5
	Over 29	30.7	18.3

(30 or more "yeses") correspondingly declined. There seems to be no question of the improvement in this area, considering prevalence of symptoms as an evidence of illness, and reduction of complaints as active improvement.

Yet in 9 out of 12 evaluation areas (Table 9) the control families seem to have done better than the study families. This finding is highly implausible — aside from our natural desire that it should be otherwise — because it is unlikely that families not receiving counseling services, public health services, and added physician services, should have done better than families that did. It is possible that the old statistical devil of "biased runs" which upsets random sampling may have been at work, or that the samples were not rigorously matched nor identical in health status at the outset. And again it should be emphasized that closer acquaintance may well have biased our observations against the study families. It is certainly not due to loss of differently constituted groups from the study families. If the families who did not complete the study were markedly different (that is, better) from those who remained, this would account for the final difference between study and control families at the end. However, Table 24 indicates that this is not so. In the areas where the scores are markedly different — Housing and Occupational Adjustment of the Father — those dropping out were in the lower weighted average range, which would tend to reduce somewhat the impact of the improvement noted in these areas for the study families; but since all the other areas are quite similar, it would not explain the discrepancy in study and control scorings in the area of emo-

Table 24. Comparison of ratings of persons remaining in the study and those who dropped out, by staff member and evaluation.

Staff member	Evaluation	Average of initial rating[a]	
		Remained in	Dropped out[b]
Physician	Family medical history	2.40	—
	Physical condition	2.67	2.56
Public health nurse	Nutrition	3.12	3.16
	Sleep and rest	3.32	3.37
	Educational achievement of children	3.50	3.43
	Recreational adjustment	3.51	3.50
	Housing	2.69	1.84
Social worker	Personal adjustment	2.91	2.89
	Family relationship of		
	Husband and wife	3.02	2.93
	Father and children	3.20	3.30
	Mother and children	2.96	3.32
	Occupational adjustment of father	3.26	2.94

[a] Weights: excellent, 4; good, 3; fair, 2; poor, 1.

[b] "Remained in" indicates that both initial and final ratings are known, while "Dropped out" indicates that the final rating was unknown.

tional relationships. Speculation is idle and rationalization all too easily in accord with our own interest, but it is reasonable to state that a judgment of comparative improvement of the control families in the emotional area should be suspended at this time.

To conclude, with another of Bacon's comments: "If we begin with certainties, we shall end in doubts; but if we begin with doubts, and are patient in them, we shall end in certainties." [5]

-VIII-

UTILIZATION OF SERVICES

I have been particularly impressed in the course of my anthropological and historical studies by the degree to which even the notion of disease itself depends rather on the decisions of society than on objective facts.

— Erwin Ackerknecht, "The Role of Medical History in Medical Education"

The "notion of disease" is the prerequisite for using medical service. No one deliberately seeks out medical care for prevention or treatment without feeling that the request is appropriate. However, even if all agreed on a definition of disease and the proper circumstance for consulting a physician, some people would go and some would not. "Effective demand" is the term used to measure services requested. Where a need exists — commonly agreed and defined illness — yet the individual does not seek care, this is defined as "latent demand." The removal of economic barriers often will translate latent into effective demand.[1] The Demonstration study families had no economic barrier to seeking care as Group patients, and there should have been no latent demand when they came under scrutiny in the Demonstration. There was a difference in access to medical service, however, because of the availability of nurse and social worker, and there was a difference in approach due to the health team's encouraging of educational and promotional activities. What was the influence of this different medical-care organization and approach on patients' use of medical services? A variety of interesting data on utilization of services helps to answer this question in a number of ways. Not only can we identify the total volume of care given, but we can relate this volume of use to characteristics of the study families and sort out those who use more services under the same conditions that others use less. Having examined the families, we could recognize, professionally, what their needs were. From the record we could then see how much demand was made to satisfy this need. It is not often that the opportunity is offered to study need and demand in the same population. Usually one estimates need, and studies demand in selected groups to measure against this. Here, we have both data for the same group, and we may go beyond simple relations between utilization and socio-economic characteristics to chart the relations that exist between illness and utilization.[2]

USING THE PHYSICIAN'S SERVICES

Since it is part of a prepayment plan with ready and easy access to medical care, the effective demand for service in the Montefiore Medical Group would be expected to be higher than in the United States as a whole.[3] As far as we can tell, the demand is indeed higher. The average annual number of physician visits per person in the United States during 1957–58, as obtained from a household survey of a national sample of the noninstitutional population, was 5.0. The comparable figure for the urban population was 5.4, or about 8 percent higher.[4]

THE PHYSICIANS

While the 1957 figure for the entire membership of the Health Insurance Plan of Greater New York (HIP) was 5.1, or about the same as for the United States, for the Montefiore Medical Group it was 6.6. These figures are not entirely comparable. HIP figures, for example, do not include telephone "visits," as the national data do, but they do support our expectations.

The methods of practice in the Montefiore Medical Group are different from those in other medical groups in HIP, even as group practice on the HIP model is different from the standard solo practice in the United States. Furthermore, the influence of cultural and class factors cannot be eliminated as an underlying force for higher utilization since these may vary even with the removal of the economic barrier in a prepayment group practice

Table 25. Utilization of physicians' services by contractor groups in the Health Insurance Plan of Greater New York (HIP), 1957.[a]

Contractor group	Average annual number of visits per person
New York City employees:	
Board of education	6.0
Police department	4.7
Fire department	4.1
Transit authority	4.9
Housing authority	4.2
Other city departments	4.8
Total	4.8
Family contracts:	
Motion picture machine operators	6.4
Local 65 security plan	5.7
Baker and confectionery workers	3.7
Machinists welfare fund	3.4

Source: Health Insurance Plan "Utilization Experience by Contractor Groups."
[a] Average number of visits per person to physicians for entire HIP membership in 1957.

plan. Table 25 gives startling proof of this. The average annual number of visits to physicians fluctuated rather widely about the HIP average of 5.1 visits. New York City employees averaged somewhat less, but even within this group there was wide variation, ranging from the average high of Board of Education employees to the low of the Fire Department. In other contractor groups the same variations occurred, ranging from 6.4 for the Motion Picture Machine Operators to 3.4 for the Machinists Welfare Fund. These occupational factors, which are influenced by class and ethnic components in employment practice and occupational selection, strongly affect utilization.

This is not to say that ready and easy access to medical care will not also increase utilization. If more disease is found, more treatment becomes necessary. Evidence for this is provided in Table 26 where case finding of serious disease (on arbitrary categories including selected diseases diagnosable by laboratory or X-ray findings) is higher in the Montefiore Medical Group than in HIP as a whole. For each of the diseases the number of cases observed in the Montefiore Group during 1955 exceeded the number expected on the basis of the average annual experience of the Health Insurance Plan of Greater New York during 1948–1951.

125

Table 26. Cases[a] of illness in selected diagnostic categories of illness by category, Montefiore Medical Group, 1955.

Disease category[b]	Number of cases		Ratio of observed to expected
	Observed	Expected[c]	
Tuberculosis	62	30	2.1
Malignant neoplasms	158	67	2.4
Benign neoplasms	663	476	1.4
Neoplasms unspecified	75	41	1.8
Diabetes mellitus	171	126	1.4
Chronic bronchitis and other diseases of lung and pleural cavity	104	94	1.1
Ulcer of stomach or duodenum	299	188	1.6
Ulcerative colitis and chronic enteritis	61	23	2.7
Diseases of gall bladder	166	156	1.1
Arthritis (rheumatoid, osteo, and unspecified)	819	476	1.7
Disorders of the back	548	351	1.6
Congenital malformations	99	94	1.1

Source: HIP Bureau of Research and Statistics.

[a] A case is here defined as the illness of an individual for which one or more physicians' services were utilized by that individual in the course of the year.

[b] The disease categories were selected because objective criteria such as X-ray or laboratory studies were available.

[c] Expected on the basis of the average annual experience of the Health Insurance Plan of Greater New York (HIP), 1948–51.

For some disease categories the observed number of cases was more than double the expected: for ulcerative colitis, the 61 cases observed was 2.7 times as high as the 23 expected, while for malignant neoplasms the 158 observed cases was 2.4 times as high as the 67 expected. In other disease categories observed and expected were much closer (although for *all* disease categories shown here observed exceeded expected).

Factors influencing utilization of medical services are not too well recognized, but variations in demand, as well as evidence of need, and access to medical care, will influence the volume of medical care provided. One may go on from these facts to assume that demand in the Demonstration for physician services would exceed demand in the Group despite an already high level of utilization, because there was more case finding in the Demonstration than in the Group.

In the Family Health Maintenance Demonstration, utilization did exceed that of the control families for the same period of time.

In part this may have been due to increased case finding, in part to the awakening of previously unexpressed demand by the Demonstration's educational program, and in part to the completely open access of the Demonstration. Whatever the reason, Table 27 indicates higher utilization in the Demonstration.

Table 27. Utilization of physicians' services[a] (annual average per person) by adults[b] and children by type of physician.

Type of physician	Study families			Control families		
	All persons	Adults	Children	All persons	Adults	Children
All physicians	5.8	5.9	5.8	3.5	2.7	5.1
Family physician or pediatrician	4.2	0	0	2.5	0	0
Family physician	0	4.0	0	0	1.6	0
Pediatrician	0	0	4.5	0	0	4.2
Specialist	1.6	1.9	1.3	1.0	1.1	0.9
Ratio (percent) of specialist to nonspecialist	38	48	30	40	69	21

[a] Includes home or office visits but not in-hospital services or telephone consultations.
[b] All persons over age 13 in study families and over 9 in control families.

Actually, the study families used almost twice as many physicians' services as did the control families. They averaged 5.9 annual services per person compared to 3.5 per person in the control families, an excess of about two-thirds. (The average annual services compared do not include hospital services, and so are lower than the HIP average.) This excess was constant regardless of whether the service was rendered by the family physician, pediatrician, or specialist. The larger number of visits per person by the study families was particularly evident in the case of adults. The average annual number of physicians' services utilized by adults in the study families was more than double the corresponding figure in the control families, as was the annual average for services of family physicians. When only children are considered the margin of excess was not as great. The effects of the Family Health Maintenance Demonstration on utilization were most evident in the provision of physicians' services to adults.

127

Specialists

When all persons are considered together, the study families used comparatively few specialist services. Table 27 shows that the annual average number of visits per person to specialists by members of the study group was only 38 percent of their visits to family physicians or pediatricians, while for the control families it was 42 percent. This is not an especially large difference, but it assumes significance when we recognize the fact that it conceals within it conflicting tendencies in specialist utilization. Taking adults alone, Demonstration patients used specialists considerably less than they used family doctors. Their use of specialists was 48 percent of their use of nonspecialists compared to 69 percent for adults in the control group. The magnitude of this difference is almost canceled out in over-all family statistics by the opposite tendency among children, since Demonstration children used specialists somewhat more often than control children.

These statistics involve averages for the entire 4 years. In Table 28 the first and fourth year are contrasted to indicate changes in

Table 28. Utilization of physicians' services[a] (annual average per person) by study-family adults[b] and children by type of physician during first and fourth follow-up years.

	First follow-up year			Fourth follow-up year		
Type of physician	All persons	Adults	Children	All persons	Adults	Children
All physicians	6.2	7.0	5.2	5.6	5.1	6.1
Family physician or pediatrician	4.5	0	0	4.0	0	0
Family physician	0	4.7	0	0	3.5	0
Pediatrician	0	0	4.2	0	0	4.6
Specialist	1.7	2.3	1.0	1.6	1.6	1.5
Ratio (percent) of specialist to nonspecialist	38	49	24	40	46	33

[a] Includes home or office visits but not in-hospital services or telephone consultations.
[b] All persons over age 13 in study families and over 9 in control families.

the pattern of utilization. The utilization of physician services by the study families decreased through the years, although their average annual utilization was still substantially higher than that of the control families.

This relative decrease of use with time was no statistical arti-fact. It did not result from any increase in the utilization of serv-ices by the control families, for the control families remained relatively unchanged, showing no consistent trend downward. It resulted from a steady and consistent decline in average use of services by the study families, which was considerably more marked in family physicians' or pediatricians' services than in specialists' services.

The patterns of change in average utilization of physicians' services by adults contrasted sharply with those by children. While adults in the study families markedly decreased their use of services with the passage of time, children increased their an-nual averages. The ratio of use of specialist services to non-specialist services remained almost unchanged for families as a whole and for adults. However, for children it increased from 24 to 33 percent.[5]

Was There Abuse of Demonstration Service?

Study families used the services of family physicians to a much larger extent than did the control families, regardless of whether visits were made for a routine check-up or for nonroutine pur-poses. Study-family adults averaged 4.0 visits per person annually, 2½ times as many as the adults in the control families (see Table 29). When these visits were for a routine check-up, the compara-ble figure for the study families was 2¾ times as high as that of

Table 29. Utilization of family physician and pediatrician by reason for visit.

| Type of physician | Reason for visit | Average annual number of visits per person[a] | | |
		Study families	Control families	Ratio of study to control
Family physician	All visits	4.0	1.6	2.50
	Routine check-up	1.1	0.4	2.75
	Nonroutine	2.9	1.2	2.42
Pediatrician	All visits	4.5	4.2	1.07
	Routine check-up	1.9	1.2	1.58
	Nonroutine	2.6	3.0	0.87

[a] Annual average computed over a 4-year period, based on the number of adults for the family physician, and the number of children age 13 or under for the pediatrician in the study group, age 9 or under in the control group.

the control families; and for nonroutine visits, the study families' average was almost 2½ times as large as the average for the control families.

The situation was somewhat different for visits to the pediatrician. The study families' annual average of 4.5 over the entire period was only 7 percent higher than the comparable figure (4.2) for the control families. For routine check-up it was about 60 percent higher, but for nonroutine visits it was actually lower.

Among the study families visits to the family physician decreased between the first and fourth follow-up years, regardless of whether they were for routine check-up or nonroutine purposes. As Table 30 shows, for all visits they dropped 26 percent;

Table 30. Utilization of family physician and pediatrician by reason for visit during first and fourth follow-up years.

| | | Average annual number of visits per person[a] | | | | | |
| | | Study families | | | Control families | | |
Type of physician	Reason for visit	First year	Fourth year	Percent change	First year	Fourth year	Percent change
Family physician	All visits	4.7	3.5	−26	1.6	1.8	+13
	Routine check-up	1.4	1.0	−29	0.4	0.5	+25
	Nonroutine	3.3	2.5	−24	1.2	1.3	+8
Pediatrician	All visits	4.2	4.6	+10	4.1	4.1	0
	Routine check-up	2.3	1.8	−22	1.2	1.3	+8
	Nonroutine	1.9	2.8	+47	2.9	2.8	−3

[a] Utilization rates are computed on population served: in study group this means pediatrician services per population age 13 or under; in control group, population age 9 or under.

29 percent for routine check-up visits; 24 percent for nonroutine. Among control families there was a rise in each instance, 13 percent for all, 25 percent for routine and 8 percent for nonroutine visits, respectively. However, the increases were small in absolute numbers, if not in percentages.

For the pediatrician, there was a rather mixed-up situation. Among study families all visits increased by about 10 percent. However, for routine check-up they decreased 22 percent, while for nonroutine purposes they increased 47 percent. Among control families all visits to the pediatrician remained unchanged at 4.1

between the first and fourth follow-up years, with a slight increase for routine check-up visits and a decrease for nonroutine visits. It may be surmised that use of pediatrician services was at a uniform level for study and control families because of the equally child-centered attitudes of both groups, and because the social and psychological factors that influenced parent use did not influence the child's use of medical care.[6]

In considering the increased use by study-family parents we must be wary of concluding that "more" means "better."[7] The fact that more services were required or provided does not indicate that patients got better care as a result. However, we can ask whether our utilization statistics show that when our patients received the permissive and encouraging services of the Demonstration they proceeded to abuse the system by "overutilization." The increased use does not seem to have been abuse. When we note that the study families made more visits to physicians than the control families (and of course visits to other workers not available to the control families), we must remember that better case finding and annual examinations enter into the calculations. If one subtracts the routine visits (annual examination and immunizations, which comprise the 1.6 visits to the doctor each year for each study-family member), not *necessarily* made by the control families in the fourth year, when case finding had leveled off, then the study families obtained only slightly more doctor's service than the control families. In the successive years this increment definitely declined. So much for "abuse" of an "open" system!

Some of the greater number of visits were due to greater real need. Participation in the Family Health Maintenance Demonstration helped uncover a much larger number of new conditions (medical diagnoses) by the physicians than was the case among nonparticipating families. Table 31 shows that the annual average over the 4-year period of 207 new conditions per 100 family members (more than 2 per person) discovered among study families compared to 154 among control families. This rate was about ⅓ higher among study families than the corresponding rate for the controls.

Among the study families, more than 9 in 10 of these conditions were classified as "minor," while the remainder were "major." The

131

Table 31. Annual number of new conditions (medical diagnoses) discovered per 100 families by type of condition and follow-up year.

Follow-up year	Condition	Study families	Control families
First	Major	19	12
	Minor	234	162
Fourth	Major	13	11
	Minor	160	138
4-year annual average	Major	14	11
	Minor	193	143

proportions to the total constituted by minor and major were identical among the control families, but the number of conditions per 100 family members was smaller — 143 minor and 11 major of the total of 154 new conditions discovered.

For both study and control families, the rate of new conditions discovered declined between the first and fourth follow-up years, but the decline was more consistent and larger in magnitude for the study families. In the study families there were 253 new conditions of all types per 100 family members discovered in the first follow-up year, 19 of which were major. In the fourth follow-up year the comparable figures were 173, of which 13 were major, a drop of 32 percent for all diagnoses and minor diagnoses, and 36 percent for major diagnoses. Among control families, however, the comparable declines were only 15, 8, and 15 percent, respectively.

In this same connection, reviewing Table 32, which shows the ratio of diagnoses made in the two groups, it can be seen that the

Table 32. New diagnoses[a] found by source of diagnosis and type; ratio of study to control family members.

Follow-up year	All services		Routine		Nonroutine	
	Major	Minor	Major	Minor	Major	Minor
First	1.6	1.4	3.8	5.1	1.0	0.9
Second	1.1	1.4	2.8	3.9	1.0	1.1
Third	1.1	1.4	0.8	4.7	1.1	1.1
Fourth	1.2	1.2	0.8	1.4	1.4	1.1
4-year annual average	1.3	1.3	2.3	3.5	1.1	1.1

[a] Total new diagnoses in 4 years: Study, 2020; Control, 2407.

greater case finding in the study group compared with the controls would account for the additional 1 or 1.2 more doctor visits per person in the nonroutine services that appeared in Table 32. Instead of demonstrating "abuse," that is, more services per illness, the somewhat larger number of services in the light of greater number of diagnoses recognized for treatment would almost presume an increased efficiency of method.

Furthermore, the utilization of physician services in the Demonstration reversed the customary ratio of group specialist to family doctor. Here, time available to the doctor would seem to be the dominant factor, for advice and reassurance take time. Explanations must be given to help a patient understand and cope with symptoms that may or may not require a specialist's consultation. Time is needed for the physician to listen, and time was more available to the Demonstration physician. He could elicit more symptoms, see the need for more tests, make more diagnoses: *find* more. Conversely, it was also less necessary for the patient to seek the security of a specialist consultation for confirmation.

Hasty office visits without the opportunity for full expression of deep-seated fears make patients uneasy. The ready access to specialists in group practice may reinforce rather than reduce this uneasiness. The specialists may become more necessary to the patient, under such circumstances. On the other hand, when the family physician has time and the necessary orientation toward family practice, the demand on scarce specialist's skills may very well be reduced. Study families may have used slightly more services, but they did obtain more diagnoses of illness, and made less frequent use of specialists to obtain these diagnoses. This paradoxical finding — more diagnoses yet less specialized services — was corroborated in another way. Among the pilot-control families in the final evaluation, 24 of the 43 individuals examined required medical care that they were entitled to and should have had, but *didn't ask for* under regular Group medical auspices. These diagnoses were confirmed by the Demonstration family doctor. This reinforces the evidence on the value of the health-team physician, since among control families with free access to the Group's medical services, with a utilization rate higher than that of the United States as a whole and with a high specialist

133

utilization, there were diseases known to the patient and his physician for which medical care was not sought.

UTILIZATION AND REPORT OF SYMPTOMS

Examining the statistics in a somewhat different way, qualities can be ascribed to the families on the basis of just how much service was used. By arbitrary classification the families could be divided into medium (40 percent of the families), high (27 percent of the families), and low (33 percent of the families) consumers of medical services.

Some families were consistently high or consistently low utilizers, while others changed from high to low or the reverse in successive years. While it may be true that families experience "bad" years with more illness than usual and "good" years with less, it does not seem that the amount of actual illness is most responsible for the pattern of use so much as *symptoms* of illness. For example, as we see in Table 33, where there are many symp-

Table 33. Level of utilization[a] (percent)[b] by study-family parents of family physician's services by score on Cornell Medical Index.

Initial CMI score	High	Medium	Low
0–9	14.5	42.5	43.0
10–29	27.8	38.2	34.0
Over 29	39.9	40.4	19.7
Total	27.1	39.8	33.1

[a] Determined from median number of services separately for father and mother each year.
[b] 4-year averages.

toms or complaints as evidenced by 30 or more "yeses" on the Cornell Medical Index, there is also continuous high utilization in a family. This pattern was consistent, even when the entire duration of the Family Health Maintenance Demonstration is considered. Table 34 shows that parents with low CMI scores at initial evaluation turned out to be preponderantly in the medium- or low-utilization category, while high CMI scorers were most often medium or high utilizers.

When the data are examined in terms of follow-up years, an

Table 34. Study-family parents' level of utilization (percent) of family physician's services during first and fourth follow-up years by score on Cornell Medical Index.

Follow-up year	Initial CMI score	High	Medium	Low
First	0–9	8.2	41.0	50.8
	10–29	23.5	34.6	41.9
	Over 29	41.2	37.2	21.6
	Total	23.4	36.7	39.9
Fourth	0–9	22.4	46.9	30.6
	10–29	29.9	34.2	35.9
	Over 29	37.2	51.2	11.6
	Total	29.6	40.8	29.6

additional trend is evident. Considering the average for all parents, regardless of CMI scores, the proportions of high and medium utilizers *increased* between the first and fourth follow-up years, and the proportion of low utilizers correspondingly declined. This increase was most evident among parents with low CMI scores. The net effect was to increase the number of medium users of service, but the trend of greater use by families with more symptoms is plain.

The number of services sought from all professional staff members — not only physicians — also appeared to be strongly associated with the CMI scores at the initial evaluation. This is shown in Table 35, where we see that study-family parents average 4.1 services of the family physician annually. Parents who scored low on the Cornell Medical Index averaged a much lower figure which

Table 35. Study-family parents' annual average utilization per person of services[a] of the staff by score on Cornell Medical Index and profession of staff member.

| Initial CMI score | Staff member | | |
	Family physician	Public health nurse	Social worker
0–9	2.7	2.1	1.9
10–29	4.1	3.0	2.8
Over 29	5.8	3.4	4.6
Total	4.1	2.8	2.9

[a] Services include home or office visits but not telephone consultations.

135

rose as the CMI score rose. A similar relation prevailed for the services of the public health nurse and social worker.

Table 36 indicates that, while the use of services of professional

Table 36. Study-family parents' annual average utilization per person of services[a] of the staff during first and fourth follow-up years by score on Cornell Medical Index and profession of staff member.

Follow-up year	Initial CMI score	Staff member		
		Family physician	Public health nurse	Social worker
First	0–9	3.1	3.4	2.8
	10–29	5.0	4.3	3.9
	Over 29	6.6	4.7	5.7
	Mean: All Parents	4.9	4.1	4.0
Fourth	0–9	2.4	1.4	1.1
	10–29	3.5	2.0	1.7
	Over 29	5.8	2.8	3.2
	Mean: All Parents	3.7	2.0	1.8
Fourth as percent of first	0–9	77	41	39
	10–29	70	47	44
	Over 29	88	60	56
	Mean: All Parents	76	49	45

[a] Services include home or office visits but not telephone consultations.

staff members by study-family parents declined with the passage of time — that is, with the duration of their participation in the Demonstration — and the extent of this decline varied with the profession of the staff member, both the extent and pattern of the decline varied with the parents' scores on the Cornell Medical Index at their initial evaluation. So, even as a long-term effect, symptomatology was actively related to use of services.

Study-family parents averaged 4.9 visits to the family physician during their first follow-up year, but by the fourth year the corresponding figure was only 76 percent as high. This decline was least among parents whose CMI scores were highest. The decline was not consistent. Their average in the first year was 6.6 physician services, in the second year 5.1, but in the third and fourth years the figure rose to 5.7 and 5.8.

As with the services of the family physician, the services of

136

both public health nurse and social worker showed a decline in average use per study-family parent during the follow-up years. In both instances the decline was much more pronounced than that of the services of the family physician, and the decline was less pronounced among parents who scored 30 or more "yeses" on the Cornell Medical Index.

UTILIZATION AND STAFF EVALUATION OF HEALTH

Chapter VII showed no clear correlation between the scoring of 30 or more CMI "yeses" and a low evaluation grade in the emotional area (the theoretical index of emotional problems). As a consequence, one would expect no clear correlation between utilization of services and staff evaluation of personal adjustment: for example, those considered poorly adjusted would not be high utilizers of service. This was not true.

Table 37 shows that the ratings which individuals received in

Table 37. Study-family parents' annual average utilization per person of staff services[a] by initial evaluation ratings in selected areas.

Staff member	Evaluation	Service used	Excel-lent	Good	Fair	Total
			Evaluation ratings[b]			
Family physician	Physical condition	Family physician	1.9	3.4	4.4	4.1
Public health nurse	Nutrition	Public health nurse	2.3	2.8	3.6	2.8
Social worker	Personal adjust-ment	Social worker	1.8	2.7	3.4	2.9
Social worker	Personal adjust-ment	Family physician	3.4	3.9	4.6	4.1

[a] Services include home or office visits but not telephone conversations.
[b] There were too few "poor" ratings to be shown, but they are included in the total.

various areas of evaluation were strongly related to the use which they made of the Demonstration staff. For example, study-family parents averaged 4.1 visits to the family physician annually over the 4-year participation period. But this average varied with their rating on the family physician's initial evaluation of their physical condition. Parents rated "excellent" averaged fewest services — 1.9 annually — and, as the rating decreased, services rose, so that the comparable average for parents rated "good" was 3.3 and for "fair" was 4.4 annually.[8]

Similar relations were evident in the other evaluation areas illustrated. Study-family parents averaged 2.8 services by the public health nurse. But parents rated "excellent" by the public health nurse in her evaluation of their nutritional status used fewer of her services: 2.3, compared to 2.7 for parents rated "good," and 3.6 for parents rated "fair." (No average was computed for parents rated "poor" because they were too few in number.) Again, the average use of services rose as the rating decreased.

The same type of relation was evident in the comparison of utilization with the social worker's evaluation of the personal adjustment of the study-family parents on their initial evaluation. Study-family parents averaged 2.9 services by the social worker, but the comparable figure for parents rated "excellent" in her evaluation of their personal adjustment was 1.8; "good," 2.7; and "fair," 3.4. Comparing the use of family-physician services by the study family against the social worker's evaluation produces similar results.

Regardless of the ratings which individuals received, their utilization of services declined between the first and fourth follow-up year of the study. However, as shown in Table 38, the extent and consistency of this decline varied. For example, all study-family parents made 4.9 annual visits to the family physician during the first follow-up year, but by the fourth year the average had declined to 3.7, only 76 percent as many. Comparable figures showed that "fair"-evaluated parents declined least in use of services. Parents rated "excellent" in the family physicians' evaluation of their physical condition declined to 83 percent; "good" to 70 percent; but "fair" declined only to 96 percent. The decline was somewhat irregular from the first to the fourth follow-up year, but it is clear that those evaluated "fair" continued to use more services. Much the same pattern holds for the public health nurse.

The social worker's evaluations do not show the same clear relation of decline to ratings — either for use of her own or the family doctor's services. It is true that "excellent"-rated people declined in service use somewhat more than the average, and "good"-rated

138

UTILIZATION OF SERVICES

Table 38. Study-family parents' annual average number of staff services[a] used per person during first and fourth follow-up years by initial evaluation ratings in selected areas of evaluation.

Staff member making evaluation	Area of evaluation	Staff member used	Follow-up year	Evaluation ratings[b]			
				Total	Excellent	Good	Fair
Family physician	Physical condition	Family physician	First	4.9	2.3	3.7	4.8
			Fourth	3.7	1.9	2.6	4.6
	Fourth year as percent of first			76	83	70	96
Public health nurse	Nutrition	Public health nurse	First	4.1	3.3	4.0	5.4
			Fourth	1.8	1.2	2.1	3.0
	Fourth year as percent of first			45	36	53	56
Social worker	Personal adjustment	Social worker	First	4.0	2.7	3.7	4.7
			Fourth	1.8	1.1	1.8	2.1
	Fourth year as percent of first			45	41	49	45
Social worker	Personal adjustment	Family physician	First	4.9	5.0	4.1	5.9
			Fourth	3.7	2.9	3.9	3.4
	Fourth year as percent of first			76	58	95	58

[a] Services include home or office visits but not telephone conversations.
[b] There were too few "poor" ratings to be shown separately, but they are included in the total.

people considerably less, but the "fair" people declined exactly like the "excellent"!

In Table 39 an attempt is made to visualize usage from the standpoint of the extreme case. Very high utilizers of physicians' services (those who used more than twice the median number of services in the first year) were the same ones who scored high on the Cornell Medical Index and poor on physical condition and personal adjustment at their initial evaluations. And in almost all cases the proportion of parents who were very high utilizers rose in proportion to their ratings in these areas of evaluation.

PREDICTION OF UTILIZATION

The good correlation between the Cornell Medical Index "yeses" and utilization indicates that, the more symptoms and complaints there are, the more is the likelihood that a patient will use medical services.* The CMI was as good an indicator of

* The family's degree of utilization is really a characteristic of each member. The CMI selects a family member as a high or low scorer, family utilization statistics are amalgamated, and the family is designated as "high," "low," or "medium."

Table 39. Very high utilization[a] of physician services according to selected characteristics at initial evaluation of study-family parents.

Characteristic	All parents	Very high utilizers	
		Number	Percent
Score on Cornell Medical Index:			
0–9	61	1	1.6
10–29	136	18	13.2
Over 29	50	12	24.0
Rating on evaluation of physical condition by family physician:			
Excellent	9	0	0
Good	108	6	5.6
Fair	117	15	12.8
Poor	13	10	76.9
Rating on evaluation of personal adjustment by social worker			
Excellent	19 ⎫ 165	4 ⎫ 14	21.1
Good	146 ⎭	10 ⎭	6.8
Fair	80	15	18.8
Poor	2	2	100.0

[a] Very high utilizers (31, or 12.6 percent, of 247 parents) are defined as persons who utilized more than twice the median number of services of the family physician in the first year of their participation in the Demonstration.

potential use of services as a doctor's diagnosis of medical illness or a social worker's finding emotional maladjustment. Thus, the amount of utilization does correspond in part to the amount of illness in a family, more so to the symptoms or complaints (perceived "illness") of individual family members. Patient complaints need not necessarily correspond to the perception of illness by professional workers, for the team members see need and respond to it in terms of their own professional knowledge rather than in terms of the family's own view of its "illness." On the whole there is good correlation between the patient's recognition of need and awareness of symptoms, less with professional evaluation of condition.

Another aspect of the relation of the Cornell Medical Index to utilization is expressed in the fact that there was a smaller percentage of high-score CMI people at the end than there was in the beginning. It is true that over-all use of services also declined at the end, but this decline did not represent a shift of patients from one category to another. Two-thirds of the people had the same score at the end as in the beginning, and 81 percent of high scorers at the end had been high in the beginning. Only 8 percent deteriorated, that is, scored more "yeses" at the end than in the beginning, while 27 percent improved.*

TEAM EFFECT

As indicated earlier, high utilizers, with a high CMI score in the beginning, tended to remain high utilizers to the end and to remain in the high CMI score group. Low utilizers who may have been in the high CMI score group tended to increase their utilization. It would seem that, if people had many symptoms or complaints and were inclined to use a lot of medical services, experience with the health team did nothing to reduce either their symptomatology or demand. On the other hand, an individual with many complaints who was a low utilizer of services for whatever reason would be encouraged by the Demonstration situation to use the easily available service and consequently increase his utilization.[9]

ETHNIC FACTORS AND SOCIAL CLASS

If one considers utilization from a religious or ethnic background, Jews apparently use services more than Catholics and Protestants. This may be a class difference, and our sample size prevents separation of class from ethnic differences.[10] No final conclusions can be drawn from our data on this interesting topic.

Social class is closely connected with utilization — as shown in Table 40. Parents in the study families used the services of family physicians more than they used the services of public health nurses and social workers, regardless of social class, follow-up year, or educational grouping. But social class (based on occupation of family head) was important in determining how much use was made of family physicians' services by parents in the study families. Middle-class parents averaged the highest number of services annually, 4.5, compared to 4.0 for lower-class parents and an even lower figure, 3.6, for upper-middle-class parents.[11]

Middle-class parents also used the services of public health nurses most, but their excess over lower-class parents was relatively slight. However, these figures exceeded the comparable

* Based on an analysis of 159 initial and final CMI forms from that number of parents.

141

Table 40. Study-family parents' annual average utilization per person of staff services[a] by social class of parent and profession of staff member.

Social class[b]	Number of parents (annual average)	Staff member		
		Family physician	Public health nurse	Social worker
Upper-middle	59	3.6	2.3	2.9
Middle	86	4.5	3.1	3.0
Lower	88	4.0	3.0	2.9
Total	233	4.1	2.8	2.9

[a] Services include home or office visits but not telephone consultations.

[b] Social class is here defined in terms of the occupation of the family head. In very general terms, upper-middle class includes proprietary, managerial, and professional occupations; middle class refers to lower professionals and skilled workers; and lower class means semi-skilled and unskilled workers. The rating scale represents a modified version of one originally developed by W. Lloyd Warner in *Social Class in America*.

average for upper-class parents by a considerable margin. Class did not appear to be an important factor in the use of services of social workers, since all groups averaged nearly the same number of services.

Without exception the average decrease in use with time was consistent. Table 41 indicates that the study-family parents'

Table 41. Study-family parents' annual average utilization per person of services[a] by follow-up year and profession of staff member.

Follow-up year	Number of parents (annual average)	Staff member		
		Family physician	Public health nurse	Social worker
First	248	4.9	4.1	4.0
Second	237	4.0	2.7	3.1
Third	232	3.8	2.3	2.6
Fourth	213	3.7	2.0	1.8
Mean: All Parents	233	4.1	2.8	2.9

[a] Services include home or office visits but not telephone consultations.

average annual number of visits to family physicians declined from the first follow-up year to the fourth, as did their visits to the nurse and social worker.

In addition, the volume of demand for medical service by a

142

UTILIZATION OF SERVICES

Table 42. Study families' annual average utilization of services[a] by social class of father and by profession of staff member.

Social class[b]	Staff member		
	Family physician or pediatrician	Public health nurse	Social worker
Upper-middle	18.6	10.5	10.5
Middle	19.7	12.2	9.6
Lower	16.5	11.7	8.3
Total	18.1	11.9	9.3

[a] Services include home or office visits but not telephone conversations.
[b] Social class is here defined as in Table 40.

family was positively correlated with social class (Table 42). Table 43 shows that for each year and for each professional worker high use is a function of the middle class and low use a

Table 43. Annual average utilization per study family of services[a] of staff during first and fourth follow-up years by social class of father and by profession of staff member.

Follow-up year	Social class[b]	Staff member		
		Family physician or pediatrician	Public health nurse	Social worker
First	Upper-middle	19.2	16.6	12.3
	Middle	20.6	18.7	10.6
	Lower	17.1	20.0	10.2
	Total	18.8	18.6	10.9
Fourth	Upper-middle	17.5	6.0	7.2
	Middle	19.3	8.3	5.6
	Lower	16.2	7.5	5.9
	Total	17.6	7.4	6.1
Fourth as percent of first	Upper-middle	91	36	59
	Middle	94	44	53
	Lower	95	38	58
	Total	94	40	56

[a] Services include home or office visits but not telephone consultations.
[b] Social class is here defined as in Table 40.

function of the lower class.[12] Since the distribution of illness and diagnoses in these groups is about the same, the social class seems to be the important factor in the difference.

143

Parents in the study families who were classified in the low-education category exceeded those of other education categories in their use of services (see Table 44). They averaged 4.4 annual

Table 44. Study-family parents' annual average utilization per person of services by education[a] of parents and profession of staff member.

		Staff member		
Education[a]	Number of parents (annual average)	Family physician	Public health nurse	Social worker
High	83	3.8	2.4	2.5
Medium	96	4.2	3.0	3.2
Low	54	4.4	3.3	3.2
Total	233	4.0	2.8	2.9

[a] High, College graduate or higher; medium, High school graduate and some college; low, Less than high school graduate.

services per person by family physicians, compared to 4.2 among parents in the medium-education group and 3.8 in the high-education group. The use of the services of the public health nurse followed a similar pattern, being highest in the low-education category but dropping in the medium- and in the high-education group. In the use of the social worker's services there was some variation. Here the low- and medium-education groupings averaged an identical amount, 3.2 services annually, compared to the smaller average annual use by the highest education category, 2.5 services.

FAMILY ROLES AND UTILIZATION

There is a suggestion of other correlations, mostly well known. Adult women, who live longer and suffer less from serious illness such as duodenal ulcer and coronary disease, paradoxically use more services than adult men. This is not true for female children, whose utilization is identical with that of the boys.

The average annual utilization of services of the team members varied by family role (whether parent or child, and by the age of the child) and by the profession of the staff member.

Whatever the family role, however, the physician was used more than the public health nurse or social worker. Parents averaged 4.1 in their use of physicians' services, compared to the use of 2.8 services of the public health nurse and 2.9 of the social worker. Among children under 13 these annual averages were: 4.2, 2.7, and 1.3 respectively. The average annual use of physicians' services by children was highest in those under 6, dropping sharply in older children. The same was true for the use of the public health nurse by the children. But for the services of the social worker, the average annual use by children was understandably at a maximum at ages 6–12, the early school years (Table 45).

Table 45. Annual average utilization by study families of staff services[a] by family role and sex.

| Family role | Sex | Staff member | | |
		Family physician	Public health nurse	Social worker
Parent		4.1	2.8	2.9
	Male	3.2	1.3	1.7
	Female	5.0	4.3	4.2
Children 13–16		3.4	1.3	0.6
	Male	3.7	1.2	0.4
	Female	3.1	1.9	0.9
Children 6–12[b]		3.2	2.3	1.9
	Male	3.2	2.2	2.3
	Female	3.2	2.5	1.4
Children under 6[b]		5.9	3.6	1.5
	Male	6.3	3.3	1.8
	Female	5.8	3.5	1.1

[a] Services include home or office visits but not telephone conversations.
[b] Served by pediatrician.

Also, although the parents' use was almost identical for public health nurse and social worker, the children used the services of the public health nurse far more than those of the social worker. In children under 6, and 13 and over, the margin of excess was over 100 percent; even at ages 6 to 12 (when use of social worker was at a maximum), the margin of excess was substantial.

When the data dealing with utilization of the services of team members are analyzed according to sex and age, many of the same relations continue to be evident, but the patterns of use by males vary somewhat from those of females. For both males and females, regardless of age the physician was used more than the public health nurse or social worker. Among parents the services of all 3 professional staff members were utilized substantially more by females than males. This was true for the services of the family physician, and even more so for the services of the public health nurse and the social worker. However, children differed somewhat from the adults. Use of the family physician was somewhat higher among males, while the female parent was a far greater user of services than the male parent. The public health nurse, on the other hand, was used less by male children. Older girls used the services of the social worker more than older boys, but 6- to 12-year-old boys saw the social worker most of all the children. Mothers used social service most of all.

When the data are analyzed for individual follow-up years

Table 46. Annual average utilization by study families of staff services[a] during first and fourth follow-up years.

Follow-up year	Family role	Sex	Staff member		
			Family physician	Public health nurse	Social worker
First	Parents		4.8	4.1	4.0
		Male	3.9	2.4	2.7
		Female	5.8	5.8	5.3
	Children 13–16		3.4	3.1	0.6
		Male	4.1	2.2	0.2
		Female	2.6	4.3	1.0
	Children 6–12		3.2	4.7	1.6
		Male	3.1	4.4	1.4
		Female	3.3	5.0	1.9
	Children under 6		5.1	5.0	1.2
		Male	5.0	4.6	1.3
		Female	5.2	5.4	1.1
Fourth	Parents		3.7	2.0	1.8
		Male	2.7	0.9	1.1
		Female	4.5	3.2	2.5
	Children 13–16		2.8	0.7	0.3
		Male	2.8	0.6	0.2
		Female	2.8	0.8	0.4
	Children 6–12		3.4	1.3	1.5
		Male	3.5	1.3	2.0
		Female	3.3	1.3	0.9
	Children under 6		6.6	2.1	0.8
		Male	7.1	2.1	0.7
		Female	6.1	2.2	0.9

[a] Services include home or office visits but not telephone conversations.

(Table 46), the average number of services from each professional staff member declined between the first and fourth follow-up years. This was true for parents and for children over 13. The use of physician services did not decline for children in the age groups under 12. Adult use of physicians declined in the fourth year to 77 percent of the first year, of the public health nurse to 49 percent, and of the social worker to 45 percent. The upward trend in use of physicians' services by the younger children is undoubtedly a function of the health education focus on young mothers. More preventive services in the younger years was characteristic of the Demonstration, and the increased use is evidence of the success of this health promotional activity.

USE OF SOCIAL WORKER AND PUBLIC HEALTH NURSE

Different factors affected the differential use of these paramedical workers. While physician utilization follows the "inverted-U" curve with its highest point in the middle class, the curve for the paramedical workers varies. The upper middle class is the greatest user of social work, the middle and lower class of nursing. The nurse is used a great deal more by those families with less education, and the social worker is used as much by medium-education families as by the low-education ones.[13]

In comparing the utilization of physician services with that of nurse or social-work services, except for the variations noted the pattern is virtually the same. The fact that different people used the social worker from those who used the nurse may indicate that the value of service was recognized, and the need met, at different levels. It may be that almost everyone wanted help of some kind and the unfamiliar structure of the team did not keep them from reaching out for it, so that they took what they wanted at the source they considered helpful. The nurse was visited by people who would not have gone to the social worker, and vice versa. Thus, having the nurse and social worker on the team had the positive value of making available services that people needed and wanted and could usually get in no other way.

DENTAL CARE

The data on dental service are restricted to children. We found out very little about adult conditions except that there is great

147

need for dental care. In line with the program objectives (and in view of the potentially very high cost of adult dental care), we confined dental services to the children. The families were delighted with this service and often gave it as an important reason for participation in Family Health Maintenance. Table 47 shows that they used it freely.

Table 47. Annual average utilization of dental services among study-family children one year and over according to age and sex.

Age (years)	Sex	Number	Services per person
1–5		92	2.6
	Males	49	2.4
	Females	43	2.7
6–12		120	5.2
	Males	63	4.7
	Females	57	5.8
13–16		46	5.0
	Males	26	4.7
	Females	20	5.4
Total		258	4.2
	Males	138	3.9
	Females	120	4.6

Children in the study families averaged 4.3 dental services annually for the entire period of the study, but use varied by age, being highest over 6 years of age and higher among females than males at each age. Children under 6 averaged only 2.6 services annually, but this average doubled for the older children. This is not unexpected, since for some years under 6 there are fewer teeth to give trouble. By sex, the average for boys was only 83 percent as high as the comparable average for girls, and this obtained at all ages.

Children at all ages averaged fewer dental services during the fourth follow-up year of the study than during the first. Considering the fourth year as a percentage of the first, services declined to 71 percent (see Table 48). For children aged 1–5, the comparable figures were 83 percent as high; for children aged 6–12, the drop was sharpest, only 53 percent as high; and for the older children, much less change was seen, at 87 percent. This may be related to improvement of mouth condition from the services

Table 48. Annual average utilization of dental services per person among study-family children one year and over during first and fourth follow-up years, by age.

Age (years)	First follow-up year		Fourth follow-up year		Fourth as percent of first
	Number	Services	Number	Services	
1–5	108	3.0	69	2.5	83
6–12	113	7.2	127	3.8	53
13–16	30	5.2	60	4.5	87
Total	251	5.1	256	3.6	71

given, but the numbers are small and the percentage difference equivocal.

The use of dental services by children varied according to the social class of their fathers. Table 49 shows that, in contrast to

Table 49. Annual average utilization of dental services per person among study-family children one year and over by social class of father[a] and follow-up year.

Follow-up year	Number of children's visits	Social class			
		All	Upper-middle	Middle	Lower
First	251	5.1	5.1	5.4	5.0
Fourth	256	3.6	3.3	3.8	3.6
Fourth as percent of first		71	65	70	72

[a] Social class is here defined as in Table 40.

the average of 4.2 services annually for the children of all classes, children in the upper-middle classes averaged only 3.9, with those in the middle and lower classes 4.3 and 4.4. The decline in average use during the follow-up years was nevertheless consistent, regardless of the occupational class of the father.

The benefit that accrued to the study children from the dental services is obvious from Table 50. While they had a markedly increased DMF rate (decayed, missing, and filled teeth) at the end of the study than at the beginning — 22.6 DMF per child compared with 10.9 DMF for the control children — this increase was entirely the result of dental attention and due to the number of filled teeth. At the end of the Demonstration study children of all ages had practically no decayed teeth and relatively few

Table 50. Rate of decayed, missing, or filled teeth (D-M-F)[a] among children of study and control families.

Age of child at exami- nation (years)	Study (initial)				Study (final)				Control (final)			
	Number of children examined	D	M	F	Number of children examined	D	M	F	Number of children examined	D	M	F
6–9	67	4.2	[b]	3.6	63	0	0.1	17.3	22	4.1	0	3.2
10–12	37	4.5	0	5.8	40	0	0.2	21.9	12	4.8	0	3.9
13–16	11	5.7	0.1	5.8	41	0.1	0.1	31.1	7	5.7	0	20.6
Total	115	4.5	[b]	4.5	144	[b]	0.1	22.5	41	4.5	0	6.4

[a] D = decayed teeth; M = missing teeth; F = filled surfaces.
[b] Less than 0.05.

missing (extracted) teeth, while the control children had a high rate of decayed and low rate of filled teeth. Filled-teeth rates were 4.5 in the beginning and 22.5 at the end of the study. As would be expected, the greatest number of fillings was in the older children.

At the end of the study the control-family children showed a distribution of DMF teeth similar to the distribution in the study-family children at the beginning. These findings graphically underline the value of routine dental care in childhood for maintenance of dental health.[14]

Utilization of medical services results from a combination of forces, acting on the members of a family with individual factors, social or personal, exerting a cumulative effect.

The use of a physician's services is based partly on his accessibility, in both the physical and psychological sense, and partly on patient conception of use and need of doctor's services. This latter element is conditioned by sex (greater female use), by social class (greater use by the middle class), by educational attainment (greater use by less educated people), and perhaps by ethnic factors as well.

Special medical needs certainly influenced utilization, but, by and large, the complex of factors indicated was more important in setting the pattern. For example, one of the highest utilizing families in the Demonstration consisted of mother, father, and 3 children, for 2 years, and father and 3 children for 2 years (the mother died of cancer at the end of the second participating year). This family used a total of 414 services, against a Demonstration average of 155.6 for the 4 years. Of these services, 126 were physician services (the Demonstration average was 72.4). Even so, this may not be a tremendous amount of service in 4 years, considering the heart-breaking burden of illness this family carried: cancer in the mother; a complicated neurological-orthopedic disease in one child; ordinary childhood diseases in the other children; and — no surprise — anxiety and depression in the father.

On the other hand, an average service-utilizing family (221 services in 4 years) had 7 children, with little medical care given to any individual. Seven children might have been expected to call forth a great deal of service, but did not. Two smaller families demonstrated exaggerated differences in utilization not entirely ascribable to illness. In one there were 54 total services, despite an automobile accident with physical injury to the father, psychosexual and gastrointestinal complaints in the mother, and usual childhood illnesses in the child. Against this was the other family of 4 in which there were 234 services over 3 years. (This family left the Demonstration for reasons of dissatisfaction.) The mother was in psychoanalysis and was found to have a duodenal ulcer; one child had a history of rheumatic fever; and another child had eczema and enuresis.

Nor is utilization based simply on economic access or availability. In this light, one of the arguments used for (and against) compulsory health insurance loses considerable force. It isn't only economic factors that serve to deprive people of medical care, and equally it isn't true that removal of the economic barrier will inundate the doctor with unnecessary demands for service. The present organization of medical practice is defective and that is what leads to inadequate service on the doctor's part and improper use on the patient's part. Consideration should be given to restructuring medical practice: provision should be made for the added time, family interest and concern, skills in guidance, and perhaps team approach, that would enable the professional people to understand and cope with the complex variables of patient demand and use.

Furthermore, although it is necessary to remove the economic barriers to modern medical care, it is also necessary to modify medical education and add an educational program to medical practice, unrelated to medicine as presently practiced, so that doctors will give, and patients will see the value of, medical service appropriately used. In defining disease and well-being, such an educational program must consider cultural and ethnic variations, psychological factors, and social class, for all these play an important role in the utilization of medical service.

PART THREE

ASSESSMENT OF THE DEMONSTRATION

- IX -

SYMPTOMS, ILLNESS, AND FAMILY LIFE

From this [Oriental] standpoint, there is a clear absurdity in
trying to achieve the "happy adjustment" of an individual to the
convention of a society which is largely composed of unhappy
people.
— Alan Watts, "Asian Psychology"

The preceding chapters dealt with differences in improvement
and variations in utilization between study and control families
and among study families. The type and amount of illness was
mentioned as a significant variable. It is worthwhile to look a
little more carefully at the patterns of illness in the families and
explore the nature of the disparity.

DISTRIBUTION OF PHYSICAL DISEASE

The Demonstration uncovered a reservoir of illness in our families not previously known; this accounts in some measure for the
high utilization. But this is not the whole of the story. Although
some illnesses previously unknown to the individual were found
among the study families, the proportion of such was bound to be
small. With some years' previous access to a sophisticated medical-care scheme and with no bills to consider New Yorkers might
be expected to have made most of their ills known and have them
looked after. Table 31 showed how little significant (major) new
disease was found and the relatively larger amount of new minor
illnesses uncovered. What is remarkable is the total volume of
disease and symptomatology uncovered. Fully 80 percent of the
people examined had symptoms and signs of illness that required

155

professional attention or were a matter of concern to the family.

It would be interesting to compare the findings in a population of this kind, so conscientiously surveyed, with the findings of others who have examined a large number of people on a routine basis rather than for cause. Unfortunately, such data are scarce. Even the report of Pearse, who with Williamson and Crocker brought the Peckham Health Center into being,[1] is not truly comparable, because the programs' standards of measurement were quite different and because there was no medical follow-up at Peckham to verify the original diagnoses. Pearse and Williamson did introduce a useful conception of "compensated" as against "decompensated" activity. In their terminology, people with symptoms or signs of illness, who felt well despite this and were able to carry on, were labeled "in well-being," and those who had symptoms and signs and did not feel well or could not carry on were called "incapacitated." Although we could not reproduce these classifications exactly, we attempted to group our patients in a comparable way, using initial physical examination results and CMI responses as our indexes.

On the basis of the initial evaluations we divided the families into 3 categories corresponding to those of Peckham. Recognizing the great gaps in definition as well as measurement, it is nevertheless interesting to compare the distribution of categories in the groups (Table 51). In Peckham 10 percent were "without dis-

Table 51. Number and percent of individuals in categories of wellness in Peckham[a] and the Family Health Maintenance Demonstration.

Category		Peckham		FHMD	
Peckham	FHMD	Number	Percent	Number	Percent
Without disorder[b]	Well[c]	156	10	9	3.6
In well being[d]	Compensated[e]	1052	69	201	81.4
In disease[f]	Decompensated[g]	328	21	37	15.0

[a] Pearse and Crocker, *The Peckham Experiment.*
[b] No symptoms or signs of illness.
[c] Fewer than 10 Cornell Medical Index "yeses"; physical examination evaluation, class 1 or 2.
[d] Some symptoms or signs of illness found, but patient does not complain.
[e] Fewer than 30 CMI "yeses"; physical examination evaluation, class 2 or 3.
[f] Patient has symptoms and signs of illness and feels sick or is incapacitated.
[g] Thirty or more CMI "yeses"; physical examination evaluation, class 3 or 4.

order"; in the FHMD 3.6 percent were "well." By Peckham standards 69 percent were "in well being," as compared to 81.4 percent "compensated" in the FHMD. And in the Peckham group 21 percent were "in disease," while 15.0 were categorized as "decompensated" in the Family Health Maintenance Demonstration. The discrepancies are of less interest than the rough approximation of size of the categories. Illness seems to be the natural or "normal" state rather than "wellness," and a surprisingly large percentage of the population (at least 15 percent) is incapacitated for effective personal or family life. Furthermore, for whatever it may be worth statistically, the degree of correspondence in the sets of figures indicates that there is a great deal of symptomatology in presumably well people which may or may not give rise to "sickness," that is, to demand for medical care. This seems to be true both in a system in which no medical care was provided (Peckham) and in a scheme in which all physician services were offered. Utilization of medical services reflects only the visible part of the iceberg of illness in human life.

PREVALENCE OF EMOTIONAL DIFFICULTIES

More than physical illness and its symptoms is demonstrated. There is provocative evidence of even wider prevalence of the symptoms of emotional illness than is generally recognized. It may come as a surprise that there is this manifestation of emotional difficulty and disease widespread in the population — a surprise to some that so much was found, to others that so little is generally recognized. Actually, such information has been available for some time. Those who might like to believe that our findings are typical only of urban areas or reflect specifically the situation in New York City, should investigate other reports, such as the findings in a Canadian community.[2] In the detailed report of that Nova Scotia study, an expectancy of emotional symptoms in the community runs as high as 65 percent.* In active case finding in the Nova Scotia community, when a survey and psychiatric evaluation of a random sample of the community was done

* Although only 4.7 percent had clearly psychiatric complaints, the authors point out that this is of a piece with the 5.5 percent rejected as unfit on neuro-psychiatric grounds in Selective Service, with 6.1 percent in active care by social agencies in Baltimore, and with the 6.9 percent found to have symptoms in a Williamson County Study.

(checking this against physician's reports and hospital records), 37 percent were found to have had actual psychiatric complaints or symptoms. This resembles the 44 percent found in the study families in our own Demonstration.

Our own data are interesting in the light thrown on family relations as well as on prevalence of emotional difficulties. In the first place, there were more people with emotional problems,[3] both absolutely and relatively, in the study than in the control group. This can be attributed to better case finding in the former. Prior to entry into the study, only 7 percent of the group was thought by the physicians to have problems (see Table 52). Although

Table 52. Emotional problems of family members (percent)[a] by staff member and time of indication.

Staff member indicating problem	Time of indication	Study group	Control group	Ratio of study to control
Physician		30.5	18.7	1.63
	Prior to entry	7.0	11.0	0.64
	After entry	23.5	7.7	3.05
Social worker	After entry	3.2	—	—
Social worker and physician	After entry	10.1	—	—
Total		43.8	18.7	2.34

[a] 557 study-group members; 663 control-group members.

somewhat less than the amount in the control group, this is roughly comparable. After entry into the study, the picture is radically changed. An additional 23.5 percent of the study group was found by the Demonstration physician to have problems, compared with only an additional 7.7 percent in the control group (by their regular physicians in the Medical Group) during the 4 years of observation. The study group produced three times as many cases with problems in that period. If the before and after are added together — that is, the proportion of the population known to have problems prior to entry into the study added to those found after entry — the study-group proportion exceeded the control-group cases by over two-thirds. This increment represents more intensive case finding by the physician alone.

In addition, the study group was interviewed by the social

worker. Independently she found another 3.2 percent with problems; and she and the physician jointly found 10.1 percent more cases. There is no comparable control finding for this latter 13.3 percent. This increment would not be expected to show up except under the special circumstances of the study. But, putting together all cases of emotional problems found in the study group by physician, social worker, and the two combined, both before and after entry into the study, the percentage of cases rises to 43.8. This is well over twice as many cases as in the control group, and leaves us with almost half of a population intensively studied showing evidence of emotional problems. Not only were more emotional problems found in study-family members, but more families with more than one troubled individual were found among the study group (see Table 53).

Table 53. Families with children having emotional problems by emotional problems of parents.

Parent with problems	Study families				Control families			
	All		One or more children with problems		All		One or more children with problems	
	Number	Percent	Number	Percent	Number	Percent	Number	Percent
Both	45	35.7	37	82.2	12	7.6	7	58.3
One	48	38.1	28	58.3	51	32.5	15	29.4
Neither	33	26.2	16	48.5	94	59.9	21	22.3

The conclusion seems inescapable that there is a vast reservoir of difficulty in the emotional sphere, evidences of which appear in the doctor's office from time to time, sometimes masked, sometimes openly, but never in the degree and quantity that it actually exists. Also that this reservoir can be tapped by careful study.

When the data are considered in relation to individual family members, much the same pattern emerges as when all persons are considered. For each family member, the proportion of cases with emotional problems is higher in the study than in the control families, but only *after* the Demonstration activity is completed. Prior to entry, a good part of the study families' problems had not yet emerged, and there were proportionately more

Table 54. Emotional problems (percent) of study and control family members by staff member and time of indication.

Staff member indicating problem	Time of indication	Father			Mother			Children		
		Study	Control	Ratio of study to control	Study	Control	Ratio of study to control	Study	Control	Ratio of study to control
Number of persons		126	157	—	126	157	—	305	359	—
Physician	Prior to entry	27.0	21.6	1.25	46.1	26.1	1.77	25.5	14.2	1.80
	After entry	7.1	14.6	0.49	14.3	18.5	0.77	3.9	6.1	0.64
Social worker	After entry	19.9	7.0	2.84	31.8	7.6	4.08	21.6	8.1	2.67
Social worker	After entry	5.6	0	—	3.2	0	—	2.3	0	—
and physician	After entry	12.7	0	—	15.1	0	—	6.9	0	—
Total with problems		45.3	21.6	2.10	64.3	26.1	2.46	34.8	14.2	2.45

fathers, mothers, and children with problems in the *control* group (see Table 54). The use of ratios may simplify these findings. Before entry, study as a fraction of control cases was 0.49 for fathers, 0.77 for mothers, and 0.64 for children. After entry, the ratio changed to conform with the increased number of cases found in the study group. Considering the total of *all* cases found (by both doctor and social worker), and including before- and after-entry figures, the ratio of study to control is more than double for fathers, mothers, and children. In view of the similarities of the study and control families in other ways, the effect is apparently related to more intensive case finding.

Quite apart from study and control, or case-finding implications, comparisons of the family members themselves are of some interest. From this point of view, a pattern emerges that tran-

Table 55. Emotional problems in study families by family member.

Family member	All members	With problems	
		Number	Percent
Father	126	57	45.2
Mother	126	81	64.3
Children, 6–18	141 ⎱ 249	63 ⎱ 101	44.7 ⎱ 39.0
Children, 1–5	108 ⎰	38 ⎰	35.2 ⎰

scends study versus control findings (see Tables 55 and 56). In almost all cases, a larger proportion of mothers than fathers and fathers than children was found to have emotional problems. In the study group twice as many mothers as fathers were found

Table 56. Ratio of mothers and children with emotional problems to fathers with emotional problems by staff member and time of indication.

Staff member indicating problem	Time of indication	Study families		Control families	
		Mother	Children	Mother	Children
Physician		1.70	0.94	1.21	0.66
	Prior to entry	2.01	0.55	1.27	0.42
	After entry	1.59	1.09	1.09	1.14
Social worker	After entry	0.57	0.41	—	—
Social worker and physician	After entry	1.19	0.54	—	—
Total		1.42	0.77	1.21	0.66

with emotional problems at the outset, but only 55 percent as many children as fathers. The control group showed a similar excess of mothers with emotional problems over fathers with problems, and a similar excess of fathers with problems over children with problems. After entry, the pattern changed radically in regard to the children but not at all in the balance between mothers and fathers. On the other hand, if one considers the over-all picture (doctor and social worker diagnosis, before and after entry) the pattern is as originally stated: mothers exceed fathers in diagnoses of emotional problems, and fathers exceed children. This relation is consistent in both study and control families.

Not everyone with problems was referred to a psychiatrist, or to a psychiatric agency for care: about 2 out of 5 were referred. The proportion of children referred was slightly higher than the referrals of adults with emotional problems. The probability that children will have problems is greater in those families where parents have problems. This was true for both study and control families. In 82 percent of those study families where both parents have problems, one or more of the children have problems. As expected, it is less likely that the children will have problems if only one, or none of the parents has problems. This is true for both study and control families. Put another way (see Table 57),

Table 57. Children with emotional problems by parents with problems.

Parent with problems	Study families			Control families		
	Number of children	Children with problems		Number of children	Children with problems	
		Number	Percent		Number	Percent
Both	100	49	49.0	22	10	45.5
One	114	37	32.5	122	17	13.9
Neither	91	20	22.0	215	24	11.2

in study families where both parents have problems, half the children will have problems. Only a third of the children will have problems if one parent has problems, and less than a quarter of the children if neither parent has problems. The same trend is exhibited by children in control families.

Furthermore, whether or not children would have emotional

162

problems seemed to be strongly and inversely related to the size of the family (see Table 58). Of the 305 children in the study

Table 58. Children with emotional problems by family size.

Number of children in family	Study families			Control families		
	Number of children	Children with problems		Number of children	Children with problems	
		Number	Percent		Number	Percent
1–2	148	61	41.2	190	26	13.7
3–4	125	41	32.8	143	24	16.8
5–7	32	4	12.5	26	1	3.8

families, 106 (34.8 percent) had emotional problems. If they were members of small families the comparable percentage was 41.2 percent; in medium-sized families 32.8 percent; and in large families only 12.5 percent! This did not hold for the small- and medium-sized control families who were very much alike. But in the large-sized control families only 1 child out of 26 showed any emotional disturbance, which is consistent. The small size of sample and small number of cases render the meaning of the control figures equivocal.

Table 59 shows that 57.9 percent of the children in small families had problems compared with 39.5 percent of the children in medium-sized families, but there were too few cases to evaluate

Table 59. Study-family children with emotional problems by family size and emotional problems of parents.

Parents with problems	Number of children in family	Total number of children	Children with problems	
			Number	Percent
Both	1–2	57	33	57.9
	3–4	38	15	39.5
	5–7	5	1	a
One	1–2	54	18	33.3
	3–4	55	17	30.9
	5–7	5	2	a
Neither	1–2	37	10	27.0
	3–4	32	9	28.1
	5–7	22	1	4.5

a Number too small for significant figures.

the effect of large families on the children. If only one parent had problems, small- and medium-sized families were quite similar in the percentage of children with problems; again there are too few cases to evaluate the large family. Finally, if neither parent had problems, there is virtually no difference due to the size of the family, except that large families had very few cases among the children.

Not only did family size seem to protect against emotional difficulties in children, it may have helped the adults too (see Table 60). This relation was not clear or consistent and cannot

Table 60. Parents with emotional problems (percent) by family size.

Parents with problems	All families	Number of children in family		
		1–2	3–4	5–7
Study families:				
Both	35.7	39.5	30.8	a
One	38.1	37.0	43.6	a
Neither	26.2	23.5	25.6	a
Number of families	126	81	39	6
Control families:				
Both	7.7	9.4	4.5	a
One	32.9	31.2	34.1	a
Neither	59.4	59.4	61.4	a
Number of families	157	108	44	5

a Number too small for significant figures.

be confirmed until more evidence becomes available. Where the family was smaller, it appeared more likely that both parents would have problems, in families with less than 5 children, at least. Control families showed similar effects: in larger families there were far fewer parents with problems.

If these data are broken down by family size *and* emotional health of parents (Table 61), this relation still holds true in the study families for the emotional health of the children. Again, the evidence is persuasive but not conclusive. There is too large a percentage of medium-sized families whose children have problems when one parent only has problems to give a perfect correlation. Still, in the small families, where both parents have problems half of the families have children with problems; and in larger families where neither parent has a problem, only 18 per-

Table 61. Study-family parents with emotional problems (percent) by family size and children's problems.

Parents with problems	All families	Number of children in family		
		1–2	3–4	5–7
Children with problems:				
Both	45.7	50.0	39.3	a
One	34.6	30.0	42.9	a
Neither	19.7	20.0	17.8	a
Number of families	81	50	28	3
Children without problems:				
Both	17.8	22.6	9.0	a
One	44.4	48.4	45.5	a
Neither	38.8	29.0	45.5	a
Number of families	45	31	11	3

a Number too small for significant figures.

cent of the families have children with problems. Perhaps we should emphasize that parent problems depended on family size and not family size on parent problems.

Other characteristics associated with the families seem to incur a higher probability of the existence of emotional problems, especially with high CMI scores, sexual problems, "fair" or "poor" evaluation in the area of personal adjustment, and "fair" or "poor" rating on the evaluation of their physical condition. Parents who had 10 or more "yeses" on the psychological section of the CMI were highest (82.9 percent) in emotional problems. A higher proportion than average of parents with "fair" or "poor" physical condition had emotional problems, but far less than those with high CMI scores, "fair" or "poor" adjustment, or sexual problems. Of course there is an element of tautology involved in that the definition of emotional problem derived in part from symptomatology as presented in those areas. But the distribution may be presumed as evidence of association.

More than half of the parents in this study were Jewish. Among them, 62.3 percent — higher than the average for all parents — were classified as having emotional problems. In contrast, the Catholic parents, a third of the total families, had a lower proportion than average — 41.9 percent — of parents with emotional problems.[4]

If we look at fathers and mothers separately with regard to the

165

same pertinent factors, some curious and interesting associations become apparent (Table 62). Although 54.8 percent of parents

Table 62. Number of study-family parents with emotional problems by selected characteristics.

Selected characteristics	Number of fathers	Fathers with problems		Number of mothers	Mothers with problems	
		Number	Percent		Number	Percent
All parents	126	57	45.2	126	81	64.3
Scores of 30 or more "yeses" on Cornell Medical Index	13	9	69.2	38	29	76.3
Scores of 10 or more "yeses" on psychological sections of Cornell Medical Index	9	7	77.8	26	22	84.6
Sexual problem	25	17	68.0	25	21	84.0
"Fair" or "poor" rating on evaluation of personal adjustment	38	24	63.2	44	36	81.8
"Fair" or "poor" rating on evaluation of relation to spouse	31	17	54.8	33	26	78.8
"Fair" or "poor" rating on evaluation of physical condition	61	33	54.1	69	45	65.2
Catholic	42	11	26.2	44	25	56.8
Jewish	69	38	55.1	69	48	69.6

had problems, mothers led with 64.3 percent as opposed to 45.2 percent for fathers. In all the areas examined, fathers were less likely to show emotional symptoms. Clearly these factors have a greater impact on the female in the development of emotional problems.

The discrepancy in emotional problem presentation seen in Jewish and Catholic parents was still in evidence when Jewish fathers were compared with Catholic fathers and Jewish mothers with Catholic mothers. The male-female gradient was also in evidence, with Jewish fathers lower than Jewish mothers and Catholic fathers lower than Catholic mothers.

The sum of these analyses is that in almost three-quarters of the study families one or both of the parents had an emotional problem that required (although it did not always get) professional help. This was far more than was found in routine health supervision of the control families, only half of whom showed such a pattern. In both study and control families, trouble in the parents was most likely to be associated with trouble in the children. Emotional difficulties were relatively more prominent in small than in large families, for both parents and children. There was more emotional difficulty in women than in men, more in mothers than in fathers, and more in parents than in children. However, more children were referred for psychiatric care than adults, reflecting the principle of the greater utility of such help in younger people, and probably also the greater resistance of adults to accept psychotherapy. Finally, the interrelation of emotional disorder with poor physical condition as evidenced in the doctor's examination and in higher symptomatology (more than 10 "yeses" in the CMI) and with expressed or discovered sexual problems and poor personal adjustment generally was manifested.

On recognizing how widely the families varied in symptomatology, and yet how uniformly evidences of family difficulty appeared, one is constrained to review these findings from the standpoint of social functioning. Were our families more likely to appear as suppliants to social agencies? If not, was it because their symptoms or needs were not so urgent? Or, if their needs were similar and yet they did not appeal for help, what supporting structure intervened? Specific information would be extraordinarily helpful, and I must say at once that too few details of family interaction were obtained to be more than presumptive. Certain elements, however, stand out clearly.

Comparison with Social-Agency Clients

It should be emphasized that the families we studied — although we speak again and again about "normal" families, selected at random with certain similarities in background or occupation — were not colorlessly or stolidly identical. They were of innumerable variety, almost as many types as there were study families. Concerning occupations, the records show that we had a police lieutenant, a fire chief, a professional wrestler, a short-order cook, and a former literary editor of a left-wing newspaper, as well as salesmen, timekeepers, motormen, taxi drivers, schoolteachers and principals, and auto mechanics. And, since some wives worked, there were a number of other jobs listed: clerks, secretaries, waitresses, social workers, and baby sitters. Among the otherwise innocuous and law-abiding citizens there appeared alcoholics, a high-school dope addict, and a compulsive gambler. A number of abortions appear in the record (self-performed or performed illegally by some practitioner). There is an incident of attempted murder, of rape, and of attempted rape. There were children with tremendous social and emotional problems in school and at home. Among the "adjusting" and "nonadjusting" we saw psychotic children. There were a number of people with serious and disabling physical illnesses. A wide range of conditions, social and psychological symptoms, employment situations, personal and medical history appear in these records. It cannot be assumed that, because we dealt with "normal" people, we dealt with one kind of person, or that the many people in civil service jobs had identical problems. They were individuals; but, paradoxically, in their individuality there was an amazing similarity in their difficulties and an amazing similarity in their responses. The differences for the most part were below the surface, in social relations. It was not unusual in going over family histories and reviewing interviews with fathers, mothers, or children to uncover incidents of breath-taking cruelty, suffering, even perversion. Although the face presented to the world by these normally functioning families was respectable and controlled, within the privacy of the home outrageous events could occur.

Item, a man tried to murder his wife by suffocation, but desisted. They live together still, eating, drinking, going to the movies, gravely examining the children's report cards. Item, a city official with important social responsibility brutalized his children to create "respect" for law and order. They do respect him, are obedient, model children in school. Family life goes on. Item, a devoted mother made her child drink urine to "cure" the little girl of bed-wetting. Item, a nun made a child eat his own vomit to "cure" him of throwing up in school. He stopped vomiting (he was resisting going to school) and the family accepted this as evidence that the solution was practical.

A variety of abnormal behavior patterns were revealed. In one family, mother and child dined at 6 P.M. (he before the TV set,

168

she in the kitchen). She went to bed to sleep from 7 P.M. to 7
A.M.; the child slept from 10 P.M. to 8 A.M. Father came home at
1 A.M. and slept to 10 A.M. Consequently, they saw each other as
a family only on Sundays. In this same family there had been no
sex relations between husband and wife for years. Sexual activity
naturally varied a good deal in families, and some (like this)
could be interpreted by professional workers as abnormal or frustrating. Yet no symptoms were reported, no professional person
was consulted. As a matter of record, if it were not for the Demonstration, these facts might never have come to professional attention.[5]

Bed-wetting, poor marital sexual adjustment, illegitimacy, pre-
marital pregnancy, attempted murder, brutality to children —
these are the presenting symptoms for which people come to
family agencies and psychiatrists for help, or are sent by the police or correction officers. Most Demonstration families had *not*
sought agency care, certainly not to any greater degree than the
control families did. So we are led back to the interesting, cryptic
fact that in most people, unacceptable behavior and emotional
difficulty can be observed (if you look!), and in a large segment
of the community, there may be visible emotional distress: symptomatology, obvious or concealed, for which no hand has been
lifted in help, nor any help requested.

"Coping" [6]

The question of why similarly afflicted families found different
paths to help or carried on without help is very similar to the
corollary question: what is the essential difference between 2
families subjected to almost identical influences who reach disparate goals? In individuals, heredity, a once-popular explanation
which lost favor as *the* cause in individuals as in races, now seems
to be returning to grace.[7] Economics, social forces, sunspots, and
historic trends have been favored explanations. The currently
popular psychoanalytic formulation of arrest at certain stages of
development offers an explanation which is analogous to predes-
tination. Yet, here seems to be evidence that a special, as yet
indefinable, factor is involved, so that 2 families marching along
apparently in step diverge at some point, one to "cope," the other
to fail.

169

Symptomatology. Some of the findings qualify the discrepancy between need and demand. "Need," in this context, is the professional definition of sickness; "demand" is what is felt by or known to the patient. There is another, perhaps more subtle, distinction. The families which did not go to agencies for help, despite the evidence (to us) of disordered feeling or reaction, were "coping" with their problems. It makes no difference whether they were aware of the difficulties with which they struggled to cope; the fact is that they healed themselves without outside help. "Wellness" was measurable in this coping. What constitutes this ability to cope, despite difficulties that drove others for help, and whether it is predictable is a suitable field for further investigation.

It may not be true in physical illnesses, such as cancer, that "leaving it alone" or "coming to terms with the disease" is appropriate treatment or satisfactory adjustment. But in the area of social and emotional problems it is unquestionably better to erect defenses and develop a working compensation. This is what social agencies hope to do for a client.[8] The problem is similar to "combat fatigue"; to some writers *every* soldier can be broken by stress, or is potentially susceptible to combat fatigue if the stress is strong enough and/or long enough.[9] Perhaps all families are potential clients of social agencies. If so, the amount of stress they can cope with, the innate variants in strength and resources and how they can be measured, and the ways to tell one approaching the breaking point, are still unknown.[10] Chapter VII established the fact that few people changed very much if at all during the 4 years of observation. In "physical condition," 70 percent showed no change; in "personal adjustment," 81 percent showed no change. Regardless of whether a small number benefited or suffered from our ministrations, it is most striking that the majority didn't change at all. In spite of the multiplicity of symptoms and the appalling evidences of disease and difficulty, most people did not break down, most people established compensation and maintained it. "Wellness" is a stage on a scale, not an absolute.[11]

In most families, both study and control, there were the same sort of emotional problems, implying that most families have difficulties but manage to adjust; few seek care. The "well" families, operating, functioning, and coping, displayed the same sort of

170

difficulties on investigation as the families that did go to agencies and did apply for help; any differences do not appear in our data. We may only speculate about cultural factors or postulate a mysterious "self-healing" quality.[12]

Professional Help. A step further along, compensation and functioning are also apparently independent of professional help. People with symptoms, with many Cornell Medical Index "yeses" and maladjustments, who were coping, didn't use the social worker or nurse for their troubles to any significant degree. And apparently they weren't any worse off in the long run than those who did. Conversely, the control families who received no help because they had no access to the nurse and social worker, yet had very much the same problems as the study families, weren't any worse off than the study families at the end of the survey. Whatever value the Demonstration had did not seem to extend to improving ability to cope with problems.

On the other hand, one eventuality should be considered: that is, that, while we may not have *demonstrated* improved ability to cope, it may have happened just the same. For example, take the case of a woman who had no apparent problem while participating in the Demonstration. She was well adjusted and considered one of the "excellent" people: relationship with her husband was good; relationship with her child was good (it was noted that she may have "hovered" a little too much and perhaps was a little too protective). There seemed to be no serious problem. However, within a year of the time that she left the Demonstration, she became pregnant and suffered a profound depression during that period. She required psychiatric care and made a slow recovery. Her former equilibrium was broken and there became apparent a need for service that was not visible at the time the patient was under observation. Was this evidence of broken compensation that might have been preserved within the framework of a continuing Demonstration team activity?

A possible explanation[13] for the relative deterioration of the study families in the emotional area at the end of the study may be inherent in the team's operation. That is, not only was there greater possibility of extracting symptoms in the period of intensive scrutiny, but the process itself may have disturbed an existing equilibrium.

The study families had already come to terms with their problems, whatever they were, perhaps without understanding them and perhaps without even accepting them. But by the team discussions new insights may have been offered to the families, and they may have become *aware* of the existence of problems. While they may have previously decided, or unconsciously proceeded, to heal themselves by dealing with whatever was defective, the Demonstration may have precipitated decompensation by offering assistance, which removed the incentive to help themselves. This argument is not the Darwinist argument it appears to be on the surface. The individual who compensated, who "coped" on his own, did so at some price, and from lack of knowledge of the availability of help. Making him aware, enabling him to seek help, didn't change his character or ability to cope. Like the sin in the Garden of Eden, it was the *knowledge* that created conflict. But knowledge should be a sign of health. *We* considered healthy the family which coped without help, unhealthy that which needed assistance to cope. Should the marking have been reversed? This is a serious question of social philosophy and is not answerable from any data.

Emotional Problems and Mental Illness

These symptoms and evidences of emotional disturbance should not be confused with mental illness.* There were a few people among the study families who had severe psychoneurotic or psychotic disturbances. These were unable to relate to others, let alone cope, had to be considered in a class apart, and usually were referred to psychiatrists for care. They did not develop mental illness as the end result of emotional problems such as were seen among the families generally. Apparently they were different to begin with, and one did not result from the other.[14]

To sum up: observation of a group of "normal" families over a period of time revealed serious and distressing symptoms, attitudes, and behavior among the family members. This conforms with the findings of others who have explored this particular area.

* For the purposes of the discussion, emotional illness and mental illness have been very carefully distinguished. Mental illness was defined as disturbance of thought or behavior interfering with all activity.

Nevertheless, most families were able to deal with these matters without requesting professional help and without disclosing the magnitude of the affliction publicly. In this, they differed markedly from similarly affected families which did seek professional aid. Although, even among "normal" families, certain characteristics relating to the *degree* of emotional difficulty varied — size of family, religion, age, or sex, for example — these characteristics did *not* determine whether or not the families sought help. The origin of this very important "coping" factor, which if known could be used to support the integrity of disturbed families, can not be elicited from our data. However, it is evident that emotional difficulty and mental illness are not causally related, since these factors do not follow one another in the observations.

173

- X -

FAMILY AND TEAM INTERACTION

Would the world be more beautiful if our faces were alike?
If all our tempers, talents, tastes — our forms, our wishes, aver-
sions, and pursuits — were cast exactly in the same mold? An
America without variety? Where all are to think alike?

— Thomas Jefferson, *Notes on Virginia*

The members of the health team reacted to the families according to their professional role concepts; their reactions were modified as they learned more about the families and their needs.
Similarly, the families modified their reactions to the team on the
basis of their experience with Demonstration service. This interaction is important because it brings in the verdict on the future
utility of a family health team.

SOME TEAM OBSERVATIONS ON THE FAMILIES

In addition to numerically comparable information, a good deal
of knowledge about the families was obtained and noted in the
observations of the team members. This was particularly true of
the observations of the nurse and social worker, data supplied
from the interviews and family conferences which colored the
Demonstration approach and results. These perceptions of family
patterns require presentation as a background against which
much of the tabular data can be seen in relief.

Nurses' Observations

The nurse, in addition to obtaining information on family nutrition, had the opportunity of observing the group undergoing

174

obesity-control measures. While only 7 percent of the adults in our study group were overweight, the problem existed in more than 7 percent of the families. In attempting to find out what motivates individuals to lose weight, no single reason appeared. One woman, after talking about the subject for a year, was moved to action by a neighbor's challenge. Although she had received detailed dietary instructions, she had never done anything about it. Once challenged, she took the diet sheets she had been given over a year before and put herself on a nutritionally correct diet. A man was motivated to lose weight by his young son's criticism of his figure. After receiving unfavorable comments by her husband, another woman was moved to go on a strict diet and lose the weight she had been unwilling to part with previously — apparently in order to look more attractive for him. Goal and motivation were neither clear nor long-lived in any of these instances.

The few other nutritional problems were related primarily to cultural eating habits and emotional problems inducing improper diet, neither of which could be dealt with by simply prescribing changes. Mothers who neglect their own nutritional needs while they look after the rest of the family will not respond to exhortation. Children whose eating habits are affected by the way the parents behave toward them or toward each other or by other tensions in the family require treatment more extensive than nutritional education. Food habits may also relate to factors outside the home such as problems in school or those resulting from moving into a new neighborhood which may make for changes in the eating habits of young children.

Home management in the face of overcrowding and poor housing can be a great barrier to good health practices, even though the impact on health may not be measurable. One-third of the families showed a crowding index of over 1 person per room, and about 15 percent of the families up to 2 persons per room. Since people meet problems in accordance with their character, success in coping with difficult housing situations varied. The ways in which families adapted to difficult housing situations was interpreted as an aspect of family health.

Family A adjusted to a very crowded duplex apartment, in spite of a marginal family income, by making use of the roof, recon-

175

structing the basement, and fencing in the outside yard for play space and washing space. Family B in the other half of the duplex reacted to the crowding with tension and quarreling. House B was generally in a state of confusion and disorder. Family A took practical steps to improve their housing. Although family B may have wanted to do something about the poor housing situation, its members didn't seem to know how, nor were they able to make the best of the situation as family A did.

On the other hand, good housekeeping wasn't always the best test of successful family arrangements. The compulsive housekeeper type of mother might seriously interfere with the recreational needs of her husband or play needs of her children.

Sleeping habits influenced family behavior in significant ways. Again, some of these were products of other factors such as inadequate housing and overcrowding. Sleeping in the bedroom with the parents undoubtedly had an effect on the infant's developing personality and emotional needs, which might later result in bed-wetting or temper tantrums, being unable to sleep without a light, or fears and nightmares. These latter may then have created other problems within the family as well as for the child himself. Moving a child out of the parents' bedroom may deprive the family of a living room, or force the conversion of a living room into a dual function room, limiting its usefulness as play or entertainment space. While this solution may improve the sleeping arrangements for the parents, it would still reduce privacy.

Job observations were limited, but the personality pattern behind the selection of employment could often be demonstrated in discussing the job. Dissatisfaction was frequently expressed by civil servants disadvantaged by inflation. Health Insurance Plan enrollment has a high percentage of civil servants so this is important in understanding our patients. The influences that led them to choose civil service, the search for security, a probable effect of the depression on this generation, as well as elements in their own personality, undoubtedly played a part in the reaction to their jobs.[1] But it would be unfair to say that civil servants were the only ones concerned about the rising cost of living. Two interacting elements entered into discussions about almost every aspect of family life — job selection and finances. Even though no team member observed a man at work for the record, the tyranny of the job could be recognized as a powerful motivating influence in family health.[2]

Complications resulting from the difficulties of arranging for the care of children when mothers worked (one-third of our study mothers did) and the modification of family relations under these conditions were frequently elaborated. Even among mothers who didn't work, very few women looked on their function as home-makers with interest or enjoyment. The working mother provided the nurse with the extra problem of helping to make arrangements to secure the children against possible emotional deprivation.

Fathers who had 2 jobs and spent little time with their families also presented special problems. These situations required emphasis on recreational needs in the family with its accompanying relaxation of tension. Where recreational opportunities were limited as a consequence of job requirements of either or both parents, the nurse had to consider what was to be done for children deprived of "family fun." In addition she had to suggest recreational outlets for the man who worked at 2 jobs, or for the working housewife.

Social Workers' Observations

From these interviews came the impressions that influenced much of the philosophy of the Demonstration. In addition to substance for their own evaluations, the social workers' interviews offered information which helped the team in developing attitudes toward the families and toward their jobs. The characteristics of personality demonstrated underlined the impression of critical instability of many families. It was evident that large numbers of adults failed to display the maturity necessary to support the demands of marriage. This immaturity was compounded by indications of sex-role reversal. Many men appeared passive and undependable. Many women appeared more aggressive than their husbands and unable to accept the feminine role. Both husband and wife in many instances gave the impression of being disappointed in their expectations of marriage, and resigned to the disappointment. They professed good sexual adjustment (though little activity), each ascribing lack of sexual interest to

177

the other. It might be said that a good relationship between husband and wife in general betokened a good sexual relationship. If serious sexual difficulties or bitter comments about sex came out in the interviews, one might safely predict a stormy marriage. From the historical pattern of the personalities, it may be inferred that sexual difficulties "express" marital difficulties, rather than cause them.

Information about sexual activity was, as one might expect, more amply provided by some individuals than by others. Answering truthfully or fully relates to one's experience, misconceptions, status feelings, prudery, and the like, or even unconscious vanity; therefore questions on the satisfaction of sexual relations produced contradictory and not always helpful answers. A woman might answer a *direct* question by saying she enjoys sex, achieves satisfaction, and has no complaint; but, in later questions about methods of birth control she might tell quite another story, that the sexual relation is distasteful or that she participates only out of desire to hold her husband.[3]

Other matters created difficulties between husband and wife, naturally, since they had to adjust to personality differences of response to a variety of problems. But in these other areas compromise and mutual role acceptance seemed more frequent. Money rarely seemed to be a source of conflict between husband and wife. One would take over control of the total income, a control the other seemed to relinquish willingly. Joint management of the budget was uncommon. It is a little surprising that the families as a whole showed such good management of income, sound financial status, and ability to plan, save, and carry on in the traditional "American" way. In assessing the curious similarity of the problems in the study families to the problems and conditions observed in "agency families" (families that have recognized their inability to cope with their difficulties and applied to agencies for help) this competence in financial management is an outstanding difference.

Religiosity, another area of potential conflict, did not become so. Of course, religiosity was not easily measurable and we had no measure of devoutness. But it was clear that the home tended to be something of a "united front" in religion, with both parents generally agreed on the kind and degree of religion practiced.[4]

178

Some interesting observations were made of the interaction between family members and the social workers, particularly of the response of family members to the social worker. Ambivalence toward the social worker and her position was often noted. But in some cases the social worker offered an important point of identification for the family with the Demonstration. A Negro family had agreed to participate in the program but never attempted to get any care or arrange for follow-up. Not until a year after they had come on the program did they begin to come to family conferences. The change in attitude became apparent following the initial social service interview with the wife. Later conversations confirmed that the wife found in that interview attitudes in the social worker that dispelled her suspicions and inclined her toward participation for her own sake. Previously, the idea of participation seemed to mean for *our* sake.

There were also those who felt a need but could not bring themselves to ask help directly. Such people would make indirect efforts to establish contact with the social worker, perhaps reaching out in a personal way without disclosing any professional appeal. The approach would be masked as friendship; the social worker would be invited to lunch or holiday greeting cards would be sent. Often such people chose to call the social worker by her first name immediately after the interview, in order to establish a bond so they could ask for help without seeming to ask for *professional* help. The interview offered a link between common problems of family members. In one family, during her social service interview the wife expressed dissatisfaction with her husband's lack of cooperation in matters of child discipline. The husband, in his interview, admitted these differences but stated that they had never discussed the matter. Subsequently the husband participated for the first time in a disciplinary action, to the surprised satisfaction of his wife (and probably of the child too). The social worker's efforts at play therapy with their child, who was having difficulties in school and in his social relationships with other children, was favorably supplemented by this uniting of parental responsibility.

Interestingly enough, the fact that the spouse was seen, although separately, allayed suspicion and was helpful in eliciting information. Neither husband nor wife felt "singled out," and

179

each had an opportunity to present his own argument. The fact that the spouse would be talking about the same situation led to surprising insights on the part of the person interviewed. It was as if it had been a long time, if ever, that he had thought about or looked at what he was doing.

Parental attitudes toward children and their place in the family structure were paradoxical. At the social and religious level, children were "wanted" as evidence of a complete family, but at the same time they were often resented and felt to be a burden. The complex of personal needs and identifications in the parent-child relationship resulted in many parents' concentrating on the symbolic nature of the child to the exclusion of consideration for the individual child. Parents who expressed strong feelings about caring for children, who had joined the Demonstration ostensibly to get something more and better for their children, also abused them and frustrated their psychological growth. This was not caused by ignorance. Most parents were very concerned about child-rearing and had managed to get good, modern information about feeding, toilet-training, and other aspects of child-rearing. They felt the importance of their role as parents so strongly that they were most easily approachable through the children, but this was not enough to change the basic character patterns that determine the individual parent's psychological reactions to his children.

FAMILY VIEWS OF THE DEMONSTRATION

Family reactions to this type of service and observation can best be described in terms of particular family experiences. One family was invited to participate in the Family Health Maintenance Demonstration at just about the time that this family was getting ready to leave the Medical Group because of dissatisfaction with the service. The Demonstration experience suited them admirably and they made substantial but not unusual use of the services during their 4 years on the program. Mrs. Q wrote when the program was terminated: "Everyone on the staff with whom we had any contact has been so wonderfully helpful. Whatever our problem, large or small, medical or not, we were left with the feeling that everyone was personally anxious to help us solve it, or eager to refer us to someone who could. It was indeed a unique experience for people who were not overly happy with the regular HIP Group." This was a middle-income family with a high degree of sensitivity to medical need. They were willing and anxious to make the most of the program. Actually, no serious problem was uncovered, no grave illness found or cured. Theirs was a simple emotional attachment, filling a need for a type of medical care the Demonstration was well equipped to give.

Another family record showed evidence of a very poor relationship between the father and the program. He didn't want to talk to the social worker; he never brought any problems to the doctor and he took his medical care only when he felt he needed it. He came for his annual physical examination and that was the limit of his contact; he didn't want to be involved any further. The rest of the family received an average number of services. Aside from this conspicuous evidence of nonattachment, no evidence of any great good (or harm) to the family came from contact with the program. The family was satisfied — they didn't leave — but the program apparently meant little in their lives.

The records on a third family, family "S" are voluminous. Both mother and father were in constant communication with the nurse and the social worker and leaned upon them heavily. They used the physician's services extensively. Not only medical affairs, but every conceivable kind of family problem was brought in by this family. In this high utilizing family there was no great problem; they soaked up a great deal of available service. Just as there were those who never felt comfortable in its setting and could not use the Demonstration fully, for others this type of medical-care program was ideal.

In some individuals initial hostility to a new idea was never overcome. Mr. H objected to the idea of coming into the Demonstration at the start. He was very reluctant; he didn't try to persuade his wife against it, but *he* wasn't going to participate. When he came for his first examination, he said he didn't like the questions and he didn't want to fill out the Cornell Medical Index. He didn't care for the pediatrician in the Demonstration. He announced that he preferred the more familiar medical-care pattern of the Group. He even put obstacles in the way of his wife's cooperation with the Demonstration. As time went by, he began to accept the idea that his family enjoyed participating in the program and he relaxed and became quite friendly. However, when he developed a back pain of the type for which it is difficult to prescribe therapy that will be promptly ameliorative, he was treated for a few days without too much success. After a conference with the Demonstration physician, he immediately consulted an outside specialist. Thereafter he refused to discuss the diagnosis or treatment with the Demonstration staff. Clearly, the Demonstration was on trial as far as he was concerned. Failure confirmed his skepticism and sent him out of the program.

Dissatisfaction with the Program

Three families dropped out of the Demonstration because of dissatisfaction. In 2 of these the breadwinner had, or was suspected to have, ulcerative colitis. This is not too common a disease and, inasmuch as these were the only cases in the Demonstration, it provides food for thought. There is a good bit of speculation about the character and emotional constitution of ulcerative colitis cases.[5] Could there be something special in the emotional need of an individual with ulcerative colitis of which the Demonstration gave too much, or not enough? Do colitis patients need the opposite of what in the Demonstration satisfies other patients?

In another case dissatisfaction with the program derived from a man's fear of exposure, that is, that his wife would reveal shameful facts about him. This was a particularly hostile family situation in which the husband was very antagonistic to the program and entered it unwillingly, trying to prevent his wife from discussing any problem with the social worker. Eventually he came in himself in order to present what he called "his side." In this family Mr. T was chronically angry with his wife and hateful to her. He had an immature need to be in control and to him his wife's discussion of any problem was defiance. He did everything possible to reduce her to the status of a servant. Their financial situation made him irritably penny-pinching and, when his wife became pregnant, he acted as if this were deliberate spite on her part. In a very angry episode (described to the social worker by Mrs. T, and confirmed sheepishly by Mr. T) he almost murdered her, holding a pillow over her face until she lost her breath before letting up. This man must have hated his wife with real passion. He was ashamed to have this, or any other of his problems or attitudes, discussed.*

Conflict between family members could strain relations between families and the Demonstration. For example, the common conflict between husband and wife as to who was "boss." In conference after conference the note appears that: "The woman dominates the family." In some instances the father felt that any questioning of his authority constituted insupportable defiance or rebellion. In other families in which the father was unable to dominate, his rebellion assumed the form of bullying the children or resisting anything his wife wanted done. Under such conditions, if one spouse favored the Demonstration, the other was apt to be hostile.

When Mrs. N was in the hospital, her husband was unable to make an independent decision about getting the children to a summer camp. He had never driven the car alone. He had to ask her advice about what route to take and where to stay, even though she was just recovering from a serious operation. This husband worked a night shift and did all the housework in the daytime. He washed the dishes, prepared the meals, changed the linen. Mrs. N taught school. Their sex relations might have given valuable information, important to an understanding of their situation, but they were unwilling to give sex information in the interviews. While Mrs. N was a loyal Demonstration supporter, Mr. N considered it "for the women," was skeptical of its objectives, uncooperative, and rarely used the services.

The Demonstration might fall into the family's bad graces for similar intrafamily problems. Team suggestions regarding treatment of children — which sometimes parallels the way in which husbands and wives treat (or mistreat) each other — sometimes led to resentment. One mother, desperate to stop her child from wetting the bed at night, rubbed the child's nose in the wet bed as if he were a puppy. A corollary of this story is that of the teacher

* It will come as no surprise that friction is common in many families, and that the storybook pattern of love, respect, and affection is offset by other storybook patterns of wicked sisters, brothers, mothers, fathers. No doubt this is what led Shaw to observe that the almost universal taboo against incest must be attributed to a hearty natural aversion toward relatives.

in the parochial school who made a child eat some of his vomit in order to stop him from vomiting and wetting himself in school. The child did stop vomiting in school, but a variety of illnesses kept him out of school almost half the following year. When it was suggested to the parents that the child might be transferred to a public school, this was construed as unwarranted interference; the parents indignantly canceled all their appointments, and there was little further contact with the Demonstration.

Family Adaptation to Difficulty

Families did not necessarily react so rigidly, avoiding the Demonstration rather than modifying their pattern. In a family where a remote, disinterested father was grinding down a passive, fearful boy who was having severe difficulties in school, the mother used the team to help her buffer the child against the father. He was sent to bed early so that he wouldn't get into difficulties with his father. Or he got up early and had breakfast with his mother, so that he would get off to school and spend less time in frictional contacts with his father. A good deal of open tension and frustration in another family was avoided by a schedule in which the husband and wife reduced their contacts to a minimum. The woman went to bed before her husband came home (he worked evenings), and got up in the morning before he did, leaving to teach school. Such family functioning which might seem unsatisfactory to an outsider represented a successful adjustment to them.

In the area of sexual behavior, adaptation through avoidance was evident in some families, sometimes providing the clue as to how bad relations were between the parents.[6] For example, the woman just mentioned effectively eliminated any sexual contact with her husband as well as other contacts that might have caused conflict. In some families, the husband and wife did not even share the same room, very often using inadequate housing as an excuse. One would think that if there were too few bedrooms the parents would use the bedroom and the children sleep in the living room, but in one case arrangements were made whereby the mother slept with the female child in the bedroom and the father

184

slept with the male child in the living room. In another instance, the husband slept in the living room while the mother shared the bedroom with the child. The avoidance character of such an arrangement is obvious.

The varieties of adaptation are numerous. It is amazing to what extent men and women will adjust to sexual difficulties, compromising and accepting, without exploding or breaking down because of denial or frustration. One man, well-educated, in a professional job at a fairly low salary, was squeezed by financial need, and burdened with a retarded boy who was spastic and required expensive equipment, a mentally retarded daughter, and a frigid wife. Helpless under these numerous pressures, frustrated, despairing, he found relief from constant tension in masturbation. In discussion he displayed some shame, but pointed out that there was no other realistic sexual outlet. This activity served as an over-all solution by reducing his tension. His adjustment would seem to be necessary and desirable.

Less adequate adaptation could be seen in the families that used the team members as support *against* each other. One man with a responsible community position whose marital problems were obvious and serious, refused all early intervention by the team and tried in many ways to keep his wife from using the team's services. When he eventually got her to stop, *he* began to come and present what he called "his side of the case!" He would make periodic visits, and asked for help in coping with his wife who was resisting his authority. Neither the husband nor the wife really used the help or the information or the services of the program. They used the individual team members as instruments to further their conflict. One would tell tales on the other; one would complain about the other. Another woman took extreme satisfaction in relating the way in which her husband "was dressed down" by a Camp Director and fired from his job because the campers had complained about how strict and unfriendly her husband had been as Head Counselor. This upset the husband very much, but it seemed to give the wife a great deal of satisfaction, and she told the story not once but many times. The team offered some release in these cases simply through their presence as sounding boards. These all can be described as the "adaptive phase" that families used, perhaps unconsciously, in order to prevent break-down that might result from constant friction.

Failure of Adaptation

Where there was no release, or no satisfactory adaptation, members of the family suffered. Even if there were not a complete breakdown, there was evidence of pain or tension. The equilibrium which healthy functioning requires could not be established without the expression of some symptomatology in a family member. In the relationship in which the mother was dominant, for instance, there may have been acceptance of the mother's dominating position, but resistance would leak out. On inspection, the family would be adequate, its members apparently functioning well in their respective roles. There might be a degree of inhibition because the mother was very moral and restrictive, but as far as the neighbors were concerned, this was a "happy" family. True, the little girl did wet the bed. The husband did indicate a rather paranoid resentment about his working situation and was suspicious in his relations with other people. He did spend a lot of time away from home, attempting to advance himself in clubs and church activities, breaking out of the pattern of female dominance. There was no obvious crack in the façade, only the symptoms in father and child revealed unresolved conflict in the family.

Where families had improved from some previous low point, the level of functioning on admission to the Demonstration might be considered comparatively good, and augur well for the future. Yet it would need to be judged, for the present, inadequate adaptation. One woman was considered a psychiatric problem in 1951, long before she came into the Demonstration. By the time we knew her she seemed to be reasonably well adjusted and it was the children who were having problems. There was tremendous psychiatric need on the part of the children so that one might have guessed that there had been some pre-existing problem in the mother, but the mother's problem did not present itself at all while the family was in study.[7]

An abrupt contrast was the family in which, with no pre-existing history of defect or difficulty in a member nor any special

186

reason for decline during the program, there nevertheless was puzzling deterioration. Such a paradox appeared in a family that had migrated to the North some few years before. On initial observation and interview they made an excellent impression. The parents seemed practical, intelligent, friendly people who had a very good relationship with one another and with the children. They were relaxed, easygoing, with a good deal of warmth expressed not only in the initial interview but in the later observations by the team members. They had problems, but they were real ones — financial problems. Mr. W was not earning enough and the family lived in thoroughly inadequate quarters. This did not seem to affect the good family feeling. Mr. W was described as "understanding" and "very warm." Mrs. W was described as "easy" and "relaxed," and it was noted that she handled the problems of the children with "initiative and tact." The Family Conference ended with this note, "The family as a whole seems to be comparatively healthy with very few manifestations of neurotic tension." The W family followed suggestions easily and made every effort to meet the problems of housing, recreation, the children, and eking out further income. When problems appeared that had not come up in the preliminary interviews, Mrs. W had no hesitation in discussing them with the workers. They took the Demonstration seriously; they were attached to the team, brought problems to them, and attempted to follow directions. Yet, by the end of 4 years the family structure was disintegrating. Mrs. W was miserable. Mr. W was thoroughly dissatisfied with what he was doing (he was working at 2 jobs), saw no future for himself, and had lost his desire to make any changes. Husband and wife were blaming each other for the financial difficulties. The children were having troubles in school and at home and a variety of neurotic symptoms had supervened. Is this an example of the evil effects of sophistication? This family, with relatively simple emotional needs, had come from a section of the country where the urban qualities of status and economic advantage did not exist. Over a period of time, did the pressure of living in the social circumstances of a New York neighborhood, with the consequent new demands made upon the parents and the children, result in acute dissatisfaction? Whatever the explanation, it was clearly a failure of adaptation.

187

Team Use Unsought

Lest it be thought that *all* families were in a "needy" state, so to speak, with regard to the Demonstration's activities, a brief review of the O family may be in order. This family, Irish Catholic with 7 children (the seventh born during the program) had problems which they had recognized and accepted before the team had made any diagnosis or recommendation, and which they proceeded to resolve themselves without requesting any help. The mother might be described as authoritarian (she would welcome the description), the father as "passive dependent" (he might resent this while admitting it), and the family's finances could only be called precarious. In addition to a city job Mr. O drove a taxi at night, but his combined earnings were insufficient to provide good housing and all the clothes, as well as the food, for 9 people. Yet neither Mr. nor Mrs. O ever saw fit to ask for help, pleasantly yet firmly declined advice, and managed to meet social, psychological, and personal problems with good sense and reasonable equanimity. The children showed few if any of the neurotic traits prevalent in most of the families. There was no school problem: the 3 school-age children attended parochial school; the oldest boy was a brilliant student, and the second an outstanding student and athlete. The O family was attached to the Demonstration, used the services as needed (such a large family was naturally a high utilizing one), appreciated what was done, but in general drew a clear line between medical services for which they sought team advice and help and personal problems, which they preferred to deal with themselves. An academic discussion of "problems" in this family would have brought out a variety of "needs" — sex education, child-rearing practices, intrafamily attitudes that might have benefited from the team's advice. However, since the adaptation to the realities of the situation were so firm and successful, it certainly appears that team intervention was unnecessary.

So there were situations in which the team's service was necessary and helpful and situations in which though necessary the team's mediation was rejected to the detriment of the family situation. And there were situations in which the family itself had struck an admirable balance and no team activity was necessary.

A lack of depth in the initial interviews sometimes misled the team and cast some doubt on the value of this brief and superficial exposure to a family as a diagnostic tool. Our family folder begins with an initial interview in which the program was explained to the mother (usually). The interviewing worker will have noted some fact about the person: that she was pleasant, had a wide range of interests, or showed fondness and respect for her husband. If the husband was seen he might be described as mild and pleasant. Or, "the child seemed bright, outgoing," or "mother spoke of him with pride," or "he scampered through the house in typical boyish fashion." Such notes will be found under "Intake."

There is an amazing discrepancy between this initial observation and what turns up in later interviews, as the team gets to know other sides of the family or as the family begins to express its feelings, needs, and difficulties. This was not always true, but there does not seem to be consistent correlation between the initial interview impression and the confirmation (or lack of it) of the impression in later interviews.

Further, it cannot be assumed that, because a family made a good initial impression which was later confirmed, it had no problems. Nor would it be possible to say that such a family would respond better when problems developed. In other words, the initial impression was dangerously fallacious in deriving conclusions about family needs, and unproductive as far as calculating program value.

Nor did observations of the home situation permit assumptions concerning school behavior. Often a child in a family with a great deal of tension would presumably need some outlet which one might expect him to find in school. Yet there would be no such evidence whatsoever.[8] That child would be bright and helpful in school, and the teachers would not feel that he was a problem in any sense or suspect that there were difficulties at home. This may well have been true of the work situation also, although since we were unable to get on-the-job views of our families we can't say. It is assumed that a man who has problems at home must carry some of them with him to the office, and that a man with

189

a certain personality trait in dealing with friends or relatives deals accordingly with his coworkers. The school experience gives one pause. Does the home situation carry over directly to the job?

Disease — physical and emotional — is widespread and prevalent in most families. While most of the symptoms do not necessarily come to professional attention, disorder in one family member takes its toll in disturbed family relationships and possibly in triggering disease or difficulty in other family members. The intensive exploration in the Demonstration revealed a great deal more emotional distress in families than is customarily presumed. Within the family, these disturbances affected adults more than children, small families more than larger ones, women more than men.

In reviewing these findings, the puzzling fact stands out that the problems, in type and quantity, uncovered in study families differed not at all from the type and quantity of disturbances found in families that appealed to social agencies for care. Yet, by and large, these Demonstration families were able to "make do," to come to terms with their difficulties, without appealing for outside help. The elusive factor which influences some families to seek help and others not to did not emerge. This "coping" is an important social factor that needs to be teased out and studied in future family investigations.

An extensive section of this chapter was devoted to statements of observations made by the nurse and social worker in their interviews and visits. These observations are unsupported by firm data; they provide sidelights rather than evidence or proof for the conclusions on family patterns. Among these observations appeared the fact that motivation, which is inextricably interrelated with personality, played an important part in altering behavior with regard to nutrition, home management, and housing. While this is almost self-evident, it is important to reiterate because health promotion programs like ours must deal more with personality attitudes and less with general philosophy. Also, the fact that many men held more than one job and many mothers worked created special problems for the children and for themselves. Broader community programs are therefore necessary for the family in recreation and education. Social-work observations into personality and personal relations brought family problems into sharper focus. The failure of many adults to accept mature roles, basic sexual difficulties, and personality conflicts distorted family relations and interfered with wholesome child care. Money and religion did not appear to be sources of conflict. And the opportunity for professional discussion of interpersonal problems between husband and wife, not overtly welcomed, was accepted and used in many instances as an opportunity to come to terms with each other.

The family patterns of acceptance and use of Demonstration services have been discussed as aspects of family interaction. Response was a sum of family attitudes, needs, and social pressures. Some families could adapt easily to this new technique of service; others could not or would not. The adaptive mechanism was not measurable by our criteria, but in many instances adaptation was evident and therefore possible. While our interviews and evaluations did not offer suitable prognostic information, they provided useful guides for working with the families, personality profiles, and areas of strength and weakness. We may be a long way from a quick test for "coping" or index of adaptation, but we have helpful indicators of the path to follow.

- XI -

PREVENTIVE MEDICINE AND
HEALTH PROMOTION

Satius est initius mederi quam fini.

— Erasmus, *Adagia*

There is such a sensible ring to the word "prevention," that to question any of the procedures sanctified as preventive must seem irrational or perverse. This is particularly true in a health program initiated with the primary purpose of introducing preventive techniques into daily medical practice. Yet many of the assumed preventive measures have been based on "common sense." Measures instituted to prevent disease altogether, if successful, are their own justification. Immunization programs, chlorination and fluoridation of water are in this category. Sometimes, too, one disease is used to prevent another — as cowpox (vaccinia) is used to prevent smallpox, or other living vaccines now in laboratory or prospective use are used, because the disease given is mild, preventing a serious, often fatal, one.

It is also reasonable to assume that to find disease early, before it can do maximum damage, is a laudable endeavor. Furthermore, early diagnosis and treatment may reduce the duration of disability and ensure prompt recovery.[1] Now the theoretical techniques for early case finding are not so easily susceptible of proof of efficacy as are the measures for forestalling disease altogether. As a consequence, a religious reverence for certain preventive procedures has grown up, so that they are treated as if they were effective, although the evidence of their effectiveness has yet to be developed.

192

Because of the nature of the Demonstration activity, with its emphasis on preventive and health promotional techniques, we were able to examine some of these techniques and reach some conclusions as to their effectiveness.

We planned a comprehensive program of prevention in the Demonstration. The commonly accepted primary measures such as vaccination and immunization against diphtheria, whooping cough, and tetanus were included. In addition, prevention was to be carried out through an annual physical examination, emotional support where family structure was considered suspiciously weakened, and general health education.[2]

Presumably, the very existence of a health team would encourage the early use of its members for problems and difficulties, and therefore act as a preventive measure. By indirectly offering a psychiatrist's services, the prevention of emotional problems was to be facilitated.

While we were able to show that the study families benefited physically from the Demonstration, the particular role that the annual physical examination and health education played in this improvement deserve consideration. And since we were not able to show benefit in the emotional area, the role of our emotional support and preventive measures in this area certainly require analysis.

PERIODIC EXAMINATIONS

To those devoted to the theoretical concept of prevention the annual physical examination is pretty much an element of dogma. In this theory the annual examination makes treatment easier and reduces the long-range effects of illness through early case finding. Often the annual examination is extended in meaning to include any periodic examination, or even any single extensive examination, performed on well persons, without symptoms of illness, all of which are customarily combined and considered "preventive examinations." It is important to separate these concepts, because they have different preventive value and different yields in cases found as well as different costs to the individual and the community. The single extensive examination, in which the individual has had no previous careful study may yield many new

193

cases, while an examination done on this group of patients shortly afterward will reveal far fewer unsuspected diseases.

Statistical analyses of periodic examinations usually list the proportion of new and previously unknown cases discovered.[3] The presumption is that these cases represent positive prevention because, if the condition had continued until brought to the doctor's attention by symptoms, its course would have been worse. It is difficult to test the accuracy of this assumption. Perhaps an analysis of cancer-survival rates of those in whom the disease was discovered during a periodic examination compared with cancer-survival rates of those treated only after symptoms appeared would be helpful. Unfortunately, the routine of periodic examination is fairly rare, and in general patients who come for a periodic examination are not symptom-free, but usually have complaints of one sort or another. This means that, even if there were a balance of survival in favor of those who had the periodic examination, it would be offset by the possibility of very early symptomatic cases being included in that category. The statistics of survival from breast cancer in the "early diagnosis" categories[4] as offered by McKinnon are not very reassuring, either.

It is very difficult, therefore, to establish the contention that the detection mechanism of an extensive examination of well people, whether on a single basis or routinely, is an effective preventive measure. One, there is no evidence that the individuals were asymptomatic; two, there is no evidence the finding of the disease (cancer, in the instance mentioned) resulted in longer life for those in whom it was found. It seems equally logical to assume that in some cases of cancer, metastasis begins with the onset of the disease and before any symptom or sign, confuting the possibility of prevention through examination while well.

Early Diagnosis and Prompt Treatment

The value of early diagnosis by means of routine examination is questioned by many physicians. Increasingly, practitioners recall the case of cancer discovered inadvertently, which although asymptomatic is already metastatic. Among the Demonstration families there was a young mother with a family history of multiple intestinal polyposis. (Her sister had died of cancer of the rectum at a young age.) This young mother was justifiably concerned about the possibility of developing cancer of the rectum. From the start of the program she was studied exhaustively.

A barium enema and sigmoidoscopy were done periodically, but there was never evidence of anything amiss in the intestinal tract. Two years after she left the program she had some slight bleeding from the rectum. She was examined, studied, and operated on within a matter of weeks. Cancer was found. She had a resection of the colon, but a year and a half later she was dead of metastases. How frequently, how carefully, how meticulously does the routine preventive examination have to be carried out to be effective? In this case there was a clear warning and special precautions were taken, but despite this the woman was doomed.

Another woman had a careful physical examination in early spring. No lumps were noted in her breast. In June of the same year she began to have symptoms (a lump in her breast) and underwent a mastectomy. There were no metastases (as of this writing it is 4 years), and she has made an uneventful recovery. This patient's treatment was initiated on the basis of her own awareness of trouble, not the preventive examination. Because some cancers may begin without symptoms, metastasizing early, while others may be symptomatic early, metastasizing late, the modest or thoughtful surgeon praises the circumstances and not his skill nor "early diagnosis." A woman who had postponed her January annual physical examination, noticed a lump in her breast in February and came to the doctor in March. She was operated within 5 days of the time she presented herself to the physician, yet she died of carcinoma within a year. Each of these cases underlines the failure of preventive measures as typified in the routine examination.

As for other diseases, we may be even more helpless in the pursuit of prevention through early diagnosis, than in cancer. The one patient who died of acute coronary occlusion while on the program had no presages that would have led one to predict the possibility of a heart attack. He wasn't fat, he wasn't a busy executive, his serum cholesterol was a normal 196 mgm., and he took his annual physical examination promptly. Or consider Mr. T, a steady, hard-working man, considered somewhat passive in our initial interview, but "warm" and a "good parent" (in fact, the better of the two). His childhood had been austere but happy, and the marital relation was apparently sound. Mr. T had left school in the seventh grade and was thought to be a bit retarded mentally, but he held a job and supported his family. He was not overtly disturbed and there was nothing in the psychological tests or interviews that predicted disturbance. Yet this man had a schizophrenic break after 3 years on the program and was hospitalized for years.

Norbert Roberts shows that for individuals who have not had a previous preventive examination, an initial physical examination is reasonably productive.[5] He also notes that as people grow older, re-examinations may be fairly productive too. In his report, 45 percent of 147 carcinomas discovered in 6754 individuals over the age of 45 were found at the time of re-examination during a 6½-year period rather than at the time of initial examination. As far as case finding of other disease is concerned, Roberts reports results similar to ours, in the *initial* examination. He concludes with (ages not given and completeness of examination not indicated) a distribution of cases in which about half have some type of illness that required looking after. This tells us nothing about those who went through the screen and what happened to them thereafter. Let us concede that a thorough examination at some time will find disease the patient knew nothing of. What of those in whom nothing was found at that time? Did they come down soon after with an unsuspected serious illness? And does periodic re-examination prevent this?

Repeated Routine Examinations

From our experience with repeated *annual* examinations, it is difficult to go along with the proponents. In fairness it should be added that the size of the Family Health Maintenance Demonstration program was a limiting factor in assessing results. Since there were less than 300 adults in the study group, the expectancy of significant new disease in any year was sharply reduced. This expectancy was still more reduced by the fact that no parent over 45 was admitted to the program.[6] In Table 31 it was seen that very little more in the way of new *major* illness was found in the study than in the control groups. Table 63 refines the data on the basis of all new disease found on annual examination.

Table 63. Number of new conditions (medical diagnoses) discovered per 100 family members on routine examination only.

Follow-up year	Type of condition	Study	Control
First	Major	9	2
	Minor	106	21
Fourth	Major	2	2
	Minor	36	26
4-year annual average	Major	4	2
	Minor	59	17

A much larger number of medical diagnoses was discovered in families participating in the study than among control families. The annual average rate for study families was more than three times as high as for control families. However, in both groups, more than 90 percent of these conditions were classified as "minor," so that the difference of 2 more cases of major illness discovered in that period in the study families is hardly significant. There was a consistent decline for both major and minor conditions in all new cases subsequently found in the study families. The increase in new diagnoses in the control families in the last year is an artifact produced by the examination of the control group in that year by the team. In Table 32 this effect is clearly indicated by the ratio of study to control diagnoses, in both major and minor conditions, and in routine (annual) examination versus nonroutine — the examination performed when the patient presented himself with symptoms. From this table it appears that the most productive source of new diagnoses for study families was the initial examination. In succeeding years, the presentation of a patient with symptoms was equally or more useful in case finding. For the control families, on the other hand, routine and nonroutine examinations were equally productive because the baseline examination had not been done.

Annual physical examinations after a single thorough examination were clearly unnecessary. The yearly Papanicolaou examination of vaginal secretions was not helpful, and the cholesterol levels bore no significant relation to high blood pressure, coronary disease, or other heart involvement. Not only were new findings meager after the first year, but the new disease that did occur was not necessarily found in the preventive examination.[7] A baseline examination may very well be a useful device, but exhaustive thorough examinations at frequent intervals cannot be said to be equally useful. Perhaps less thorough, less frequent examinations at regular intervals, aimed at specific disease finding, particularly in older females may be desirable, even though we may not yet know the components of the examination nor the appropriate intervals.

Examinations of what population groups, at what intervals, and with what tests are questions which require careful future investigation. Undoubtedly the procedure and frequency must vary with the age of the patient (for example, glaucoma examinations in those over 40) since certain diseases are more prevalent at different ages. The critical periods of life — adolescence and menopause — might be appropriate periods for a thorough overhaul. Annual re-examination using a fixed set of tests appears to be useless and wasteful. Since the control families did not suffer significantly more or graver illness, that found in the study families through the routine examination probably would have been discovered anyhow.

Symptoms and Prompt Examination

It appears that people may be aware of minor difficulties, but do not (even in a prepaid system) bother going to a physician for diagnosis or treatment. This is indicated by the high number of minor illnesses found in study families. They are relatively unconcerned about minor illness unless there is acute distress or chronic discomfort.[8] The team relationship apparently encouraged study families to obtain care for minor complaints that would otherwise have gone unnoted.

The corollary may be that in a prepaid system the ease of access to medical care can make prevention a function of *symptomatology* rather than of routine examination. Since neither cost nor any other barrier keeps the patient from the doctor, he may well report at the beginning of symptoms or change of accustomed signs. The role of the preventive program is to educate patients to an understanding of symptoms and recognition of those early symptoms for which a physician should be consulted.

In brief, the team activity and continuous observation appear to be as effective preventive measures as the routine examination

— maybe even more so. It might be valuable to institute a routine examination at appropriate intervals in order to *reinforce* continuous observation. Since it is the continuous observation which is of value, however, rather than the routine examination itself, a physician who knows the patient and his previous condition is of great importance.[9] The contribution of the Family Health Maintenance Demonstration to prevention was the team's availability and the meticulously recorded symptoms rather than its annual examinations.[10]

The Routine Health Conference

From the lesson learned in well-baby conferences, the principle of a "well-person conference" ought to be adopted, so as to provide the clues a physician or paramedical worker will need to take preventive action on a patient's behalf. Based on a health-team relation, this type of conference is a reasonable substitute for the routine examination and incorporates the best of both systems. The routine health conference has other values. It was perhaps the single most useful device employed by the Demonstration. In recommending the team conference with the family as a routine, many of the Demonstration's family conferences may be recalled, with the fascinating insights and unexpected effects they provided. It was pointed out to one father at such a conference that he was too much driven by his job, paid too little attention to his family, and needed to be more relaxed. He angrily denied the statements and implications. But following the conference, he bought a car. He acted on the implicit acceptance of the charge that he should share his time with the family and develop family recreation activities. He bought a car; another gave up a mistress; a third changed his job. Children went to camp or different schools, or psychotherapy was accepted. All these things might have occurred anyway. But they occurred after a discussion of factors that bore upon the changed situation.

Like continuous observation, the routine well-person conference is possible only in a prepayment setting and practicable only with the health team. A careful physical examination or a follow-up psychiatric consultation may be its natural developments. The routine health conference is far more useful than the routine physical examination — and more efficient and economical.

EMOTIONAL SUPPORT AS A PREVENTIVE ROLE

One of the disappointments of the Demonstration was its apparent ineffectiveness, or at least failure to demonstrate effectiveness, of prevention in the area of emotional disturbance. Theoretically, the social worker should have taken the lead. She worked with the physician and nurse in daily team practice so there was an occasion for mutual influences, but she was expected to offer social-work activity in the preventive context. The contradiction in this role is obvious. Social work, carried on through hospitals or agencies, is concerned with problems that exist in the client's knowledge. The social worker is oriented either to the function of the agency or to disease in the client. To reorient social work toward a preventive role, the social worker, on the basis of her experience and knowledge, would have to identify symptoms or behavior patterns that portended future disease or reflected present pathology. The team could then make an effort to inform the family of the presence of these problems and treat them by supporting the strengths and working to eliminate the weaknesses in the family structure. Hopefully, breakdown would be averted and the calamity foretold by the social worker's experience prevented.

In carrying out these team roles, however, the traditional role of the particular profession had to be enlarged. For the nurse, this was of no consequence, since her traditional role includes prevention. But the social worker, like the doctor, saw herself in a preventive role only conditionally. If everyone suffers from some degree of sickness, it is difficult to engage in "preventive" activities. This is mentioned to balance the picture of "role failure" against realities. The Demonstration, while modifying professional role concepts to some degree, could not alter them completely, possibly because the experimental team operated in a real world where other professionals were not changing one whit. Total commitment to prevention would have had something of the effect of abandonment of career. For the social worker particularly, the attempt to establish a preventive role was unrealistic, not only because of the difficulties she had in seeing herself in such a role but because the clients certainly could not see her that way.

It was difficult for the social worker to create a preventive role because the families too were unwilling to accept this kind of prevention. It is not hard to understand (this is not to condone) the families' reluctance to embrace prevention in the emotional area. In general in the United States families do not consider emotional difficulties "medical" conditions. Demonstration families understood the program as a step to better *physical* health, but they were unable to extend the formulation to include emotional difficulties, particularly ones of which they were not aware. As a consequence, the social worker was relegated by patients to a nonmedical role on the team. In an earlier chapter we saw that the social worker was looked upon with some degree of suspicion and hostility and this undermined the preventive role further. Failure of acceptance — like failing to keep appointments, for example — made prevention impossible. This also led to a narrowing of the social worker's role, so that she was restricted to dealing only with disturbances that the families *did* recognize and *did* accept. She was unable to reach people whose difficulties were in a relatively unorganized stage, where they might be dealt with in simpler fashion. Perhaps the social worker's experience, insights, and knowledge, coupled with the observations of symptomatology in these "normal" families, did help the other professional workers to do their own jobs better. In that sense only the social worker might be considered to have contributed a preventive function.

Other explanations of this apparent failure of prevention are possible, too. We may have given insufficient weight to the "self-healing" quality or overestimated the likelihood and degree of deterioration to be expected. The strengths in most families are such that, regardless of symptoms, deterioration to the point of seeking help does not occur anyway. We have noted the curious similarity of study families to families that are socially "sick" (who use agencies or psychiatrists). The difference may be not in diagnosis but in the family's conception of sickness. It is true that there was no less symptomatology in the study families at the end, and perhaps less evident symptomatology in the controls, with whom we had not had 4 years of probing for symptoms. Our inability to demonstrate prevention in the emotional area may not be failure to influence the emotional health of the fami-

201

lies favorably, but simply further evidence that a multiplicity of symptoms is not synonymous with sickness.

HEALTH-PROMOTION ACTIVITY

While health promotion was an integral part of what we hoped each of the team members would do in individual conferences and office sessions, we also carved out an original area of group activity for the families labeled "health promotion." The philosophy of health education in this connection gave rise to a great deal of discussion. Since we were trying to get people to do what we considered right for them to do, the question of judgment (how do we know our "right" is "right" for them?) and ethics (isn't "motivation" really synonymous with "manipulation"?) were debated constantly. The Demonstration never resolved these questions but carried on the educational activities in a common understanding. Our consensus was that "right" constituted that goal of healthy functioning which was the common goal of the Demonstration, and achieving it meant pointing the families toward health practices which in our present state of knowledge embodied this goal. It meant deciding that child-rearing should be "sensible," neither too authoritarian nor too permissive. It meant helping individual families to accept and deal with their own problems on their own terms, since no dogmatic or inflexible rule of family conduct exists. Families had doubts and fears about what they were doing and how they handled problems, so we felt that the function of our health education program was more to help them examine themselves, measure their actions against the behavior of others as well as the pronouncements of authority, and modify their own activity only as the result of their own recognition of need for change.

Motivation

The key to action is motivation, and this was visualized as a process in which the family members who attended meetings had to share. Group discussion had to mean more than simply discussion in a group, as there is a qualitative difference between a meeting in which an expert tells something and one in which the group finds out something.[11] The quality of the discussion leader is vital. Dr. Shapiro,* our health educator consultant, had enormous zest for his job and was able to establish excellent relationships with the team and with the family members in the discussion groups. In his demonstration of how a group meeting should be conducted he briefed the team frequently, and made tape recordings of the meetings which he later played back at seminars for critical discussion. The instructions he provided as a basis for the orientation of the team members in leading discussions are in the Appendix. The training and orientation of team members to keep in mind this motivational concept of "sharing" with discussion members was relatively easy. All may not have agreed on concept, but they could agree on the approach and follow through. They could offer opportunities for learning (giving information), and allow airing of opinions.

Shapiro's conception of teaching — motivation in the sense used here — was to "build a climate of learning." [12] As examples of group meetings that point up both the philosophy and the method the following brief account of a series is presented. "Discipline, Authority and the Family," was the general topic of one series. A pamphlet was distributed [13] and discussion centered around the point that families are different: some may be autocratic, others democratic. It was emphasized that democratic families tend to have happier children than autocratic families. An autocratic family doesn't always mean one in which the parents are autocratic (deciding everything for the children); sometimes the children dominate. In such a family the entire household revolves around children and the parents do everything possible to make life pleasant for them. So the idea emerged in discussion that a democratic family is one in which everyone shares in the decisions. From this the idea followed that self-centered existence is not good for children or for adults. Everybody should feel that others expect something of him. As a consequence, choices must be made and it is important to do things right.

From group responsibility (the nucleus of that discussion) the

* Irving Shapiro, Ed.D., now Director, Health Education Division, the Health Insurance Plan of Greater New York.

participants went on to discuss discipline. Discipline was seen within the frame of self-set standards, not other people's standards. Rewards (or punishment!) cannot be substituted for self-direction. Discipline was presented as the *opportunity* for choice and decision. The emphasis on democracy hinged on the fact that the parents, with greater experience, may be considered senior partners who must carry more weight in decision making.

A few large group meetings were held. One was on the topic of "A Healthy Personality For Your Child." [14] The first meeting was held in the evening. A film, "Family Circles," was shown and discussed to elicit the particular areas of interest of those who attended. As part of the discussion, various means by which understanding could be aided were illustrated: movies, puppets, panels, role playing, and so forth. The pamphlet was distributed and used as background for succeeding meetings. It was never read aloud, but was left as basic material for each participant to read, and to serve as an outline from which the parents could take their cue to ask further questions or introduce their own problems or ideas. This group met 6 times. A "meeting reaction" sheet was filled in by participants and team members, and the value to the individual assessed. All the meetings were recorded and discussed afterward with the team.

The content of the program did not include only emotional and family problems. Social factors relating to good medical care were also discussed: the need for legislation to protect working mothers so as to protect children and the family endangered by such a separation; the need for good teachers and good schools to support the home's efforts to produce sound and sturdy citizens; job protection; good housing and good neighborhoods to oppose the social tension that might disrupt family health. Obviously these were matters the Demonstration could not *do,* itself, but equally obviously these were matters the Demonstration could teach and clarify. Since "medical care" is only an aspect of health (as it is of life!), health education had to range widely. And the health education meetings and conferences were intended to support the team's teachings on growth and development, on problems of transition from infancy to school life or from puberty to adolescence, and on sex and family health.

Small Group Meetings

In the words of the health education consultant, the group meetings were designed to "enhance the learning value of the Family Health Maintenance Demonstration experience." In the process, the team members were to learn more about the families and so be able to help them better. Although the value of these meetings can be judged only within the frame of the whole health promotional activity, analysis of the meetings may offer some worthwhile clues as to the value of this process, independent of the success of the program as a whole.[15]

If the majority of the study families had frequent contact with each other and with team members in group meetings, the meetings must be considered to have offered an important educational opportunity. Few families participating, and infrequent attendance must be considered evidence of a lesser role for group meetings in assessing the health promotion activity. In the latter case, even if attitudes or behavior changed, the changes may have been due to factors other than group educational meetings.

Degree of Participation. Looked at in terms of any participation at all, the group educational meeting was a technique successfully applied. From the standpoint of numbers of meetings held, of team-member involvement, of approach to well people, and of content, the educational program was carried off as planned. However, examined from the standpoint of numbers of people involved consistently, who attended regularly and could be assumed to have obtained good "exposure" to the educational material, the program was less successful. Merely to have touched 94 people casually cannot be said to be health education, and even to have provided a regular program for a dozen people can hardly be described as an important health-promotion technique (see Table 64). Considering 1954 and 1955 representative, only 17 families participated in both years. If the meetings are examined in terms of topic and discussion leader, we see that attendance was sporadic, too, and there was considerable variation from group to group. For the social worker's play-therapy group there was 100 percent attendance at one meeting, but the average attendance of the 12 families invited was 5 in 1954, when 15 meet-

205

Table 64. Study-family attendance at small group meetings by topic of meeting, and staff member leading, 1954 and 1955.

Year	Staff member	Topic	Number of meetings	Number invited	Attending one or more meetings		Average attendance per meeting
					Number	Percent of invited	
1954	Social worker	Play therapy	15	12	12	100	5
	Family physician	Teen-age	16	20	12	60	6
	Public health nurse	Adult obese	14	25	10	40	5
	Public health nurse	Parents of pre-school children	8	82	12	15	6
	Public health nurse	Parents of school-age children	5	96	24	25	13
	Health educator	Parent-child relations	12	98	24	25	12
1955	Social worker	Play therapy	6	13	7	54	6
	Family physician	Teen-age	10	34	23	68	7
	Public health nurse	Adult obese	6	14	7	50	3
	Public health nurse	Parents of pre-school children	12	34	16	47	6

ings were held. In 1955, mean attendance was 6. The family physician held 16 meetings with the teenagers in 1954, 10 in 1955; average attendance was 6 in 1954, 7 in 1955.

The public health nurse held 3 different types of meetings: an adult obesity group, one for parents of pre-schoolers, and another of parents of school-age children. The percentage attending of those invited varied, but the average attendance was never more than 13. For the health educator's meetings in 1954, average attendance was 12.

The limited and rather selective attendance was the subject of constant discussion among team members and consultants. The topic of group meetings was on the agenda of numerous staff conferences. The attendance figures were compared with other indices (illness, utilization) in an effort to visualize the effects of attendance, but the correlations were inconclusive, principally because of the small numbers. It was pointed out by the health educator that the range of recommended group size for educational discussion purposes is from 6 to 20 people, and frequency of attendance 3 or more meetings, to be beneficial. From this standpoint, our group experience is ideal. Furthermore, it might be underlined here that the function of health education was not restricted to meetings, but permeated all the Demonstration activities. Health education was a "total push." Therefore, while only a few people may have been reached by the group meeting method, a large number was reached at least once, and at some time or other almost every individual was exposed to one or another of the health educational activities. Many health educators do feel even a few contacts may have important effects.[16]

Attendance and Utilization. The use of medical services in general was not correlated with attendance at meetings, nor was greater or lesser use of the social worker or nurse connected with attendance. Even where there seems to be some correlation between "sickness" (as evidenced by Cornell Medical Index "yeses" and the social worker's evaluation) and attendance, the numbers are too small to allow conclusions to be drawn. One might say that there was more in the way of symptoms in the attending group, more concern with the process of illness, even though there may not have been more actual illness or more use of service. In that sense the group meetings were selective; people who came needed to come or, better, recognized the need to come. On the other hand, there was a feeling on the part of the team members that the people they saw at meetings were the same people they saw in the office a great deal, and so the meetings represented duplication of effort. This was only partially true in that group meeting attenders were generally not *poor* utilizers of service, so that they would be "familiar faces." But they did not seem to represent the high utilizing families either.

Reasons for Nonparticipation. Speculating on the reasons for low attendance at meetings, it was agreed that New Yorkers are sophisticated, and have many meetings on these same topics at P.T.A., school, or church. New Yorkers have a multitude of entertainment available, possibly more stimulating and attractive than health education — and there is always TV. Baby-sitters are expensive and hard to find; and, if one parent can't go to a meeting, the other is reluctant to attend. Finally, "moonlighting" is a growing problem; the two-job father (or working mother) may make it impossible for either to attend a meeting; or, if both parents worked during the day, the evening was necessary for family life.

One parent holding 2 jobs, or both parents working, has become an increasingly important factor in American family life. In about three-fifths of our families (see Table 65), in addition to

Table 65. Number of study families[a] in which parents had extra jobs by type of situation.

Duration	Job situation	Number
Whole of demonstration	Father, 2 jobs; mother not working	6
	Father, 1 job; mother working	22
	Father, 2 jobs; mother working	1
	Total	29
Part of demonstration	Father, 2 jobs; mother not working	15
	Father, 1 job; mother working	16
	Father, 2 jobs; mother working	16
	Total	47

[a] 124 families.

the job of the breadwinner, another job was held by one of the parents. For almost a quarter of the families this "extra" job lasted throughout the entire period. In most of these families the "extra" job was held by the mother. In 1 family the mother worked *and* the father held 2 jobs, while in 6 families the father held 2 jobs all through the Demonstration. However, where the "extra" job lasted only a part of the period of Demonstration observation, the 3 conditions — mother working, father with 2 jobs, or both, appeared as a factor in an equal number of families.

Undoubtedly many things were responsible for the consistently small attendance at group meetings. Within the team there was some resistance to organizing group meetings. It meant extra evening work, new and unfamiliar forms of professional relationships, new administrative responsibilities, all of which may have reduced the effective leadership in group activity.

In general the success of the meetings lay in giving support to the participants. The mothers who came to sessions with the nurse, the children who attended play hours with the social worker, or the adolescents who met with the doctor, all gained something or they wouldn't have come. Less clear is the reason for the continuation of the obesity group in the face of very discouraging results. Its members could see that they weren't losing weight — or even gaining — but although attendance was spotty some continued to come.[17]

The response of the people who *did* attend gives an impression that all previous considerations of the reasons for the lack of widespread success and mass attendance are insufficient. The meetings were rewarding for those who attended. Extracts from a report of the team consultant in health education indicate the enthusiasm and interest of the participants:

A summary by one team member stated: "The parents expressed appreciation and interest . . . some had tried suggestions offered and others demonstrated a change from giving the answers with authority to a more objective listening and sharing of ideas."

In written comments, both after each meeting and following the series, parents said — "I liked the 'frankness and friendliness' and the discussion of the problems of our own children." "I enjoyed the informality . . . and the close relationship between the parents." "There's always a new idea — this is related to 'my feelings toward enjoying people.'" "The 'open discussion' made problems seem less difficult." "I felt more one with the other parents." The parents carried their group experience over into personal conferences, and even into family conferences.

Another commented: "The parents brought out verbally and in written comments that they liked being with people who have an understanding of their problems, and that they couldn't find such a group 'outside.' It was evident that those who attended received a good deal from the experience. But at the start the sole focus of the discussion was on calories and diet. But as the meetings progressed the members began to think in other terms. There was some recognition of the relation of tension to overeating, and in some instances an awareness of what caused tenseness. The importance of outside-the-family interests for one member was revealed and underscored by the group. Another parent said that the discussion at least had kept her weight steady. Still another had been negative and flip at the start, but altered her attitude as time went on, and lost six pounds. There was recognition of the need to lose weight for the sake of health, yet appearance loomed larger as a motivation."

A third team member described her group: "Despite the gross inadequacy of the meeting room, the lack of appropriate materials, marked success was achieved. The children expressed intense desire to continue to attend, and were enabled to express themselves freely. The reactions of parents to the experiences their children were having, and to consequent behavior changes, were revealing to the leader."

The teen-age group leader stated that parents reported "success" based upon the children's behavior at home. In the group, itself, he said, he observed improved attitudes and behavior.

Several team members stated that they got additional information and new insights into family members and their lives. They also reported more confidence in themselves as discussion leaders, increasing feelings of comfort in being with the group, and improvements in their skills of leadership.

It would seem that family members do derive benefit and can learn at such meetings. In a special study of attitudes of those who attended a series of meetings, there was indication of modification of ideas and behavior.[18]

Weakness of Individual Family Approach

As it is difficult to practice prevention in the absence of awareness on the part of the patient, it may not be possible to involve the family in a preventive regimen before there is awareness of symptoms. Two thoughts occur. In one, an analogy to public health, purification of water comes to mind — chlorination of water versus typhoid immunization. In both instances typhoid fever can be prevented. But the mass preventive mechanism of chlorination is certainly more economical and certain. To carry the analogy back to health education, we assume family difficulties have an influence on the healthy development of the children in the family; and so we want to modify family relations by supporting elements that strengthen the healthy emotional development of the children, at the same time repressing unhealthy elements. Our approach to individual families, to form educational groups, was a type of individual "immunization." The resistance spoken of earlier, arising from lack of awareness of need, would increase the certainty that the individual family approach would be relatively ineffective. Add to this the unwillingness of most families to recognize emotional problems as having medical relevance and it would seem that individual immunization techniques in influencing families in the emotional area were fated to be unsuccessful.

Family Health Education in a Social Context

Mass prevention involves treating a whole community. This we did not attempt. And as a matter of fact, we had set up our program so as to make this impossible. The Family Health Maintenance Demonstration families were not selected as neighbors or from parochial units, but as a random sample of the Medical Group population.

It seems logical to think that health education and the group-meeting procedure ran into difficulties because family selection for the Demonstration was not designed to select families who had a common basis for action of *any* kind. We know that neighborhood groups select opinion leaders for different values, such as fashion, school, politics, and presumably medical care. Our families had no community relationship with each other and did not depend on one another for guidance or leadership or diffusion of ideas. The influence structure and community power network that determines use of a community service like the Demonstration could not be tapped.[19] We were not in a position to influence the "medical opinion leader" who would accept our health education program and bring the others into this pattern. Attendance at group meetings was unstructured and probably restricted to those who in other circumstances may have been the leadership people, but leaders whose natural followers were outside the

211

Demonstration. Or those who attended may have been "isolates," outside the community influence structure altogether. Health education could not be effectively utilized as a mass prophylaxis effort for these compelling reasons.

The team structure of the Family Health Maintenance Demonstration provided a vehicle for the introduction of a comprehensive preventive service. The value of prevention is unquestioned, but the value of this particular preventive service was doubtful for 3 reasons. First, after a baseline physical examination frequent periodic examinations were not very productive. Second, emotional support was not particularly effective partly because the social worker's preventive role could not be realized. And third, the group-meeting part of the health education program did not attract a high percentage of the families nor involve them frequently.

Reviewing the prevention and health-promotion activities of the Demonstration, 2 very sharply defined conclusions of interest to future designers of Demonstrations stand out. First, the team-conference technique should be substituted for routine examinations; and second, the selection of Demonstration families should take into consideration the neighborhood influence structure. These relatively simple steps will spare a great deal of unnecessary and unrewarding medical work and still offer comprehensive preventive service.

-XII-

FAMILY HEALTH MAINTENANCE

The conceptions I have summarized here I first put forward only tentatively, but in the course of time they have won such a hold over me that I can no longer think in any other way.

— Sigmund Freud, *Civilization and Its Discontents*

Medicine's obligation to heal and allay suffering transcends its laboratory aspects. A format for medical practice that fosters this healing aspect is professionally important and socially desirable.

THE IDEAL MEDICAL SERVICE

The growing complexity of medical knowledge and the expense of medical care has impressed upon most thoughtful observers the necessity for a more efficient and carefully structured type of medical practice — namely, group practice with prepayment. A family-oriented health team introduced into group medical practice will help carry out the social function of medicine along with the scientific, creating a family medical service.

The team developed in the Demonstration was composed of a *physician*, a specialist in internal medicine (aided by a specialist in pediatrics), a *public health nurse*, and a *social worker*, who essayed this type of practice for 8 years. During that time nearly 150 families were given the unique experience of obtaining medical care in this new way, each family for a 4-year period. In addition to medical care, special attention to preventive factors, emotional support, and guidance was given. Information was collected to attempt to measure the effectiveness of the program.

213

The Health Team

The Demonstration team was satisfactory to patients because it fulfilled the ideal of medical service. The study families were interested in and liked this team operation; therefore they developed a feeling of confidence in this service. However, though the families appreciated the team as an advisory family counseling service, they continued to consider the pivotal service that of the physician. Since all the case-work and preventive activities could not be provided by the physician alone, other members of the health professions were necessary and justified the team structure to the patients. But to the patients the doctor represented medicine; the others were "helpers."

The confidence and satisfaction engendered by the team operation has to be recognized as a real instrumentality of medical service. The act of payment is said to be a significant aid to the patient in accepting treatment.[1] As prepayment plans spread, the removal of this significant ritual act of payment may interfere with acceptance of the new plans. This particular barrier may be overcome by the establishment of a strong team-patient relationship, which could substitute mutual regard for the exchange of money.

Teamwork provided a unique pattern of service which altered the growing trend toward use of specialized medical service. The team operation made some kinds of medical care unnecessary. While it may have increased the medical service obtained at the team level over what a family doctor gave in the control situation, it reduced the amount of service that the more narrowly trained, expensively equipped, medical specialist customarily gave. As with the other points made, this argument for the value of the health team is independent of considerations of measurable benefit in health.

I have said nothing about cost or the practicability of transferring the Family Health Maintenance Demonstration into wider application. This is partly because, in the mixture of research and service activity the precise dimension and cost of the service aspects of the program cannot be completely distinguished from those of research. Too, it is recognition of the inutility of offering a specific number of dollars as a base for a service, when the inflation to which we have been subjected in the past 10 years mocks the effort. Since the program began, there were 2 premium increases for HIP subscribers, several increases in Blue Cross subscription cost and sizable percentage increase in the cost of drugs and dental care. The most that can be said about the addition of the Family Health Maintenance type of team service, with the added personnel to provide family care and the added doctor's time involved (which would necessarily increase per-service doctor cost) is that it would be more expensive than the present system of medical care, although in a prepayment structure, the premium increase might not be more than 10 percent over the ordinary premium.

A BRIEF REPRISE OF THE FINDINGS

(1) A health team was demonstrably satisfactory to the families and to the professional people involved.

(2) A physician with training which gave him family orientation was necessary in this new setting in order to allow appropriate team interaction.

(3) In carrying out their tasks, the public health nurse was fully acceptable to the families as an aid to the physician, even as a substitute; the social worker was considerably less so.

(4) Under the conditions of the Demonstration the social worker's role could not be extended easily to include a preventive aspect.

(5) In general the health of the study families improved. In addition, by the end of the study, housing and nutrition, closely associated with health, were significantly better in study families than in control families.

(6) Emotional health and emotional problems showed little improvement. Some reasons for these equivocal results may be: the short duration of experiment; the probable inadequacy of instruments for measuring change; and the inadequacy of the assumptions.

(7) There was a high degree of emotional difficulty in presumably normal families. They had the same problems that one associates with families who appeal to agencies or psychiatrists for care. Since these normal families did not apply to agencies, there

may be a self-healing or "coping" factor which enables some families to compensate without recourse to outside aid.

(8) Various conclusions were reached regarding patterns of use of service. A permissive system does not lead to abuse, since use of physician's services in the study families was little greater than in control families. Over a period of time use actually declined from an early high volume. The patterns of use in this relatively open system underline the fact that under ordinary circumstances most people do not get all the medical care they need. A health team spares specialist services. Social class, ethnic and cultural factors, and multiple complaints (with or without actual illness) are associated with high medical utilization. The Cornell Medical Index is a good predictor of high utilization.

(9) The routine health examination was useful for a first or baseline examination, but frequent routine examinations were not very productive. The substituting of a routine team conference on health problems is recommended in place of frequent routine examinations.

(10) Health-education programs on a group-meeting basis were not very successful. The community network of influence related to medical care in families might be examined as a future study of appropriate health educational methods.

NOTES ON THE CONCLUSIONS

In certain areas the lessons learned may be profitably underlined. The unusual character of the team operation in daily medical practice and the opportunities presented for observation of patients and professional people in this setting should be emphasized. Whatever the future of medical practice, a glimpse of the possibilities was obtained in the Family Health Maintenance Demonstration.

Professional Roles

When Carl Binger devised the title for his book, *The Doctor's Job,* he had in mind sharpening the focus of the doctor's *view* of his job by adding psychiatric insights to laboratory methods. Through the health-team structure we had hoped to add a family orientation. And we hoped that the doctor would gain personal and professional satisfaction from this new way of practicing. In discussing this, the internist who spent 7 years with the health team summed up the experiences this way. There were advantages in this method of practice, in the broader range of information available (psychiatric and social), in the ability to deal with more aspects of family need (again psychiatric principally), in the emphasis on prevention, and in the satisfactions of teamwork. The disadvantages were chiefly the laborious details of records and examinations attributable to the research: heightened consciousness of sickness on the part of the patient occasioned by the concentration on health and sickness implicit in the research; and the ambivalence of "family practice" in which not he, but a pediatrician, was responsible for half the family members.

The pediatrician, relegated to a consultant status in that the internist was *the* family adviser and senior medical member of the health team, felt this latter disadvantage, but mentioned identical advantages, emphasizing the indispensable character of the information offered by the nurse and social worker. The positive values emphasized by both physicians: broader knowledge of, and area of service in, preventive medicine and psychiatric orientation, indicate the sources of professional satisfaction.[2]

To the patients, the doctor was the top of the professional hierarchy. The nurse was considered a practitioner a step below the doctor, taking orders from him and responsible to him. This position was not unsuited to the nurse's conception of her own role, and there was no area of conflict between doctor and nurse or nurse and patient. For the doctor and nurse, except for some additional orientation, slipping into team roles would occasion no difficulty.

The social worker tended to be excluded from this hierarchical structure because she deals with emotional difficulties and problems which are not as yet included in the popular mind as part of the area of medical need. There was sharp cleavage between patient use of social work and of patient use of doctor and nurse. Social case-work skills and training do need to be brought to bear on patients at the daily medical practice level, but it was not easy in our structure. From the observations in the Demonstration, inclusion of social work into daily team service would be difficult. Certain changes suggest themselves for the social worker's characteristic role. Social workers need to take a long

217

look at the professional picture they try to maintain for themselves and foster for the public. Perhaps it is right that they should aim to be minor psychotherapists but should they then be pale copies of, or substitutes for, psychoanalysts of a rather lesser order of training and competence? Perhaps they should be office workers rather than field workers, but who will do the home visiting and home care? There is clear necessity for the development of *family* casework more closely related to medical practice, particularly to help people see their own need in the family situation. A good bit of self-study would seem to be indicated from the findings about patient reactions to social work.[3]

Other efforts to involve case-work concepts may progress in another direction. If casework is necessary because of patient needs, perhaps it ought to be added to public health nurse qualification, since the nurse is accepted so well by families. By broadening the capability of the nurse, it may be possible to carry on the desired activity without adding a social worker to the team. The factors which appear to militate against the social worker's being used as part of the team could thus be bypassed. The necessity for revising social-work curriculums or reversing the trend to psychotherapy would be obviated. The suggestion that public health nursing include case work as a function to make a combined worker available for a health team is not novel. Tentative steps toward this end have been taken in many places.[4] Furthermore, since serious study is currently being given by social workers themselves to a definition of their role, it may be that the profession may want to move into a more circumscribed area of activity and detach part of their presently jealously guarded province for the nurses' use.

A serious effort at popular education to alter attitudes relating to emotional disorder is also indicated. Emotional disease must be recognized as a medical problem. Furthermore, somewhere in that educational process popular acceptance of preventive intervention — before the awareness of need — will have to be pressed. It is almost hopeless to look forward to dealing with crises as the only technique in mental hygiene. If we can only wait for people to "ask" for, or "accept" help, we are already far behind in our efforts and without much chance of catching up.[5] As with the

218

previous suggestions, huge tasks confront those who would implement them.

Psychiatry and the Team Operation

The presence of emotional problems and difficulties made a resource such as the health team desirable and useful to the families. Within presumably normal families, there is a reservoir of emotional disturbance, of personal and family difficulty that constitutes a plea for professional help. As a rule these families do not go to professional agencies or persons for help. The family physician, who could be a natural resource to whom the families would turn, is declining in availability. In addition, the skills for this kind of professional help are diminishing parts of the doctor's role as he becomes more laboratory oriented. The provision of such help through the health team was accepted and welcomed by families.

One of the key people in the development and extension of the family health service was the psychiatrist. He helped the team achieve its goal of raising the level of health in families by lowering tension states and altering attitudes and behavior that might predispose to psychopathological conditions. An important added facet of the psychiatrist's role was in the mediation of the roles of team members in their team activity. When patients with overt mental illness were carried by the team because they refused other care or psychiatric hospitalization, the team could be very helpful to the family by explaining and supporting the other family members. The psychiatrist could be of extraordinary help to the team by "controlling" their activity, giving them support in carrying the patient.[6]

This aspect of service to the team may also have been helpful in resolving intrateam conflict, particularly in mediating potential conflict when areas of interest of the professional workers in the emotional problems of patients overlapped.[7]

So much psychiatric need was found during the baseline examination and interviews of the study families, that, while efforts were made to deal with the problems within the structure of the Demonstration itself, many family members were referred to other agencies for care.

219

There is a further implication in this use of psychiatric consultation. Today, pressures for psychiatric service are enormous. Some 10,000 to 20,000 additional psychiatrists[8] would be necessary at present apparent rates of morbidity. At no point in the whole structure of medicine could there be more effective substitution for the scarce psychiatric skill than at the family practice level. Efforts to develop attitudes and skills of family doctors in this respect have been mentioned and also the attention that is being given to the idea of using medical workers of all kinds to look after emotional disturbance.

The health team in family practice, using a psychiatric consultant, could serve brilliantly to fill this need.[9] Prepayment programs do not now generally include the cost of psychiatric care, with one or two exceptions,[10] partly because it is difficult to include psychiatric care in insurance programs in view of the shortage of psychiatrists. Provision of a substitute service at the family-practice level, siphoning off the demand for the scarcer and more expensive service, offers social, economic, and professional gains. On the evidence that over a third of the population suffers from symptoms of emotional disorder at one time or another, and that some accommodation is made without recourse to professional help, the availability of team guidance might serve to backstop the "self-healing" factor. As an example of such activity, there is the evidence of those individuals actually considered by the team as patients, "counseled" rather than treated, for long stretches. These were cases in which referral for psychotherapy may have been refused or commitment deemed undesirable or unnecessary. These patients were helped to carry on and function as family members and community members, without damage to the family structure, in this modestly protected way.[11]

Prevention and Health Promotion

An important lesson drawn from the Demonstration's essay into prevention is that continuous observation by a health team is at least equal to, and probably superior to, routine "preventive" examination. The routine family conference should be a regular part of continuous observation, paralleling such accepted preventive measures as the well-baby conference. A routine family conference within the framework of continuous observation would support case finding for early diagnosis and at the same time offer opportunities for the control of chronic disease. The family conference offers more time for professional conversations and more time to obtain otherwise unknown information about the patient, as well as an occasion to furnish educational information to the patient. It allows the patient to relieve himself of information he may consider trivial and develop confidence in the team.

Social Influences Affecting Provision of Medical Care

Factors outside medicine play an important part in healthy living and cannot be ignored — world peace, economic security, and housing, for example. Recognizing that home–job–social relationships play a more significant part in the modification of life behavior than does access to medical care alone, it is still evident that at certain critical times the availability or *type* of medical care may be crucial. This is not only true in matters of life and death, but in those situations profoundly affecting family life that improperly or inadequately cared for illness imposes. In examining the dynamics of health and illness it is evident that people should be able to get prompt help of a kind they want in time of illness. But the best of medical care cannot substitute for adequate wages, better economic opportunities, good housing, or the abolition of racial and religious discrimination. Correction of housing defects alone may make for improvement in family life and perhaps alter the very nature of the problems brought by families to medical-care agencies. Conversely, reducing the economic burden of sickness and the unpredictable cost of medical care may make it possible to divert social capital to improvement of housing and economic security. This interaction was evident in the study, but outside the framework of evaluation.

FOR FUTURE REFERENCE

The time we devoted to the examination and improvement of the lives of the study families is a very short period within the life span of an individual. Four years may not be a sufficient period of observation to establish that family life was strengthened by the concentrated efforts of the health team; nor with any certainty that within this period there could be observable the maximum effect of the Demonstration. There are too few people in the various categories where changes might be highly visible: too few menopausal people, too few children in adolescence. Since the total observations cover too short a period of time and too few people in the critical periods of their lives, we must be very cautious as to the conclusions drawn and as to what is meaningful in the emotional and physical lives of people based on our findings. Results must be regarded as tentative and inconclusive.

Exploration of different team structures are clearly indicated: a doctor qualified in internal medicine *and* pediatrics for example; or a doctor-nurse team in which the nurse has case-worker qualifications. The development of a social questionnaire on the order of the Cornell Medical Index would be inordinately helpful in providing necessary insights at intake and establishing the groundwork for team–family interaction. Many other suggestions appear in the body of this book relating to the specific findings — the structure of health-promotion activities, use of a psychiatric consultant, and so on.

One basic type of trial experience will require deft political management and tact: the introduction of the family health team into school and job health services. Health services for the schools should be in the hands of the family physician or health team, and this may be extremely difficult to initiate. Family physicians have intimate knowledge of the child's problems and medical care. Either a school health service should be established that would be intimately associated with the family health team, or the family health team should be the school health service. Present school health services are inadequate and inconsequential. They pay attention to episodic events and do not concern themselves with the characteristic continuity of the child's life in which medical or psychiatric care may be needed and in which the observations and attitudes of the teachers and mothers are equally important. Similar considerations hold for on-the-job medical care.

The health-team approach needs to become a part of the educational activity of professional schools.[12] The isolation of the medical student from the problems of medical practice can be overcome completely by giving him an opportunity to learn clinical medicine, not in the isolated, fragmented, out-patient department, but in the family health team. Social workers and nurses can come to recognize roles in family practice through student experiences on such a health team. From newly trained professional workers, sensitized through health-team teaching, other and more fruitful demonstrations will be staffed. From the report of this "reconnaissance in force," perhaps a strategic attack to advance social medicine can be launched.

A family health team operating within a group-practice unit and practicing preventive as well as therapeutic medicine is a viable model for our society. It will require shaking people's minds loose from old stereotypes and helping them to recognize the new possibilities. It may turn out that, attractive as the model is, other forms of medical practice, as yet unsuspected, may be even more attractive, simple, and useful. Only by systematic study of various prototypes can this be determined. If we initiate developments, taking advantage of our knowledge of what patients want, and introduce elements that meet these wants, we can accelerate the trend toward new types of practice. If, at the same time, we meet professional needs for new working forms, the trend will be accelerated further. The correlation of these factors will produce the most desirable type.

Many significant problems must be resolved before final answers can be given. We must learn a great deal more about patients' notions of effective service and demand patterns, about professional needs and satisfactions. We must begin to learn about the causes of neurotic behavior and mental illness and what can be done to prevent or ameliorate these widespread disorders. However, investigation should and must go on to explore the aspects of administration and organization of medical care developed in the Demonstration. In historical perspective, offsetting specialism, orienting medicine toward families, and wedding health promotion to disease treatment is a valuable contribution to medical-practice organization. Much remains to be done.

And so we actually begin to see the outlines of a new physician. Scientist and social worker, ready to cooperate in teamwork, in close touch with the people he disinterestedly serves, a friend and leader, he directs all his efforts toward the prevention of disease and becomes a therapist where prevention has broken down — the social physician protesting the people and guiding them to a healthier and happier life.

— Henry Sigerist, "Trends in Medical Education"

PART FOUR

SOCIOLOGICAL OVERVIEW

- XIII -

SOCIAL SCIENCE RESEARCH
IN THE FAMILY HEALTH
MAINTENANCE DEMONSTRATION

by Eliot Freidson

The Family Health Maintenance Demonstration was set up as a controlled experiment in which the experimental group of patients obtained health services provided by a professional team in a medical group and the control group obtained health services provided by individual practitioners in the same medical group. In initial plans the sociologist, like the psychiatrist and health educator, was assigned a consultant role. In this role he could on occasion contribute to the enlightenment of the members of the team, but he was not expected to introduce changes into the Demonstration.

Rather than intervention, his role required gathering data independently of the Demonstration's already established program of data-collection. He set himself the task of broad exploration of the social context within which health practices take place, attempting to locate and define the significance of the Family Health Maintenance Demonstration within that context. In studying the patients he used a variety of methods — observation at the Demonstration offices, intensive interviews in the home with 71 adult members of 36 subscribing families, 3 separate questionnaire surveys of the Demonstration families, and a questionnaire survey of 676 subscribers to the Montefiore Hospital Medical

227

Group. In studying the professional staff he used the methods of participant observation and interviewing.

One way to introduce and organize the context within which the health practice described in this book takes place is to ask what patients want from health services. Of course they want to feel well, and when they feel ill they want to be made to feel well again if possible, but what else do they expect? The patients seem to use 2 interlocking criteria in evaluating health services: first, they feel, good medical care requires what they assess as *technical competence;* second, they feel, good medical care requires taking *interest* in the patient such that the patient not only obtains emotional satisfaction from the practitioner but also that the competence will be exercised in a more than routine way.

A practitioner need not have both qualities. He can be perceived as a "good" doctor but a "cold fish," "impersonal," or "mechanical," which is to say possessing an adequate degree of technical competence but an inadequate degree of the characteristics that imply interest in the patient. And he can be perceived as "very nice" but not "up-to-date," which is to say having an adequate degree of interest in his patient but somewhat lacking in technical competence. In general, questions of competence are raised far less than questions of interest, for most patients seem to assume adequate competence on the part of individual doctors.

What is meant by "interest?" Superficially the patients seem to be saying that practitioner interest involves his treating them as a person rather than as an object, but this is not really what they are saying. They do approve of an egalitarian sense that the practitioner is willing to recognize that he too is human but none of them really ask for a fully egalitarian relationship. They recognize that there is a point beyond which the doctor is "taking liberties," such as in "joking too much," or in "getting too personal," and another point beyond which he is "cold," "impersonal," and disinterested. Between these extremes is a considerable range, from genial and friendly to "reserved but nice," which represents the range of "appropriate" professional interest that patients want.

The criterion of technical competence can be kept separate from that of interest. For example, in discussing a physician one patient said: "He wasn't bad. He knew his business, but I think he wasn't interested. When he came into the office he never said, 'Hello, how are you?' he just went about his business. But he knew his business." On the whole most doctors are presumed to "know their business," but the technical facilities at their disposal, the use of such facilities, and their attitudes are critical to the exercise of competence.

The matter of technical facilities and their use is quite simple. What makes the difference is the extent to which doctors have available and use laboratory and testing facilities. The more such facilities are available and used, the greater is the patient's sense that "good" medicine is being practiced. It is this *activity* as such that impresses the patient, not only in the use of technical facilities but also in the behavior of the practitioner himself. In some cases the perception of such a superficially simple and obvious matter as effecting cure seemed to hang precisely upon such activity on the part of the physician, whether it is prescribing medication, ordering a diagnostic test, or making a thorough-looking examination, for it was only through tangible activity that the patient seemed able to get the impression that the physician was working diligently on the case and that the physician himself rather than time or "nature" was responsible for cure.

In spite of "interest" and "competence" being distinguished separately by the patients, however, it is the rare and peculiar patient who chooses one of these criteria rather than both. It was an extreme and probably rhetorically motivated patient who said, "Sometimes I think it's a lot more important to me that I be treated as a person when I go to the doctor than that I get the best medical care of all." Most patients insisted on good technical care, but also insisted that without personal interest the practitioner cannot use his full competence. As one said, "If he isn't interested, he just won't do careful work even when he's a good doctor." The two together are what the patients seem to want from health services.

HOW THREE MODES OF PRACTICE MEET PATIENT WANTS

In interviews and questionnaires the patients were asked to discuss and evaluate their experience with the individual entrepreneurial practice they used before joining Montefiore Hospital

Medical Group, with the Medical Group, and with the Family Health Maintenance Demonstration. By such comparative data one may gain some sense of the significance of the Demonstration to the patients.

But in these comparisons we do not have a random sample of Bronx laymen. Rather, we have comparatively few families who, insofar as they are subscribers to the Montefiore Hospital Medical Group, have signed a contract that formally precludes the use of neighborhood practitioners. In this sense they are likely to be biased. Perhaps symptomatic of this self-selection is the fact that of the 36 families interviewed, 25 either had no regular relation with an independent physician before they joined the Medical Group, or had experiences with an entrepreneurial practitioner that seriously annoyed or frightened them. Four liked the practitioners they had before subscribing to HIP, but had no special commitment to them. Seven families had, on the whole, highly satisfying experience with entrepreneurial practitioners.

In spite of this fact that less than a third of the interviewed patients had any extended or satisfying experience with "private" medical practice, most of them felt that more personally satisfying care was likely to be found in entrepreneurial practice than in the Montefiore Hospital Medical Group. They believed that the independent physician is in a better position to take an interest in his patient than is the group physician. On the other hand, most of the patients did not believe it was possible for the independent physician to give them "good" medical care — they felt that the technical facilities of the Medical Group combined with the availability of diagnostic and treatment services given by a prepayment plan allowed group physicians to practice "better" if not "nicer" medicine.

It is in this context that we may place their responses to the Family Health Maintenance Demonstration. They felt that the Demonstration had the virtues of both independent and Medical Group practice and the deficiencies of neither: it provided them with technically good medical care, like the Group, and like entrepreneurial practice it provided them with the feeling that personal interest was being taken in them. The technical quality of Demonstration care was seen to stem largely from its connection with the Medical Group, with an extra push being provided by what they believed to be its preventive orientation. Thus, only the impression of "personal interest" distinguished the Demonstration from the Medical Group. What hints do the patients give us about the way in which interest was communicated?

The fundamental difference between neighborhood practice and Family Health Maintenance Demonstration practice is organization. In the former it is the behavior of the physician alone that is important — the practitioner often has an aide, receptionist, or nurse working with him, but it seems significant that none of the interviewed patients made any spontaneous mention of such an assistant. In discussing entrepreneurial practice the patients used the third-person singular; in discussing the Demonstration practice the patients largely used the third-person plural. While in one fundamental sense Demonstration practice can be seen as a physician with a few specialized assistants, the patients did not perceive this; they perceived a plurality to be responsible for their care, and they responded to it as such. Indeed, it was the plurality, not the physician alone, that seemed to communicate a sense of interest.

The Demonstration communicated a sense of interest to the patients in a variety of ways. All workers contributed to the climate of friendliness by their cordiality to the patient when he entered the waiting room. In dealing with the physician the patients did not feel rushed and felt free to ask questions. The physician's perceived willingness to make house calls as well as his occasional telephoning of the patient to inquire after the course of illness also contributed to the patients' feeling that the staff was interested in them. And as special professional workers, the nurse and the social worker acted as resources for aid and advice for things that the patients felt were too minor to trouble the doctor with, or inappropriate for the doctor's attention. Giving aid and advice in marketing, visiting the children's schools, contacting agencies for medical or dental care for an indigent relative, trying to obtain low-cost housing for them, and making occasional home visits are examples of services that patients did not expect of a physician, but that when performed by the public health nurse or the social worker contributed to the patients' sense that interest was being taken in them.

It was this perception of personal interest that seemed to

transform the patients' conception of the quality of care they were getting. On the whole, Family Health Maintenance patients did *not* seem to think they obtained care that was *technically* superior to that obtainable in the Medical Group. Rather, it was the addition of personal interest to that high technical quality that made Family Health Maintenance Demonstration care seem superior. One patient said that the interest shown in her encouraged her to bring her problems in for care, and because she brought her problems in for consultation and treatment she got better care. Thus, the patients believed that the staff's interest motivated them to use facilities that they would ordinarily avoid or "never get around" to using.

We may summarize this view of the patients' response to the Family Health Maintenance Demonstration with their answers to a questionnaire that was administered to them after they had left the program and returned to Medical Group services. Of those responding ($N = 213$, 81 percent returns), 89 percent felt that the Family Health Maintenance Demonstration had either improved their health or prevented it from deteriorating. In "its effect on the general health of you and your family," only 1 percent felt that the Medical Group was superior to the Demonstration and only 5 percent felt that the "private" care they have had was superior to the Demonstration. Further, only 2 percent felt it was "more pleasant" to be a Medical Group patient than a Demonstration patient and only 3 percent felt it was more pleasant to be a patient of a "private" doctor than of the Demonstration. It is quite clear that most of the patients believed the Demonstration to be superior both to the Medical Group and to the entrepreneurial practice they have known.

SOME PROBLEMS OF ANALYSIS

Once it was quite clear that the patients liked the Demonstration, and once hints were uncovered that suggest why this kind of organization of health services was more attractive to them than two other types of organization, the task was to determine how patient behavior accords with patient attitudes. In other words, did such expressed satisfaction manifest itself in a high degree of cooperation with the professional workers of the program, both in the "appropriate" degree of utilization of Demonstration services and in following through the prescriptions of their professional consultants?

There is no objective criterion of such cooperation, but from the point of view of the professional workers the patients' behavior left something to be desired. Attendance at health education meetings, success in the reduction of obesity, and above all utilization of the social worker was disappointing. It was also discovered that some of the patients were going to "private" doctors for some of their care. In a survey of the Family Health Maintenance Demonstration patients (92 percent returns, 236 individuals or 121 families), 16 percent reported that some member of the family used the services of an outside surgeon or obstetrician during the time that he was an eligible patient of the Demonstration. For medical care other than obstetrics or surgery — that is, the sort of care provided by the staff of the Demonstration — 39 percent reported use of the services of an outside physician "quite a bit" or "occasionally."

Two of those problems were chosen for intensive analysis because of their strategic importance: the utilization[1] of the social worker because it allows us to attack the problem of the organization of team practice itself; and the utilization of outside services because it allows us to refine our view of the relation of the organization of practice to patient behavior.

SOCIAL CLASS AND PATIENT BEHAVIOR

The concept of social class was found to order both sets of data in a highly regular fashion. Using years of education and occupational status as indexes of social class, it was found that the middle-class group reported using both surgical and nonsurgical outside services more than the lower social-class group. But since the middle class can better afford to pay for "outside" services than the lower class, it may be not that the middle class is distinct in *desiring* to go outside, but only that the middle-class group has the *resources* to do so.

This does not seem to be the case. In a survey of Medical Group subscribers[2] who were sufficiently numerous to allow refined tabulations, it was found that high social class was associated with a greater degree of sensitivity to insult, and to feeling like a "charity case," and with a critical and manipulative approach to medical care. In contrast, the lower classes were somewhat more insensitive to their status as patients and were rather more passive and uncritical in their approach to medical care. And the higher classes were somewhat less satisfied with the Medical Group than were the lower. Thus, if we may generalize from regular Medical Group subscribers to that special group of subscribers — Demonstration patients — we may conclude that the use of outside services in the Demonstration reflects not merely the ability to pay for outside services, but as well differences in orientation to medical care that the principle of social class organizes.

Class differences were also quite clear in patient responses to the various workers of the professional teams of the Family Health Maintenance Demonstration as obtained in 2 questionnaires administered while the Demonstration was still in existence. (One with 85, the other with 92 percent returns). These questionnaires explored not only the degree to which the patients believed they utilized the various professional workers of the program but also the interpersonal context of such reported utilization and the type of problem for which they believed they would seek out individual workers.

The over-all view obtained from these responses is one in which the priority of the physicians over the other professional workers is manifest. The patients valued their relationships to their physician more than anything else in the Demonstration. For a variety of problems he was the consultant they chose first. But it is significant that they perceived their contact with him to be largely within the framework of formal visits scheduled by advanced appointments. The nurse, identified with the physician as a medical worker, was considered second in importance to him — the alternative to him for a wide variety of problems but, very importantly, more accessible than the physician, far more likely to be consulted in a highly informal, personal context. The social worker, finally, was seen to be accessible in the same sort of informal context as the nurse, but was most often third choice for consultation and indeed reported to be seen on a formal consultative basis to a lesser degree than either the nurse or the doctor. She was first choice only for problems connected with children's schooling, and shared first choice with the doctor for problems connected with adult personal adjustment.

Social class proved to be a major variable in differentiating responses *within* this general pattern. In the perceived use of the physician, neither middle nor lower class was much different, but there was a consistent tendency for more of the middle class to report that they use the nurse less and the social worker more than the lower class. Further, more of the middle than the lower group considered the social worker an important addition to the staff. And for most of the hypothetical problems posed by the questionnaire the higher class group was more likely to choose consultation with the social worker than was the lower group. The lower group emphasized the role of the more accessible, lower status, and culturally familiar nurse in their response to the Family Health Maintenance Demonstration team services.

THE CONCEPT OF LAY REFERRAL SYSTEM

Use of the social class as a variable introduced some order into our understanding of the patient's behavior. Those who go outside the Demonstration for some medical services are more often from the middle class than from the lower class. Those who feel more prone to consult the social worker tend to be middle-class and those who feel more prone to consult the nurse tend to be lower-class. Also, use of the variable of social class gives us some impression of fundamental differences in attitude toward health care as such, leading us to understand that while one is more "up-to-date," more "scientifically" oriented, more prone to accept the psychiatric orientation of the social worker, it is also more prone to be critical of services and to seek other care if Demonstration services are deemed inadequate. Not only attitude but status difference seems significant, in that the lower-class patients were more reluctant to "bother" the doctor and more eager to accept the substitute services of the lower status nurse.

Social class is not in itself enough, for, while it does imply important attitudinal and behavioral differences between patients, it tells us nothing of the interpersonal mechanisms by which these differences are communicated between individuals and sustained among them. During the course of the investigation it became clear that a further concept was needed to organize the data to the greatest effect.

In the intensive interviews with patients it seemed that the decision to see a professional practitioner took place through a process that was by no means automatic even when, as in the case of seeing a Medical Group Demonstration doctor, cost was eliminated from consideration. At the very least the prospective patient had to wait for a period of time to make sure that his difficulty would not pass away unaided. This wait was followed by self-diagnosis and self-prescription of home remedies, or of left-over drugs from a doctor's previous prescription. At this point of realization that the symptoms are not merely fleeting, a certain amount of discussion with other members of the family tended to occur — discussion of the symptoms and of the propriety of what was chosen from the medicine cabinet or the stock of aphorisms about diet, rest, and the like. Very often, before seeing a doctor the advice of relatives, friends, and colleagues was solicited casually, in the course of everyday small talk, and sometimes, depending on the patient, the neighborhood druggist consulted for a patent remedy. If the symptoms persisted the more formal step of seeing a doctor was likely to be taken, but usually only after these lay or semi-professional consultants had been exploited.

Typically this process of consultation involved not only attempts at diagnosis and prescriptions of treatment, but also referral to other consultants in the event of ignorance of the symptoms or failure or anticipated failure at cure. Indeed, prescription itself often consists in a referral — to someone else who had the same symptom, or who was once a nurse, or to a doctor who treated the consultant for the "same thing." Assuming a process that is not stopped after taking the first aspirin, antacid, or laxative, referrals may be seen as alternatives inseparably contingent upon the perceived adequacy of diagnoses and prescriptions.

The use of the professional practitioner, then, often takes place after other lay resources have been utilized. Thus the doctor is only one step after many, one consultant out of many, and the patient often arrives at the doctor's office after having exhausted a whole network of less formal consultations. In this sense we

236

may speak of a lay referral structure, which consists in a network of consultants, potential or actual, running from the intimate and most informal confines of the nuclear family through successively more select, distant, and authoritative persons until the "professional" is reached. This network imposes form on the process of seeking help. Taking this network in conjunction with the culture or "education" of the patients we may speak of the whole as the *lay referral system*.[3]

Not only does this lay referral system impose form on the *seeking* of help — on how help is sought, and on what sort of person is asked for help — but it also validates and sustains the help after it has been sought. The patient is not passed along until he reaches a professional practitioner and, after he sees the practitioner, is after a fashion passed back and quizzed about his consultation. Retrospective approval of this nature is thus an element that sustains a consultant position in this system, just as retrospective disapproval may lead to avoiding the practitioner in the future. It is this interpersonal interaction with nonprofessional consultants just as much as the cessation of symptoms and the patients' opinions about proper medical treatment that seems responsible for not following the doctor's orders or not coming back to the doctor. In this sense, seeing a practitioner requires continuous validation by the consultants subordinate to him in the lay referral system.

It follows from this that a factor of significance to patient behavior is the kind of lay referral system in which he participates. Obviously, if the culture of the lay-referral system is based primarily on folk beliefs, the prospective patient is unlikely to use professional medical services. And if the lay referral structure is extensive, the prospective patient tempted to use professional medical services is likely to be subjected to countervailing influences. On the other side of the coin is of course patient culture stressing the overriding value of professional services in which, if the referral structure is extended, the patient tempted to use irregular services is likely to be subjected to a good deal of questioning and even ridicule. Where the referral structure is truncated, however, the patient is on his own, subjected to little control by his lay associates, and so his behavior can vary more closely with his feelings.

INTERPERSONAL RELATIONS AND THE USE
OF OUTSIDE SERVICES

Social class is related to the use of outside services. It is also related to neighborhood and familial participation, which in turn is related to the use of outside services. The number of cases is too small to allow controlled tabulations to sort out the precise relationships involved but the evidence is consistent. Typically, the middle-class patient (and the user of outside care) is not a long-term resident in his neighborhood and does not frequently participate in his extended family of parents, parents-in-law, and relatives. In this sense he is comparatively isolated and his behavior is unlikely to be controlled closely from day to day by such intimate lay associates outside of the family. In turn, he tends not to know of any relatives or neighbors who belong, as he does, to the medical group. At best he knows only of fellow-workers or colleagues. In this sense many of those who might be his consultants do not share his experience in the medical group and are likely to refer him outside. Insofar as his class attitudes are such as to raise occasions of doubt relatively often, there are few intimate lay consultants to dispel doubt and what consultants there are testify to the excellence of "outside" services. His lay referral system points outside.

In contrast, the lower-class patient (who does not use outside services) tends to be a long-term resident in his neighborhood and member of an extended family. Further, he has relatives, neighbors, and fellow-workers who belong to the same medical group. Thus, predisposed to be comparatively passive and uncritical in the first place, encouraged in this by an extensive network of intimates who not only share this attitude but who also share his experience in the medical group (and who like him have comparatively little experience with entrepreneurial practice), he is unlikely to be stimulated to go outside should some occasion of doubt arise. His lay referral system points to continued use of his prepaid medical services.

The Use of the Social Worker

Returning to the problem of what the professional workers judged the underutilization of the social worker, we may first contrast the role of the nurse with that of the social worker. In almost every instance involving the use of the public health nurse for aid in problems that might be considered emotional the patients explained their choice by reference to their familiarity with the nurse such that it was "natural" to see her. They believed that the problem was not "serious" enough to require the services of the social worker. The social worker's role, by its very restriction to highly specialized problems, seemed removed from the course of everyday affairs, detached, specialized, and therefore forbidding to the early, not strongly motivated search for help.[4] The public health nurse's role, however, by its very generality and second-choice accessibility was inserted into the course of everyday affairs and became a strategic point of consultation. It was placed within the lay referral system, while the role of the social worker stood outside that system.

These differences become clear when we note that the nurse's initially perceived function is embedded in homely problems of everyday life which are somewhat "beneath" the physician's concern. When the family was taken on the program she visited the home to examine sleeping facilities, crowding, diet, and the like. At that time, and of course subsequently, she dealt fundamentally with techniques of housewifery and objects of domestic consumption. To this common ground of interaction was added medical authority, albeit subordinate to the doctor's. In all, the nurse was considered the only person who knew what things were really like at home. In contrast, the social worker rarely visited the home. The nurse routinely visited the schools attended by the children of the family; the social worker rarely visited the schools. The nurse was associated with the aura of healing and could authoritatively suggest remedies for minor medical problems; the social worker was sharply segregated from medical affairs. The nurse was routinely preoccupied with the everyday manifest life of the household; the social worker was not concerned with these things unless they had a latent association with personal problems. In practice, the social worker was so thoroughly specialized in function that she was isolated from what people consider normal and everyday.

This functional isolation seemed doubly significant in that by its nature it was also ideological or cultural, for what the so-

239

cial worker was supposed to deal with—personal problems—emerges from and permeates those everyday affairs. Insofar as the social worker was perceived as a specialist, divorced from everyday affairs, a referral to her implied that the problem was not of an everyday character. These patients did not consider the emotional problems of everyday life to be distinct: they saw as everyday what the professional worker saw as neurotic or even psychotic, and so they sought the everyday aid of the generalist physician and the public health nurse. When the doctor or the nurse tried to refer them to the social worker they resisted because they did not believe their problem was so special that they must see a "special" person.

The public health nurse, by inserting herself into everyday household affairs, assumed a position in the lay referral structure that was prior to that of the physician. As such, she was highly accessible functionally. Both her traditional role as nurse and her position in the program, however, granted her less authority than the physician. Insofar as the lay referral process characteristically exploits first the less authoritative but more accessible sources of consultation, we can understand how the public health nurse could be chosen frequently for consultation but designated "first choice" infrequently.

The social worker stood in an entirely different position in the lay referral structure. As someone unconnected with the everyday she was unlikely to be chosen in the early stages of perception of the problem: if the prospective client himself was to choose her it was likely to be late, when more common remedies have failed and when his motivation has become more pressing. In turn, referral to the social worker was unlikely to be effective until the more common remedies and the more commonplace and casual definitions of the nature of the problem had been exhausted. Part of the failure of referral to the social worker seemed to stem from making the referral too early in the process of defining the problem. If the social worker were in the position of a technical aide rather than a specialist, referral might not have been so difficult.

It has been noted that the health teams were composed of internist, pediatrician, social worker, and public health nurse. While no actual directives were apparently made, these teams were supposed to operate more "democratically" than is commonly the case in medical settings. Rather than being merely the doctor's assistants, the social worker and the public health nurse were to be fully professional workers themselves, with specific areas of competence in which they have full responsibility. The physicians certainly had no over-all administrative responsibility for the program.

This led to a curious state of affairs. In essence, the teams developed three distinct types of organization. In the everyday course of giving services to patients the individual members of the teams more or less went their own ways, as they saw fit, occasionally developing a temporary, informal, cooperative relationship with one of the other professional workers when work required a deliberate division of task. If there was any administrative coordinator of this fragmented organization at all it was the secretary of the program, for she was the central point of communication in its day-to-day affairs. As the person whom every patient calls in order to get needed services, not only was the secretary likely to know more of what was going on than any other worker, but she was of necessity the only one required to know where each worker could be reached. In fact she was the only person who did know where every worker was, who was most likely to know what they were doing, and who was most likely to know how the patients were responding to their services. Simply in this she was the sole administrator of day-to-day staff activities and the sole central controlling agent. And her participation in gossip with other secretaries and with the female members of the professional staff added to the means by which she could serve as a controlling agent.

The second type of organization was observed when the whole staff had to cooperate and when patients did not have to be taken into consideration. The most common instance of this was found in staff conferences. Here was observed an at best shifting equilibrium, with lines of alliance being drawn now by status (sex and otherwise), now by professional orientation. In pressing an interpretation and diagnosis or in contradicting that of someone else, the physician did establish his authority by falling back on purely technical data. This effectively drew a line of professional competence over which none of the others could or would cross. But medical authority was quite unstable: the psychiatric interpretations of the social worker were difficult to contain and almost impossible to ignore. The net result was that in staff meetings something resembling an egalitarian, if not peaceful, climate prevailed.

It was when the staff was in conference with the patients that the egalitarian professional climate shifted. Here the task required the staff to cooperate with patients. The organization which ensued was hardly desired by all staff members but was necessary. Time and again the social worker tried to take the lead in discussing with the patient a problem that her training equipped her to deal with authoritatively, only to find that the patient ignored her and addressed his questions to the physician. The general insistence of patients on the authority of the physician forced the staff to develop the strategy by which the physician acted as "chairman" of the meeting, occasionally turning the floor over to one of his associates. Indeed, recognition of this problem led to the development of conscious prearrangement of the strategy of dealing with particular patients: before meeting with the patient the members of the staff decided how the physician should discuss "delicate" problems with the patient, and how and at what point in the discussion he could invite the comments of the other professional workers. Clearly, the patients themselves forced the development of an authoritarian structure centered around the physician.

In this variation in team organization, the nature of the task to be performed played a considerable role in determining the organization of services. Where activities had to be coordinated, authority of some sort seemed inescapable, even if it had to be authority by default. Where activities hinged on the participation of "outsiders," and where those outsiders were voluntary participants whom the staff wanted to hold, organizations shifted to conform to the preconceptions of those outsiders even though that shift was against the grain of the staff participants.[5]

In sum, the Family Health Maintenance Demonstration patients seemed to want medical care which they can consider technically competent and in which practitioners are personally interested in them. Most of them believed that the Demonstration provided both features, unlike the regular Montefiore Medical Group which provided primarily the former, and "private" practice which provided primarily the latter. In spite of their remarkably high level of general satisfaction, however, they avoided the use of social workers in the Demonstration and many reported that at one time or another they had used "outside" medical practitioners. If there is a moral in this, it is that expressed satisfaction is neither the most accurate index of what people actually do nor of the value of a medical program.

Pursuing the circumstances in which the patients rejected the social workers or avoided the Demonstration to use an outside physician, social class proved to be an important source of order. More refined as a source of insight, however, was the observation of a course of self-perception, self-diagnosis, self-treatment, and lay consultation which preceded the seeking of professional services. Conceptualizing that career preceding professional care, health services could be seen to vary in their position in the "lay referral system." Compared to the public health nurse, the social worker was relatively distant from that system. More precise investigation of lay referral systems might allow future medical programs to adopt strategies which can extend care even further and more effectively than could the Family Health Maintenance Demonstration.

APPENDIXES

BIBLIOGRAPHY

NOTES

INDEX

APPENDIX A.

Members of the Operating Board

George Baehr, M.D.	1950 - 1959
Frederick R. Bailey, M.D.	1950 - 1959
E. M. Bluestone, M.D.	1950 - 1952
Bailey B. Burritt	1950 - 1954
Martin Cherkasky, M.D.	1950 - 1959
Samuel W. Dooley, M.D.	1954 - 1956
Stanley P. Davies	1950 - 1959
Richard L. Day, M.D.	1950 - 1954
Guy Emerson	1950 - 1959
John W. Fertig	1950 - 1959
Frank Hertel	1959
George G. Kirstein	1950 - 1959
Sheridan A. Logan	1950 - 1959
Henry L. Moses	1950 - 1959
Conrad M. Riley, M.D.	1954 - 1959
Robert D. Steefel	1950 - 1959
Aura E. Severinghaus	1950 - 1959
George A. Silver, M.D.	1951 - 1959

247

APPENDIX B.

Personnel of the Program

Robert S. Aaron, M.D.	Internist	7/1/52-----7/31/58
Hannah Bamberger	Psychiatric Social Worker	10/13/52----6/15/54
Albert S. Beasley, M.D.	Pediatrician	7/1/53------8/31/54
Emanuel Chusid, M.D.	Pediatrician	2/1/57-----9/13/57
Carol Creedon, Ph.D.	Sociologist	7/1/52-----6/30/53
Martin Cherkasky, M.D.	Physician-in-Charge	10/1/50-----7/31/51
Elizabeth G. Estrin, M.D.	Pediatrician	9/1/54-----7/28/58
Eliot Freidson, Ph.D.	Sociologist	10/1/55-----5/30/60
Bertha Kahn	Public Health Nurse	9/2/52-----9/30/57
Donald Gibbons, M.D.	Internist	7/1/57----11/15/57
Robert N. Ladenhaim, D.D.S.	Dentist	2/54--------6/58
Miriam Tanzer McKenzie	Psychologist	10/1/52------6/1/55 10/1/55-----7/31/57
Anna Mink	Nurse	12/18/50-----3/1/51
Charles Orbach, Ph.D.	Psychologist	2/1/52-----7/1/54
William Pollack, D.D.S.	Dentist	9/52-------6/56
Alan S. Pomerance, D.D.S.	Dentist	6/54-------4/58
Jeanette Quinn	Nurse	4/4/56-----2/7/58
Helene L. Ringenberger	Public Health Nurse	3/15/51----7/31/58
Amy L. Rosebury	Psychiatric Social Worker	12/11/50-----3/1/51
Isadore Rossman, M.D.	Internist	12/1/50-----10/1/52
A. B. Siegelaub	Bio-Statistician	3/15/54--12/31/60
Howard H. Schlossman, M.D.	Consulting Psychiatrist	2/1/51-----9/30/57
Leon Schneyer, D.D.S.	Dentist	7/51--------6/52
Irving S. Shapiro, Ph.D.	Health Educator	10/1/52-----5/30/57
Estelle Siker, M.D.	Pediatrician	1950-----6/30/53
George A. Silver, M.D.	Physician-in-Charge	8/1/51-----5/30/60
Charlotte Stiber	Psychiatric Social Worker	3/1/51-----7/31/57
Alice L. Thompson	Psychiatric Social Worker	6/1/54-----9/30/57

APPENDIX C. RECORD FORMS

Family Health Maintenance Demonstration
Administrative Record System

April 1952

After the families have been selected, entries will be made
of all families, study and control, into the Family Health Maintenance Registry. This lined journal will list all families as
entered, by FHMD member, as follows:

Journal

FHMD #	Family Name	Date of Entry	Household Persons Total Family Others			Remarks

Item	Explanation
FHMD #	Prenumber last 3 digits in consecutive order beginning with 100,101, etc. Enter year of acceptance in front of number as 2 for 1952, 3 for 1953, etc., e.g., 5th household 1952 - FHMD # 2105. (Controls - odd FHM Nos. Direct participants - even FHM Nos.)
Name	HIP Family - Surname
Date Entered	Month and year household (direct participant only) joined study group.

Household Persons

Total	Number of persons in household
Family	Number insured by HIP
Other	Number of others in household
Remarks	Specify others - uncle, grandmother, boarder

At the same time, a linedex alphabetical listing of families and family members in the study group, as well as family listing of the control group should be set up as follows:

249

FHM M2 No.	FHM Yr. No.	Insured Family Name	Person (First & Last Name) if different from household	Address	Birthdata HS Mo Yr	HIP No. Disposition	Persons M	Persons F	M/Y	Family Household Strip / Direct Study Person Strip
2	100	Abercrombie		2620 Decatur		9001624	4	4		Service House-hold
2	100		George		11 08 08					
2	100		Joan		51 10 14					Household Members
2	100		Mary		61 09 36					
2	100		Harold		32 06 38					
2	303	Arnold		1820 Gr. Conc.		8003602	4	4		Control
2	154	Baker		2620 Marion		8162040	6	4		Service House-hold
2	154		Joseph		11 06 07					
2	154		Lillian		51 11 10					
2	154		Josephine		61 09 41					Household Members
2	154		Sylvia		62 11 43					
2	154	Lewis	John		21 06 84					
2	154	Lewis	Catherine		41 08 88					

Strips

Households - Buff with transparent yellow sleeve
Household Members - Buff

Filing

Section 1 - Active Households: Alphabetically by surname of insured
family
    Person: Immediately following household strip, head,
        spouse, children (eldest first, others).

Section 2 - Lost - By month within year - alphabetically for family
        strips, person strips immediately following.
Family Strip

ITEM: FHM - year of entrance and FHM No.   (see FHM #1)
        insured family name - surname of HIP insured family
    Address - complete in pencil
    HIP No. - HIP certificate or policy number
    Persons - T - total in household. F - No. in insured family

Signals:
    Colors
Red   1. New this month
Blue   2. Lost this month
Green 3. Served this month

Person Strip

ITEM: FHM - year of entrance and FHM No.
    Person Name - First name, if surname is same as family name,
            if not same, full name.
    Birthdata - Household status, sex and month and year of birth

    Calculation of Birthdata:
        Six numbers are used. First two numbers represent
        household status, derived as follows:

Status	Male Pers. No.	No. in House	Female Pers. No.	No. in House
Head	1	1	-	-
Spouse	-	-	5	1
Children	3	1, 2, etc.	6	1, 2, etc.
Other relations	2	1, 2, etc.	4	1, 2, etc.
Other residents	7	1, 2, etc.	8	1, 2, etc.

So, male head of household is 11, 2nd female child is 62. The last
four digits are month and year of birth - 0812 for August, 1912.

        Male head of household born in August 1912
                110812

APPENDIX C.

Signals:

Colors

Red   1. Entered this month
Blue   2. Lost this month (record reason under "Disposition")
Yellow   3. Death - this month
Orange   4. Cases of special significance (diabetes, epilepsy,
                 tuberculosis, etc.)
Green   5. Served at least once this month.

FHM #1

At the same time, a Monitor Sheet (FHM #1) will be kept as a running record of progress in taking on families. Only study families will be entered.

FHM #1   Monitor

Item	Explanation
HIP No.	Subscriber number (1, 2, 3, 8, or 9 million)
Household Name	Subscriber Name (Last)
Dates	Letter, interview, or other means used.

Disposition Dates
   Not Accepted
   Accepted
	
	Give reason under "remarks"
	Assign FHM No. as follows:
	   First digits year entered - 2 ('52)
	                             3 ('53)
	                             4 ('54)

FHM #2

The household record form is to be kept as a front sheet in the family folder. The front of the form will include the following information:

FHM #2 - Household Roster

Item	Explanation
Surname	HIP subscriber
Color	W-white, O-other
Religion	J-Jewish, C-Catholic, P-Protestant, O-Other
Date Entered	Mo/Yr accepted FHM
FHM No.	4 digits, e.g., 6th household 1952 - 2106
HIP No.	Subscriber No. (1, 2, 3, 8, 9 million)
Total Household	No. persons in household
Total HIP insured	No. HIP insured persons

Household Composition

Person	First and last name (if different from HIP family surname)

252

| Relationship | Wife, son, daughter, aunt, or exact relation, or no relation. |

| Dates and Reasons for Changes | Explain changes, if any, and give dates |

On the back will be entered the services as rendered, according to the following:

Service Record

Date	Date seen
Place	1 - office, 2 - home, 3 - hospital, 4 - telephone
Name and Birthdata	List in each column name and birthdata for each household person - begin with HIP insured family (male head, wife; first child, second child, etc., other direct family, others)
Date Entered	List in each column the household status, month and year each person entered study.

| Item | Explanation |
| Services | A letter to designate the person rendering the service is prefixed to the number. |

Letters:
P - General physician
C - Consultant physician
S - Social worker
N - Nurse
X - Psychologist

Numbers:
1 - Routine or study visit
2 - Immunization only
3 - Teaching service - individual or group
4 - Illness (new)
5 - Illness (continuation or follow-up)
6 - Informal (contact out of office, or in office in conjunction with other family member contact)
7 - Telephone communication with study family
8 - Staff meeting on behalf of family
9 - Miscellaneous - Telephone or letter to other agency or other agency conference on behalf of family.

Examples:
"X 1" - routine psychological test
"P 4" - physician first visit for an illness.

253

APPENDIX C.

FHM #3 (Workers Daily Report)

Fill in one sheet for each family on the day seen. Check the appropriate service space. The carbon should be used by the worker for rough notes preparatory to entry on the clinical record.

From the original, the clerk will make an entry into the "Daily Log." This journal will contain the lists of daily services. (The carbon of FHM #3 can be destroyed, the original filed.)

FHM #4

Monthly summary of the workers daily reports.

Evaluation Form and Procedures

* * * *

Montefiore Hospital
INDIVIDUAL EVALUATION SUMMARY

3M 7-57   DATE

Family Member   Birth Data   Initial   Subsequent   Final

    AREA   SCORE   C O M M E N T S

   I. Family
      History

  II. Physical   A
      Condition   B

 III. Nutrition

  IV. Sleep and
      Rest

   V. Personal
      Adjustment

  VI. Relationship
      with
      (Husband),
      (Father)

      (Wife)
      (Mother)

      (Children)
      (Siblings)

 VII. Occupational   A
      Adjustment   B

VIII. Education

  IX. Recreation

   X. Housing

* * * *

Instructions for Completing Individual Evaluation Summary (FHM #5)
   Insert the appropriate number in the column marked "SCORE".
   Underline or circle appropriate answers in check sheets.

APPENDIX D.

1. Family history of longevity, parents and grandparents lived to be over 75.

2. No family history of major diseases; however, there may be a history of minor illnesses including those of a hereditary nature that are not life-shortening, such as allergy or otosclerosis, in one or both lines.

3. Family history of disease with hereditary aspects, life shortening major illness, restricted to one side of family.

4. Family history of disease, with hereditary aspects, in many members of both lines, life-shortening, disabling, major diabetes, cancer or recognized familial diseases.

II. PHYSICAL CONDITION (See Appendix A - Work Sheet "Outline for Routine Physical Examination")

    A) PAST MEDICAL HISTORY

        1. Previous medical history negative.
        2. Medical history of minor disease only.
        3. History of major disease.
        4. Many major illnesses, continuous pattern of illness.

    B) PRESENT PHYSICAL CONDITION

        1. Excellent physical condition, skin and muscle tone good.

        2. Physical condition good, no defects, a previous illness controlled or halted.

        3. A major disease susceptible of improvement, control possible, or minor remediable defects. Also where major diseases previously not under control, are now under control.

        4. More than one major disease. Uncontrolled or uncontrollable, progressive major illness.

        Major defects must include irremediable conditions of such a character as to shorten life or threaten disability even if perfectly compensated at the time of examination; remediable defects, if so long neglected as to constitute a hazard to life or longevity (for example, marked overweight, over 25 per cent) and psychosomatic illnesses.

        Minor defects include diet, remediable defects of vision, hearing, tonsil enlargement, mild obesity (under 20 per cent), posture or musculo-skeletal defects as well as those irremediable defects that do not threaten life (for example, psoriasis).

History of rheumatic fever, for example - 11 A 3, B2
With mitral stenosis, never in failure -   "   " B3
   "   "   "   decompensating -   "   " B4
   "   "   "   compensated   -   "   " B3

III. NUTRITION (See dietary history)

    1. Excellent. Good eating habits and food selection. Nutritional status, excellent.

    2. Adequate. Weight and nutrition good but
      A) Defective eating habits.
      B) Past history of nutritional disorder

    3. Overweight, or underweight (20 per cent) or (B) Nutritional deficiency with poor eating habits or history of a nutritional disorder.

    4. Irremediable physical defects associated with nutritional defects and poor eating habits. (Here, we must include clinical vitamin deficiencies -- anemias, and serious disturbances of eating patterns.)

In arriving at the score, the following check sheet can be used:

    Degree to which diet selection conforms to standards of N.R.C.[+]:

      Entirely   Marginal   Unsatisfactory

    Degree to which eating habits are satisfactory:

      Entirely   Marginal   Unsatisfactory

    Weight limits according to M.L.I.C. Tables[++]:

      Normal   5% over or under   20% over or under

    Muscle tone: Excellent Good Fair Poor

    Vitamin or iron deficiency noted. Yes No

IV. SLEEP AND REST:

    1. Excellent. Energy level high; rest adequate (approximately ten hours per day for children under twelve or approximately eight hours for adults and children over twelve).

    2. Good. No impairment of function. Some irregularity of rest and sleep hours.

    3. Fair. Disturbance of sleep in rest hours; impairment of function; complaints of lassitude or mild insomnia or sleep disturbances.

    4. Excessive impairment of function. Severe insomnia or sleep disturbances.

+ Recommended dietary allowances, National Research Council Publication #129, 1948

++ Metropolitan Life Insurance Co. Publication, "Overweight and Underweight", 1950

APPENDIX D.

In arriving at the score, the following check sheet can be used:

Feels rested on rising: Yes   No

Fatigue in middle of day: Usually   Sometimes   Never

Insomnia or other sleep disturbance: Yes   No

Amount of rest needed: Below   Above
                          Average   Average

V. PERSONAL ADJUSTMENT

1. Excellent. Constructive responses to reality, adapta-
     bility. Satisfaction derived from several aspects of
     living. Solid self-esteem, long range goals capable
     of fulfillment. Expanding areas of satisfaction.

2. Adequate adjustment. Mild tension or anxiety may be
     present. Satisfaction derived from some aspects of
     living. Fluctuating self-esteem. Little expansion of
     areas of satisfaction.

3. Emotional disturbance severe enough to interfere with ac-
     tivity. Severe difficulties in one particular area of
     function[+] and mild curtailment of several other areas,
     or overt anxiety which creates difficulties in func-
     tioning in any one area. Exaggerated positive or nega-
     tive self-evaluation.

4. Emotionally disabled. Severe impairment of function. In-
     ability to work (attend school). Social isolation.

     (Under (4) major defects would include severe neurotic
     behavior or psychosis.)

In arriving at the score, the following check sheet can be used.
   (Adult)

1. Life is generally regarded as worthwhile: Yes   No

2. Feelings of inferiority: Widespread   Limited   Absent

3. Compulsive or ritualistic behavior: Marked   Moderate
     Little or None

+ Definitions: "Areas of Function" are those having to do with
     the carrying out of (1) adult responsibilities (relating
     to job, home, community), and (2) pleasure giving activi-
     ties (sex, recreation, etc.).

     (Interpersonal relations, as an area of functioning, sub-
     sumed under both (1) and (2).

258

4. Manifest anxiety or tension: Marked   Moderate   Little or None

5. Aware of anxiety: Yes   No

6. Social isolation: Complete   Partial   Not at all

7. Parents (dead or alive) seem to play a controlling role:
   Markedly   Moderately   Little or None

8. Physical illness disturbs functioning: Markedly
   Moderately   Little or None

9. Sexual relationship is a source of friction between the
   partners: Markedly   Moderately   Little or None at all

10. Sexual problems can be discussed by partners: Yes   No

(Child)

1. Emotional disturbance in school adjustment:
   Markedly   Moderate   Little or None

2. Usually plays with older or younger children (even when
   children of own age are available): Yes   No

3. Has friends: Yes   No

4. Sees his parents as approving and supportive:
   Usually   Occasionally   Rarely or Never

5. Physical evidences of emotional disturbance: Yes   No

6. Speech disturbances (not organically based):   Yes   No

7. Sleep disturbances (nightmares, sleepwalking): Yes   No

8. Disturbances in elimination: Yes   No

9. Compulsive or ritualistic behavior: Marked-Moderate
   Little or None

10. Nailbiting (including tics) or thumb sucking inappropri-
    ate to age: Yes   No

11. Negativism or stubborness (if inappropriate to age):
    Usually   Occasionally   Rarely or Never

12. Withdrawn: Markedly   Moderately   Little or not at
    all

13. Fear of physical injury: Marked   Moderate   Little
    or not at all

14. Provokes hostility from others (teases, ridicules, etc.):
    Frequently   Occasionally   Never

15. Hostility or aggression: Marked   Moderate   Little
    or none at all

16. Feelings of inferiority: Widespread   Limited   Absent

APPENDIX D.

VI. FAMILY RELATIONSHIPS

1. Wholesome relationship. Shared interests, supportive in crisis situations, acceptance⁺ (of spouse, child, sibling, parent) as an individual with those rights culturally defined as belonging to spouse, child, sibling, parent.

2. Some evidence of maladjustment in relationship. Some dissatisfaction with functioning (of spouse, child, siblings, parents), limited shared interests, insufficient support in crisis (for spouse or siblings), too demanding of performance (of children or parents) in some areas.

3. Hostility, unusual attachment, undue dependency, detached relationship with spouse, or self abasement. Harsh punitive relationship or lack of interest.

4. Indifference or extremely limited emotional relationship. No areas of shared interest or communication, complete rejection (of parent, child, sibling, or spouse).

In arriving at the score, the following check sheet can be used:
(Spouse)

1. Work schedules or outside interests interfere with contacts: Markedly   Moderately   No more than customary

2. Shared interests: Many   Some   Few or none

3. Dissatisfaction or depreciation: Marked   Moderate   Little or none

4. Communication: Considerable   Limited   None

5. Dependency: Marked   Moderate   Little or none

6. Controlling or demanding: Markedly   Moderately   Little or not at all

7. Emotional support in crisis situations: Dependable   Variable   Absent

8. Valuation of spouse: Essentially positive   Mixed   Essentially negative

9. Feeling of acceptance: Usually   Occasionally   Seldom or never

10. Expression of hostility or aggressiveness: Direct (in behavior)   Mixed   Indirect

⁺ Acceptance refers to sympathetic understanding and a capacity to identify with another person. Acceptance in this sense is to be distinguished from acceptance of responsibilities with respect to another person.

260

11. Hostility or aggression: Marked   Moderate   Little or none at all

12. Submissiveness: Marked   Moderate   Little or none at all

(Parent - Child)

1. Parent is remote or detached: Markedly   Moderately Little or not at all

2. Parent is interested in the child's activities: Considerable   Moderately   Little or not at all

3. Parent spends time with child: Frequently   Occasionally Rarely or never

4. Parent is controlling and demanding: Markedly   Moderately Little or not at all

5. Parent's discipline: Harsh   Moderate   Absent

6. Parent rejects child: Yes   No

7. Parent's valuation of child: Essentially positive   Mixed Essentially negative

8. Parent recognizes achievement: Considerably   Moderately Little or not at all

9. Parent gives emotional support in critical times: Considerably   Moderately   Little or not at all

10. Parent encourages assertiveness and independent action: Yes   No

11. Child is loved and accepted: Yes   No

12. Child feels loved and accepted: Yes   No

(Siblings)

1. Excessive sibling rivalry: Yes   No

2. Valuation of sibling: Over-valued   Appropriate   Under-valued

3. Submissiveness or complaint behavior with respect to sibling: Marked   Moderate   Little or not at all

VII. OCCUPATIONAL ADJUSTMENT   (Enter score for adjustment to second job, if individual is carrying such, or role of housewife, under "B").

1. Constructive adaptation to the reality of the work situation.⁺   Assumed responsibilities appropriate to the

+ Definition: The "reality of the work or job situation" refers to (A) the content of the work itself (tasks, activities related to the job) and (B) the social relationships (employer-employee, employer-supervisor, employee-employee, employee-union) on the job.

APPENDIX D.

job. Shows planfulness; is efficient and well-organized with regard to expenditure of time and energy. Experiences considerable satisfaction in connection with the job.

2. Good adjustment with some difficulty in adapting constructively to one or more reality aspects of the job situation. Some inefficiency and lack of planning exists. Experiences satisfaction in connection with the job, although some dissatisfaction is definitely present.

3. Inadquate adaptation to the requirements of the job. Assumes some job-connected responsibilities, but is erratic and unstable in this respect. Planfulness is not coordinated with reality. Inappropriate investment of time and energy. Few satisfactions found in work.

4. Poor adjustment to the job situation, or failure to accept the responsibilities inherent in the job. No planfulness. Strong dissatisfaction is present.

In arriving at the score, the following check sheet can be used:

Satisfaction derived from work: Considerable   Moderate   Little or none

Would prefer some other type of work: Yes   No

Place of work is physically satisfactory according to patient: Yes   No

Salary is source of job dissatisfaction: Markedly   Moderately   Little or not at all

Limitations on advancement are source of job dissatisfaction: Markedly   Moderately   Little or not at all

Relations with boss or supervisors: Excellent   Fair   Poor

Relations with co-workers: Excellent   Fair   Poor

Relations with subordinates: Excellent   Fair   Poor

Job changes within past 5 years: Many   Some   None

Fatigue after working usual hours: Marked   Moderate   Little or none

Expenditure of time and energy on job: Appropriate   Inappropriate

VIII. EDUCATION (Children only)

1. School grade of age. Participates actively in classroom. (Educational activities).

262

2. School grade of age. Adequate participation in class-room activities.

3. Some failures, or moderately below age level of accomplishment. Little or no participation in classroom activities.

4. Failing, serious educational problem.

IX. RECREATION

1. Engages in recreational activities in accordance with needs.

2. Recreational activities are not entirely satisfactory in kind or amount.

3. A) Recreational activities are distinctly unsatisfactory in kind and amount.

   B) No recreational activities but recognizes great areas of need.

4. No recreational activities and no recognition of need.

Note: "Activity" as used here means game, sport or hobby, and need not involve physical exercise.

Community activities and educational or cultural interests would be considered recreational. The area of recreation should be noted under "remarks".

List below organizations and if active in them.

X. HOUSING (See Appendix D "Housing")

1. Excellent - Positive advantages in space, ventilation, lighting, lack of hazards and defects. Community facilities available.

2. Adequate - No hazards, but one or two non-basic deficiencies such as:

   Walk-up above second floor or
   Crowding index 1 per/room or
   No play space or
   No laundry facilities on premises or
   No sunlight, but daylight in at least one room or
   No grocery store or playground in neighborhood.

3. Inadequate - No hazards, but several deficiencies as listed below:

   Crowding index 1.5 persons/room or
   No room for general living purposes or

APPENDIX D.

> Psychologically poor sleeping arrangements[+] or
> Daylight obstructed by adjoining buildings.

4. Poor - Basic deficiencies such as:

> Crowding index above 1.5 persons/room or
> Less than 40 sq. ft. sleeping area/person or
> Basic sanitary facilities lacking or shared or
> Outside window lacking in any room or
> Major maintenance defects or accident hazards.

Criteria derived from A.P.H.A. Committee on Housing (1946) Standards.

+ "Psychologically poor sleeping arrangements" includes (A) arrangement in which parents and child over 1 share bedroom, (B) siblings sharing bedroom where age disparity exceeds 5 years, (C) siblings of different sexes sharing bedroom.

FAMILY HEALTH MAINTENANCE DEMONSTRATION

Outline for Doctor's Interview

Man as an Individual

  I Sexual History

    1. Age of first sexual experience
    2. Circumstances
        a) Older girl
        b) Girl procured by older boy
    3. Sexual Dysfunction
        a) Impotence
        b) Premature ejaculation
        c) Retarded ejaculation
        d) Hypersexuality
            1. Repeated need for intercourse during each ex-
               perience

  II Marital Relationship

    a) Does he get permission from his wife
    b) How much control does wife exercise over sexual contacts

Woman as an Individual

  I Sexual History

    1. Age of first sexual experience
    2. Circumstances
    3. Sexual Dysfunction
        A. Sexual inhibition
            1. Shyness or fear of men
            2. Phobic fear of venereal disease or cancer

        B. Frigidity
            1. Inability to achieve orgasm
            2. Inability to enjoy sexual act
            3. Feelings of disgust, shame and self devalua-
               tion

        C. Fear of Injury

        D. Painful coitus or vaginismus

  II Marital Relationship
    1. How much control does husband exercise in relationships
    2. Does wife ever initiate contact

  III Menarche

    1. Age of onset
    2. Preparation by mother or other figure
    3. Difficulties if any and when occurred
        A. Soon after menarche
        B. Marriage or when

265

4. Duration of flow
    A. Woman's estimation of flow
5. Feelings
6. Periods missed or unusual
    A. Any change in life situation at that time
7. Euphoria or depression associated with menstruation

FAMILY HEALTH MAINTENANCE DEMONSTRATION

Outline for Routine Physical Examination Procedure

1. Cornell Medical Index

2. History

3. Complete physical including rough visual and auditory

4. Complete blood count including sedimentation rate, urinalysis

5. Chest x-ray

6. Electrocardiogram

If over 30

    1) with family history of early cardiovascular disease
        Blood cholesterol

If over 40 (not mandatory)

    1) Every six months - breast examinations in women

    2) Every year proctoscopy

    3) Every year electrocardiogram

If over 40

    1) with family history of diabetes - 2 hr. glucose tolerance

If over 50

    1) Routine ocular tension every year

(Chart Form)

THE MONTEFIORE HOSPITAL

Medical Group

G.A.

Height: Weight:

Head: Skull: No abnormality. No tenderness.

         Eyes: External.
                    Pupils round, regular, equal, react to L and
                       A.

                    Conjunctivae   Sclerae
                    No exophthalmos, lidlag, or stare. EOM
                       normal.

         Fundi:

         Ears: Hearing normal.
                    Canals,   drums,

         Nose: Externally neg.
                    No sinus tenderness.

         Mouth: Teeth

                    Tongue

         Pharynx:

                    Tonsils

                    Mucous membranes

Neck: Trachea in midline, freely movable.
         Thyroid

                              Pulsations

         Cervical Veins

Lymph Nodes:

Chest: Configuration.
         Breasts.

         Lungs: Resonance unimpaired.
                    Breath sounds unaltered
                    Fremitus normal.
                    No rales.
                    Bases move freely.

         Heart: PMI
                    No enlargement.
                    Sounds of good quality
                    No murmurs or thrills.
                    A2   P2.
                    Rhythm regular.

267

APPENDIX D.

Pulses: Equal, synchronous, regular, of good quality.
                   B. P.

Abdomen: Soft. No distention.
                   No tenderness or rigidity.
                   No masses or viscera felt.
                   No hernia.
                   No CVA tenderness.

Genitalia:
Pelvic:

Rectal:

Skin:

Extrem.:   No clubbing, cyanosis, or edema.
                   No tremor.
                   Peripheral pulses patent.

Skeletal: No percussion tenderness.   No deformity.
                   Joints.

Neurol: deep reflexes

                   Superficial reflexes.
                   No pathological reflexes.
                   Muscular and sensory status neg.
                   Cranial nerves intact.

Psychic:

IMPRESSION:

FAMILY HEALTH MAINTENANCE DEMONSTRATION

Functions of the Psychiatric Social Worker

I   Collect data (see outline of social worker's interview) on past and present functioning of families in the areas of work history, relationship between husband and wife, of parents to children, etc.

II   Interpret the above data to other team members in order to elicit a more complete understanding of the family, the individuals within the family, and to help the team use this knowledge as a basis for realistically meeting the needs of the family.

III   Help families or individuals within the family in the particular area of inter-personal functioning with which they are dissatisfied and where they recognize the need for change.

IV   Help families or individuals within the family to recognize those areas of which they are not as yet aware in which they could use help in order to function at a more satisfying level.

V   Interpret need for and help families to seek help from already existent community resources which would best meet their need as in the case of psychiatric treatment.

VI   Assist families in securing specialized services from other community resources such as home-maker services, day-camp, adult education, etc.

VII   Interpret to the family the results of psychological testing, particularly in the case of children and to assist them in working out a plan, which will best meet the needs of the child.

VIII   Participate in research aspects of the program such as development of criteria for measuring family changes; team relationships; and group education.

FAMILY HEALTH MAINTENANCE DEMONSTRATION

Outline for Social Worker's Interview

I Woman as an Individual

Background Information

1. Birthplace
2. Family composition
3. Family background - social, cultural, economic, etc.
4. Education
5. Relationship to siblings
6. Relationship to parents

269

APPENDIX D.

II Relationship to mother

    A. Doll play
       Amount and duration

    B. Perception of mother –
       interested in her or not

III Relationship to father

    A. Perception of father

       1. Interested in her
       2. Consulted about problems

    B. Opinion of father's relationship to mother

       1. Good husband and father or not

IV Pattern of discipline in own childhood

    A. How
    B. By whom
    C. Parent feared more and why

 V Dating – Practice and Procedure

    A. How permitted and under what circumstances by woman's
       own mother

VI Courtship

    A. How much control exercised by woman's mother in selec-
       tion of marital partner
    B. Where met husband
    C. Duration of courtship
    D. Why and how decision to be married
    E. Perception of courtship – as contrasted with actuality
       of marriage
       1. Happy or not, difficulty, etc.
       2. Pre-marital relationships
    F. Opposition or acceptance by fiancee's family

VII Marriage

    A. Circumstances
       1. Large wedding, church, etc.
       2. Who wanted it, bride, her family, groom, etc.
       3. Forced
    B. First or second marriage and circumstances
    C. Importance of man's economic role in the marriage

VIII Children

    A. How feel about raising a family
    B. How long need to wait for children
       1. Need for money in bank, etc.

 IX Pregnancy

    A. How long felt necessary to wait before becoming pregnant
       and why

B. Reason for having children
    1. accident
    2. planned
    3. social or religious pressure or own desire
C. Reaction to Pregnancy
    1. Weight gain
    2. Nausea
    3. Sexual contact - continued or not
    4. Fears about possible injury to child or self
    5. Suicidal impulses or aggressive feelings toward
       child
    6. Presence of hypochondriasis or depression
       A. Extreme concern over body and functioning
D. Delivery
    1. Instrument, "natural" childbirth, caesarian, etc.
    2. At time of delivery - feelings about having an-
       other child
    3. Fears if any about dying or child's dying
    4. Sex of child
       A. What hoped for
       B. Feelings re sex after birth of child
       C. Freedom in affection in relation to sex of
          children
    5. Labor - prolonged - how many hours and reasons

X Feeding

A. Breast Feeding
    1. Experience with own pediatrician
    2. Feelings about breast feeding
       a) Devaluation of self - reference to self as cow
       b) Child taking good out of mother
B. Bottle feeding
    1. Difficulties in formula
    2. Colic
    3. Schedule of feeding - demand, regular, etc.
    4. Weaning
       a) age
       b) how accomplished
       c) difficulties
C. Introduction of coarse foods
    1. At what age
    2. Difficulties in chewing, etc. How met.
D. How long did mother feed child
    1. Reasons for so doing
       a) easier
       b) kind and extent of interference with child's
          learning motor skills
       c) concern regarding dropping food and getting it
          on himself
E. Present status of child re eating
    1. Anorexia

        a) Does child refuse all foods or just certain type
        b) Will child eat other places beside home, only at home, not at home but outside
        c) Was child recently ill
        d) Is there any recent or present cause for tension in household or in past of child

  2. Vomiting
        a) At what time of day
        b) Relationship to meals or bed-time
        c) What member of family has been concerned with child at time of vomiting
        d) Reaction of mother or other person to vomiting
            1. disgust
            2. punished for it

  3. Overeating
        a) Child eats fairly continuously

XI Toilet Training

  1. At what age introduced
        a) feces
        b) urine
  2. Method used
        a) potty
        b) How approached - reward, punishment
        c) Mother's reaction
        d) Child's reaction
            1. Fear of toilet, dirt, etc.
            2. Constipation
                a) If child does not have daily excretion is he considered constipated or only if stools dry, bulky and produce discomfort or pain.
            3. Smearing of feces
                a) Age of onset and cessation
                b) Mother's reaction

XII Motor Development

  1. Sitting up, walking
        a) Age of onset
        b) Parents' evaluation
            1. Early or late
            2. Comparison with other children
  2. Speech
        a) Age of onset
        b) Parents' evaluation
            1. Early or late
            2. Worried over late learning
            3. Attempts to teach child
        c) Stammering or stuttering
            1. Age of onset
            2. Precipitating factors if any
                a) fright, etc.

3. Parents' handling of problem

XIII Temper Tantrums, Breath-Holding, etc.

    1. Age at which present
    2. Parents' reaction
    3. Can child be readily checked
    4. Will child accept substitute
    5. Under what circumstances do they appear

XIV Thumb Sucking, Nail Biting, Tics

    1. Onset
    2. Parents' reaction
    3. Parents' attempts to deal with habits

XV Nightmares and Fears
    1. Onset
    2. Frequency
    3. Precipitating situations
    4. Parents' reactions

XVI Accidents and Operations

    1. Proneness to injury
    2. Age and circumstances of injury or operation
    3. Preparation of child for surgery or hospitalization
    4. Reaction of child to experience

XVII Relationship to parents

    1. What opportunities for shared play or recreational ac-
       tivities with parents
          Example - story-telling, games, excursions, etc.
    2. Discipline
       a) Method
       b) Effectiveness
       c) Parent administering
       d) Situations calling forth discipline
    3. Favored parent
    4. Feared parent

XVIII Relationship to siblings

    1. Jealousy
    2. Aggressive
    3. Submissiveness and subjugation
    4. Derogatory

XIX Relationship to 3rd person in home such as grandparent

    1. Resentful or accepting of grandparents' authority
    2. Grandparent regarded as court of appeal
    3. Parent's evaluation of presence of grandparent in rela-
       tion to bringing up of own child
       a) Resentment
       b) Jealousy

APPENDIX D.

XX Child's adaptation to world outside family
  1. School
     a) Age when started
     b) Reaction to first experience
        2. Attitude toward school now
           a) Eager to go
           b) Unable to get up in time
              1. Parents' role in this
           c) Learning ability
              1. Disturbed
              2. Average or above
              3. Parental pressures
           d) Adjustment and personality
  2. Playmates
     a) Accepted by other children or not
     b) Bossy or submissive
     c) Fearful of fights
  3. Social groups - Scouts, clubs, etc.
     a) Why attend
        1. Parental wish or own desire
     b) Extent of participation
  4. Hobbies or other interests
     a) Music, reading, stamp collecting, etc.

XXI Marital Adjustment
  1. Is relationship mutually satisfactory or not
  2. If not - to whom and why
  3. Cultural attitudes which may influence lack of adjustment or attitudes about it
  4. Is there conflict between husband and wife in this area
  5. How free are they to discuss difficulties with one another

XXII Parentally
  1. How do they share responsibilities for children
  2. Is there conflict between them in the carrying out of their respective roles in the rearing of the children
  3. How does each see his role in relation to his own experience as a child
     a) Need to make up to the child for lacks in own childhood
     b) Emulation of patterns observed by own parents in relation to self as child
  4. Are they in agreement as to hopes and plans for children
  5. What is their conception of parental role
     a) Authoritarian, patriarchial, etc.

XXIII Work History
  1. If works - from conviction, necessity or both

274

2. How resolves problem of care of children
3. Type of work
4. Satisfactory or not in terms of what would like to do or would have liked to do
5. How arrived at choice of work
   A. Special education or apprenticeship
   B. Choice predicated on strong interest or not
      1. When developed and how manifested
         A. Hobbies, association with adults in field, etc.
      2. Influence of parents or other "key" adults
6. With whom does she work
   A. Fellow workers and feelings about them
   B. Relationships to those responsible to and responsible for
7. Does she feel her work is as important as husband's
8. Does she feel her work is meaningful
   A. Distinction between money, status, and work satisfaction
9. What is her idea of success
10. What types of work would never do and why
11. Strain of job regarded as injurious to health and life
12. Is she tired when gets up in morning
13. Is she exhausted at night
14. If housewife - does she feel work as homemaker important or not
    A. Overwhelmed by work
    B. Plans to return to work or not
       1. When and why
       2. Husband's feelings regarding this

XXIV Aspirations and Goals

1. Does she have a goal toward which working
2. Does she feel these are possible of fulfillment
3. Are these goals realistic
4. Are these goals acceptable or usual in terms of culture
5. Does she feel her husband and family are helping or hindering her in realization of goals

I Man as an Individual

Background Information

1. Birthplace
2. Family composition
3. Family background: social, cultural, economic, etc.
4. Education
5. Relationship to siblings
6. Relationship to parents

II Relationship to Mother
   A. Maternal control

        1. Interference with physical activities
          a) Prevention of participation in "dangerous" activities such as football, bicycling, etc.
    B. How father regarded by mother
        1. Change in status if European born father
        2. Emphasis by mother on not being like father

III Relationship to Father

    A. Interest in boy's educational and vocational plans
    B. Consulted in relation to sexual information
    C. Was he perceived as someone interested in boy's problems and was he supportive
    D. Did he spend time with boy in leisure time activities

IV Pattern of discipline in own childhood

    A. How
    B. By whom
    C. Parent feared more and why

V Dating - Practice and Procedure

    A. How much did mother interfere

VI Courtship

    A. How much control exercised by mother in selection of marital partner
    B. Where met wife
    C. Duration of courtship
    D. Why and how decision to be married
    E. Perception of courtship as contrasted with actuality of marriage
        1. Happy period, difficult, etc.
        2. Pre-marital relationship
    F. Opposition or acceptance by fiancee's family

VII Marriage

    A. Circumstances
        1. Large wedding
        2. Who wanted it
        3. Forced
    B. First or second marriage
    C. Importance of man's economic role in marriage

VIII Children

    A. How did he feel about raising a family
    B. How long need to wait for children
        1. Need for money in bank, etc.
    C. Reason for having children
        1. Accident
        2. Planned
        3. Social, religious, pressure or own desire

IX Work History

A. What does he do
B. Satisfactory or not in terms of what would like to do
C. How arrived at choice of work
    1. To what extent did his mother shape his choice
    2. Special education or apprenticeship
    3. Choice predicated on strong interest or not
        A. When developed and how manifested
            1. Hobbies, association with adults in field of work, etc.
        B. Influence of parents or other "key" adults
        C. Long range goal or one of many jobs
D. With whom does he work
    1. Fellow workers and feelings about them
    2. Relationships to those responsible to and those responsible for
E. If wife works, does he feel his work is as important as wife's
F. Does he feel his work is meaningful
    1. Distinction between money, status and work satisfaction
G. What is his idea of success
H. What kind of work would he never do and why
I. How does he feel he can get a better job
    1. Being sponsored
    2. Through pull
J. How much fear does he have about losing his job, not being able to support family, being unemployed
K. Is he tired when he gets up in morning to go to work
L. Is he exhausted at night on return
M. Is strain of job and work environment regarded as injurious to health and life

X Aspirations and Goals

    1. Does he have a goal toward which working
    2. Does he feel these are possible of fulfillment
    3. Are these goals realistic
    4. Are these goals acceptable or usual in terms of our culture
    5. Does he feel wife and family are helping or hindering in realization of goal

Relationship Between Husband and Wife

I Socially

    1. Do they go out together
    2. Has there been a change since marriage
    3. What is the family's cultural pattern in relation to this
    4. What is their place in the community
       Church affiliation and activity

School - PTA, etc.
Other groups - political, neighborhood, scouts, etc.
5. Is their present life satisfactory to both
6. Extent of visiting friends and relatives
7. Have children, if any, changed social picture and what is attitude of parents to this.

II Marital Adjustment
1. Is relationship mutually satisfactory or not
2. If not - to whom and why
3. Cultural attitudes which may influence lack of adjustment or attitudes about it
4. Is there conflict between husband and wife in this area
5. How free are they to discuss difficulties with one another

III Parentally
1. How do they share responsibilities for children
2. Is there conflict between them in the carrying out of their respective roles in the rearing of the children
3. How does each see his role in relation to his own experience as a child
   a) Need to make up to the child for lacks in own childhood
   b) Emulation of patterns observed by own parents in relation to self as child
4. Are they in agreement as to hopes and plans for children
5. What is their conception of parental role
   a) Authoritarian, patriarchial, etc.

FAMILY HEALTH MAINTENANCE DEMONSTRATION

Outline for Nurse's Interview

I Family as a Whole

Eating
1. Meal Pattern and behavior
2. Atmosphere at table
3. Forcing of foods, etc., with children
4. Anorexia (of any member)
   a) Times and circumstances

II Rest
1. What is pattern of sleep for all members
2. If children wake at night
   a) Get into bed with parents
   b) Other results
3. Hours and type of sleep
4. Difficulties in relation to bed time
5. Difficulties in arising
   a) Husband, wife, children
6. Feelings on arising

III Recreation
    1. Do family have any activities as group

IV Domestically
    1. How is the work around the house apportioned
    2. If wife works outside home, how does this affect the situation
    3. If they have help - what type
    4. Is there a third person in the home such as mother-in-law, and how does this enhance or detract from the total situation
    5. Finances
        How apportioned
        Division of responsibility
        Are expenditures discussed jointly or how
        Is there any open or concealed difficulty in this area

Woman as an Individual

I Recreation and Interests
    1. What does she like to do
        a) hobbies
        b) sports
        c) travel and vacation
    2. Does she do it
    3. Has marriage changed interests and how
    4. Are her interests source of conflict between husband and self

Man as Individual

I Recreation and Interests
    1. What does he like to do
        a) hobbies
        b) sports
        c) travel and vacation
    2. Does he do it
    3. Has marriage changed interests and how
    4. Are interests source of conflict between wife and self

FAMILY HEALTH MAINTENANCE DEMONSTRATION

Outline of the role of the public health nurse in the joint
evaluation of the health of families

I Pertinent observations of health aspects of physical home environment

    1. Housing
        a) Location and type
        b) Adequacy of space, light, ventilation, heat and sanitation
        c) Safety measures and accident hazards

279

APPENDIX D.

        d) Living arrangements with relation to health limita-
           tions of individuals in family

II Evaluation of family's knowledge and practices of basic principles of healthful living with regard to changing needs of
  infants, children, adolescents, adults and aged persons.

    1. Nutrition
      a) Knowledge of nutritional requirements
      b) Adequacy of diet
      c) Cooking skills and facilities
      d) Food selection - cultural patterns
      e) Eating habits
      f) Meal planning
      g) Availability and use of marketing resources
      h) Budgeting

    2. Sleep and rest
      a) Facilities available
      b) Arrangements
      c) Adequacy of established routines

    3. Posture - Knowledge of body mechanics in relation to
      basic principles of good posture.

    4. Personal hygiene
      a) Personal habits with regard to care of skin, hair,
        elimination, etc.
      b) Individual habits with regard to use of stimulants,
        tobacco and drugs.

    5. Dental hygiene
      a) Dental care
      b) Knowledge of relation of nutrition to dental hygiene

    6. Recreation
      a) Type and amount
      b) Facilities and equipment available in home and com-
        munity

III Pertinent observations of health practices with relation to
  home management
      a) Knowledge of application of homemaking skills
      b) Housekeeping facilities
      c) Knowledge and use of basic principles of body
        mechanics in housekeeping activities
      d) Planning of household routine to permit rest, relax-
        ation and recreation

IV Evaluation of family's knowledge of community medical, social
  and recreational resources and ability to use these wisely for
  promotion and maintenance of health.

280

V Evaluation of family's knowledge and application of basic principles of first-aid and home nursing care in illness and accident situations.
   1. Medicine chest supplies for first aid.

VI Observation of the supervision and care of children

VII Observation of general atmosphere in home with regard to the family's interpersonal relationships in action.

VIII Occupational health hazards
   1. Type and conditions of work with regard to fatigue, accident hazards, smoke, fumes, noise, intense heat or cold, etc.

APPENDIX D.

TABLE OF DESIRABLE WEIGHTS
FOR MEN of ages 25 and over*

HEIGHT (with shoes on) 1-inch heels		SMALL FRAME	MEDIUM FRAME	LARGE FRAME
Feet	Inches			
5	2	116-125	124-133	131-142
5	3	119-128	127-136	133-144
5	4	122-132	130-140	137-149
5	5	126-136	134-144	141-153
5	6	129-139	137-147	145-157
5	7	133-143	141-151	149-162
5	8	136-147	145-156	153-166
5	9	140-151	149-160	157-170
5	10	144-155	153-164	161-175
5	11	148-159	157-168	165-180
6	0	152-164	161-173	169-185
6	1	157-169	166-178	174-190
6	2	163-175	171-184	179-196
6	3	168-180	176-189	184-202

FOR WOMEN of ages 25 and over*

2-inch heels		SMALL FRAME	MEDIUM FRAME	LARGE FRAME
4	11	104-111	110-118	117-127
5	0	105-113	112-120	119-129
5	1	107-115	114-122	121-131
5	2	110-118	117-125	124-135
5	3	113-121	120-128	127-138
5	4	116-125	124-132	131-142
5	5	119-128	127-135	133-145
5	6	123-132	130-140	138-150
5	7	126-136	134-144	142-154
5	8	129-139	137-147	145-158
5	9	133-143	141-151	149-162
5	10	136-147	145-155	152-166
5	11	139-150	148-158	155-169

For girls between 18 and 25, substract 1 lb. for each year under 25.

*These tables are based on numerous Medico-Actuarial studies of
   hundreds of thousands of insured men and women. Weight given
   in pounds according to frame (as ordinarily dressed).

FAMILY HEALTH DEMONSTRATION
Directions for Diet Questionnaire

PART I on Page One -

Please record all the food you ate for one 24-hour period.
Read carefully the following instructions before you start:

1. Write down everything you eat or drink. Remember to include candy, soft drinks, ice cream, cookies or crackers.
If you skip a meal, write in "nothing" for that meal.

2. Be sure to say how the food is cooked -- for example,
fried or broiled meat; baked, mashed or french-fried pota-
to. When food is eaten raw, be sure to say so.

3. When two foods are eaten together, write down both -- like
this:
1 piece whole wheat toast spread heavy or light with
margarine or butter.

4. Write down how much you eat of each food -- tell as near
as possible how many teaspoonfuls or tablespoons, or 1/4,
1/2 or 1 cupful.

5. Name the kind of food you eat -- that is, if you eat
cereal, write oatmeal, cornflakes, or whatever the kind.
Other examples might be split pea soup, mixed raw vegetable
salad, 2 slices enriched white bread, etc.

6. Please list the amount and kind of food supplements, such
as 1 teaspoon cod liver oil, 1 vitamin capsule, 10 drops of
vitamin preparation, 1 tablespoon wheat germ, 1 yeast tab-
let, etc. If you take none of these, write in "nothing".

7. Be sure to write down the approximate time of the three
regular meals and the in-between meals.

PART II on Page 2 -

Please record the number of times a week you eat the various
foods listed. Please note that:

Green and yellow vegetables include such foods as kale, lettuce,
chicory, escarole, spinach, string beans, broccoli, green pep-
pers, beet tops, asparagus, green peas, squash, carrots, sweet
potatoes.

Other vegetables include: Corn, lima beans, beets, cabbage,
brussel sprouts, cauliflower, cucumbers, onions, turnips.

Food supplements include cod liver oil, vitamin preparations,
iron, iron and liver preparations, wheat germ, yeast.

283

APPENDIX D.

DIET QUESTIONNAIRE

Food Record for 24 Hours

Name

Date   Day of the Week

Breakfast   Time

Between breakfast and noon meal   Time

Noon Meal

Between Noon and Evening Meal   Time

Evening Meal   Time

After Evening Meal: Time

Food Supplements:

Medications:

1. What foods disliked:
2. List foods which cause rash, other allergic reactions, or any
   distress:
3. Do you consider your food pattern good   fair   poor
4. Have your eating habits changed recently
5. What is your usual weight   . Any sign of change recently?
6. Have you ever been on a special diet?
7. How many glasses of water do you usually drink daily
8. Do you take laxatives?   If so, how often:
9. Tobacco, amount used daily
10. Average hours sleep daily   . Rest periods
11. Average hours fresh air and sunshine   weekly.

Weekly Food Record

Milk   glasses per day
Milk (in cooking)   X per week.
Cheese   X per week. Kinds

Oranges, grapefruit or juice of   X per week.
Tomatoes or juice of   X per week.
Dried fruit (raisins-prunes, apricots, etc.)   X per week.
Fresh fruit   X per week.
Canned or frozen fruit   X per week.

Cereal (cooked)   X per week
Cereal (dry)   X per week
Bread, white   slices per day. Rye sl. per day. Wh. wheat sl.
  per day.
Spaghetti, macaroni, or rice   X per week.

Vegetables, cooked   X per week
Vegetables, raw   X per week
*Green and yellow vegs.   X per week
*Other vegetables,   X per week
Potatoes   X per week.

Eggs   No. per week.
Meat or fish   X per week. Liver or kidneys   X per month
Dried peas, beans or lentils   X per week.
Nuts, peanut butter   X per week.

Butter or margarine, on bread. Heavy   Light
  As seasoning - Yes   No
Mayonnaise on bread   X per week: In salads   X per week.
Fats and oils in cooking   X per week.
Other fats (cream, sweet or sour, etc.)   X per week.

Sugar   Tsp. in beverages per day.   Tsp. on cereal per week.
Cake, pastry, cookies.   X per week.
Ice cream   x per week.
Syrups, honey, molasses, jam, jelly   X per week.
Candy   Amt. per week.

Coffee   cups per day
Tea   cups per day
Soft drinks   amt. per week.
Beer   amt. per week.
Other alcoholic beverages   X per week.

*Food Supplements   X per week.

Note: See explanations on instruction sheet.

APPENDIX D.

Date

Evaluation of Housing

Apartment #

Name

Rent

I. Family Composition:

_____ Adults
_____ Children
_____ 2 or more basic family units

II. Location:

_____ Congested   _____ Semi-Suburban
_____ Residential   _____ Business District

III. Type of Building:

Apartment House
_____ Floor elevated
_____ Floor walk-up
_____ Central heating
_____ Cold water flat

Private House
_____ Apt. in private house
_____ Attached house
_____ Detached house
_____ 2 or more stories
_____ Bungalow

IV. Size of Family Unit:

_____ Rooms to Unit

Dimensions in square feet:	Kitchen	Dining Room	Foyer	Living Room	Sun Porch or Den	Bed Rms.
						__ __ __

V. Crowding Index:

_____ one or less persons per room.
_____ 1 - 1 1/2 persons per room.
_____ more than 1 1/2 persons per room.
_____ 1 room for general purposes.
_____ no room for general purposes.

Sleeping area:

_____ 40 or more square feet per person.
_____ Less than 40 square feet per person.

Sleeping Arrangements:

_____ parents have own room.
_____ each child has own room.
_____ children same sex share room.
_____ children under 6 yrs. of opposite sex share same room ___ own beds, ___ same bed.
_____ children over 6 yrs. of opposite sex share same room ___ own beds, ___ same bed.
_____ child over 6 mos. share room with parents.
_____ child or children share bed with adult.

286

Play space in unit

_____ definite play space provided in the home.
_____ definite play space not provided in the home.

VI. Household Facilities:

Standard sanitary facilities (toilet, wash basin-tub or shower)

_____ family
_____ shared

Standard kitchen facilities (installed sink - stove - refrigerator)

_____ family
_____ shared

Laundry facilities

_____ installed tub or washing machine on premises.
_____ No facilities on premises.

Closet facilities

_____ 1 closet for every room
_____ Less than one closet in every room
_____ No closets

VII. Light and Air

_____ at least one outside window in each room
_____ exposure affording sunlight part of day in at least one room
_____ exposure affording daylight part of the day in at least one room
_____ daylight obstructed by adjoining structures

VIII. Maintenance (major defects such as broken plumbing; falling plaster, large holes in floor or walls)

_____ bathroom
_____ kitchen
_____ other rooms

IX. Accident Hazards

_____ cluttered fire escapes
_____ cluttered or unguarded stairs (including cellar stairways)
_____ stair treads in poor repair
_____ hand rails present at staircases
_____ dark hallways or staircases
_____ no protection at staircase for toddlers
_____ cluttered halls or rooms
_____ highly waxed floors
_____ defective electric wiring
_____ gas leaks

287

APPENDIX D.

Neighborhood Resources:

Stores

_____ Grocery stores (including large chain stores) in immediate neighborhood (within 6 blocks)
_____ No Grocery stores (including large chain stores) in
immediate neighborhood (within 6 blocks)
_____ No Grocery stores (including large chain stores) in
immediate neighborhood, but family use car for shop-
ping.

Elementary School

_____ Number of blocks from home
_____ Bus provided
_____ Bus not provided
_____ Car pool

Play Area

_____ Play area or park in immediate neighborhood (within
6 blocks)
_____ No play area or park in immediate neighborhood (within 6 blocks)

PSYCHOLOGICAL TESTING

Thematic Apperception Test, Children's Apperception Test and Per-
ceptual Test material will be classified in the following terms:

1. Function carried out with tension associated with it.
   Marked   Moderate   Mild

2. Distortions in function: Marked   Moderate   Mild
   (Included under distortions of function are instances where
   a variety of precautionary practices are necessary before
   activities can be carried out.)

3. Curtailment of function: Marked   Moderate   Mild

Areas of Functioning:

4. Self-Esteem: Adequate   Inadequate

5. Interpersonal: Dependency   Hostility   Empathy

6. Authority: Usually submissive   Usually rebellious
   Generally appropriate

7. Sex: Acceptance   Aversion   Ambivalence

Reaction to Testing:

8. Behavior: (a) Relaxed   Tense
              (b) Hostile   Friendly

288

9. Voice: (a) Relaxed   Tense
          (b) Friendly   Unfriendly

10. Reaction time: Abnormally fast or slow
                   Consistent or inconsistent

11. Speech flow: Free   Varying   Hesitant

12. Language: Concrete   Abstract
          (b) Appropriate effect   Inappropriate effect

APPENDIX E

Educational Program

PART I

(This section adapted from "Parent Group Education & Leadership Training - Three Reports", Child Study Association of America, 1952").

A. - Basic Goal

A better understanding of children's needs at different stages of development and of the parents' role and feelings toward their children during the process of growth, in order to bring about modification of parental attitudes.

There is evidence that in group meetings parents seem to gain (a) in understanding their children, (b) changed responses on their part to their children's behavior, (c) changes in their feelings about themselves in their parental role, and (d) changes in the behavior and feelings of the children. As parents gain insight they become better able to answer their own questions and find greater ease and satisfaction in their home relationships.

B. - Basic Technique

The sharing of ideas around common problems; conscious exposure to varied experiences from which choices suitable to individual needs and situations may be made. The focus is on exploring and learning from the common parental experience rather than discussing and working through individual problems.

C. - Education - Not Therapy

Therapy directs itself to the deviant aspects of personality, the symptoms or the character disturbance, with a view toward effecting change in individual pathology. Making use of a specific technique consciously applied, it approaches conflicts in order to free the energies bound within them, thus making these energies available for healthy growth.

Education is aimed at those faculties of the ego which are undisturbed by conflict. It is oriented toward the healthy factors of the personality, and appeals to the ability to judge, to learn by experience, to gain understanding, to plan, to make choices, to adapt to changing circumstances.

The term education, in connection with group experiences, is not used in the traditional sense of applying only to the intellectual capacities of the group members. Here the educational experience takes on a broader meaning. It recognizes the importance of feelings and attitudes and uses emotional mobilization as well as intellectual stimulation. It uses all the potent psychic factors of the educational process while maintaining an awareness of the difference between education and therapy.

290

And while in group education there is an awareness of individual problems and their effect on the parents' functioning,
the unconscious motivations of emotional problems are not explored nor are attempts made to resolve these problems.

D. - Content

Group discussion should concern itself with:

(1) An understanding of the growing child and his needs.
Increased understanding of the child's needs at different
stages of development, gained through sharing the experiences
of other parents, will help lay the groundwork for more adequate parent-child relationships. It will strengthen the
parent's knowledge that growing up is accomplished with much
experimentation on a trial and error basis, and will help him
view this experimentation with less anxiety.

(2) The conscious feelings of the parent toward the
child. The fullest expression of the parent's feelings of
pleasure and disappointment in the child gives him an opportunity to examine these feelings in comparison with those of
other parents and to shift his feelings and reactions as he
gains new recognition of his child's needs and of his response. Encouraging the expression of these feelings is
based on the belief that there is sufficient health for such
modification.

(3) Choices of reactions to the child. As suggested,
these open the way for modification of attitudes and behavior. In the give-and-take of the group discussion, the
parents will offer many explanations of any one situation,
and will give many reactions to one parent's way of handling
the child. A parent then can often come to see that his way
of reacting is really only his way; and the road is open for
further investigation of the many ways in which situations
can be met. The consideration of choices, their advantages
and disadvantages, should be encouraged continuously by the
leader. Each parent may not find the most suitable choice
immediately, but tentatively and with hesitation he explores
the many possibilities presented by the group until he comes
to the position in which he feels comfortable.

E. - Role of the Leader

(1) The group leader sets up a framework of discussion
in which the content is drawn from the members' own experiences. Thus the discussion is not developed in reaction to
theoretical questions but is an expression of the real-life
situations experienced by the members.

(2) The leader encourages the members to express their
feelings as well as their ideas, so that the group experience
becomes both emotional and intellectual, and thus one in
which thinking and feeling come to be clarified and inte-
grated.

291

(3) The leader serves to help the individuals in the group move together in their relationship to each other. Recognizing that they first come together to solve a common task or problem, he acts as a catalyst, helping the process to develop, giving them encouragement to share experiences they face and to make significant contributions to one another.

(4) The leader's contribution is to help the group toward its own independent thinking, rather than to take it upon himself to answer questions. He should not lecture, but should summarize here and there, building up general statements and formulating principles of agreement out of the material and experience presented by the group. The group leader thus helps the group members to come to formulations of their own, developing specific ideas which they can translate into their attitudes and relationships.

(5) He guides the discussion by selecting points from the material produced by the group to which the group is helped to react in a more adequate way. It is here that the leader has the responsibility of underlining those contributions of group members which evidence strength and healthy attitudes.

(6) He brings out from the group again and again that there are many different ways in which one can react to situations, in the light of the best understanding of the child and family relations. These choices are reassuring; they need not be threatening. They can also lead to a fuller awareness of a child's real needs, since inevitably they lead, not just to other answers, but to better answers, made on the basis of more selection.

(7) The leader meets all the material directly. He does not avoid a topic merely because it reveals anxiety; his very avoidance would indicate that the topic is dangerous and would tend to increase the parents' anxiety.

(8) Material introduced by group members as a minor point or side issue may suggest to the leader a significant area for further exploration; this, however, should be encouraged only when the group is ready to relate to it, to absorb it, and not before. Furthermore, the group dynamic process is such that a group may introduce too many questions and bring up too many problems, stimulating more response in each member than can adequately be met. The task of the group leader is to limit the number of questions so that those that are raised can be developed to the point where the problems are understood emotionally and intellectually. In this way he avoids the creation of additional anxieties.

(9) If the leader postpones discussion of a topic suggested by the group, he should share with the group the

reasons for this, and get their consent. Otherwise the group
will feel that (a) the leader is too controlling; (b) too re-
jecting and/or (c) the leader is reacting in personal terms
to the subject, rather than responding to the ability of the
group to understand and deal with it.

PART II

A. - Method

All families on the program will be invited to a first meeting
October 29, in the Patients' Library at the hospital. Return
postal cards will be enclosed. The general purpose and procedure are to be announced. A film (probably "Family Circles")
will be shown and discussion stimulated so as to demonstrate
the essential nature of the educational program, and to define
a particular area of discussion for the subsequent meeting.
The actual mechanics will, to some extent, be influenced by
the number of persons attending and the room arrangements.
Various discussion aids may be employed, ranging from movies
to puppets, from parent panels to role-playing. For the first
meeting sufficient copies of the pamphlet "A Healthy Personality for Your Child" will be available for distribution.

B. - Staff Involvement

It is expected that various key members of the service team -
family doctor, pediatrician, nurse, social worker - will become intimately involved in the discussions either as leaders
or straight discussants. Benefit to the F.H.M.D. will be
fourfold. (1) The experience and understanding of these
staff members will be available for pooling in the discussions. (2) Parents may reveal in speech and attitude aspects
of family health of importance to the staff but which might
not as readily be made evident elsewhere. (3) Patients may
be encouraged to seek counsel and guidance from the staff
more readily, or more often and in areas previously avoided.
(4) Staff members may become more sensitive and effective
educators.

Before the first meeting the staff will receive copies of
"Parent Group Education and Leadership Training" issued by
the Child Study Association of America, "A Healthy Personality
for Your Child" (a booklet based on the 1950 Midcentury White
House Conference on Children and Youth, and intended for
parent groups), and a "Discussion Aid" for this pamphlet, both
issued by the Children's Bureau, Federal Security Agency.

The Staff will also preview "Family Circles", and as before
each meeting to be held, will discuss procedures and materials

APPENDIX E.

to be used. It is also expected that an evaluation will follow each meeting.

Irving Shapiro
September 24, 1952

* * * *

No. _____   Date _____

FAMILY HEALTH MAINTENANCE DEMONSTRATION
Meeting Reaction Sheet

What did you think of this meeting? Please be frank. Your comments can contribute a great deal to our future meetings. You will
receive a copy of the summary of all the comments.

1. What did you like about today's meeting?

2. What did you dislike?

3. What improvements would you suggest in the operation of the
   next meeting?

4. Of the times you wanted to talk but did not, how many were
   because-------
   a. You couldn't break in when you wanted?   About____ times
   b. On the whole it didn't seem worth while? About____ times
   c. The group might not accept the contribution well?
                                                About____ times
   d. It would not have helped the group at that
      moment?   About____ times
   e. You couldn't phrase it well enough?   About____ times
   f. Someone else said it?   About____ times
   g. Reasons other than those listed here
      (please specify):

      _____   About____ times

      _____   About____ times

5. On the whole, how do you rate this meeting? (Check One)

No Good Mediocre All right Good Excellent

You do not need to sign your name.

* * * *

LIST OF MEETINGS CONDUCTED BY INDIVIDUAL TEAM MEMBERS

Obesity Clinic   Public Health Nurse
                                (Helene Ringenberger)

Teenagers Meetings   Doctor
                                (Dr. Robert S. Aaron)

294

Meetings With Mothers
   of preschool Children   Public Health Nurse
                       (Bertha Kahn)

Play Therapy Sessions   Psychiatric Social Worker
                       (Charlotte Stiber)

Meetings with Mothers   Psychiatric Social Worker
   of school children   (Hannah Bamberger)

* * * *

LIST OF GROUP MEETINGS AND DISCUSSION LEADERS

April 1, 1955

   About the Family Health Maintenance Demonstration

     Participants: George A. Silver, M.D.; Team Members;
               Irving Shapiro
     Questionnaires distributed.

December 5, 1955

   About the Family Health Maintenance Demonstration

     Film: "The Cure" (with Charlie Chaplin).

March 5, 1956

   PARENTS HAVE RIGHTS TOO

     Pamphlet: You Don't Have to be Perfect...even if you are
           a Parent, by Jean Schick Grossman

May 8, 1956

   YOUR CHILD IN YOUR FAMILY, Physical, Social, Emotional Growth
   (first of series of 3 meetings).

     Discussion Moderators: E. G. Estrin, M.D.; Bertha Kahn,
           Public Health Nurse

     Film: "Children's Emotions"

     Pamphlet: A Healthy Personality for your Child

May 22, 1956

   ELEMENTARY SCHOOL AGE CHILDREN

     Discussion Moderators: E. G. Estrin, M.D.; Bertha Kahn,
           Public Health Nurse

     Film: "Noisy 6's, Sociable 9's"

June 5, 1956

   ADOLESCENCE

     Discussion Moderators: E. G. Estrin, M.D.; Bertha Kahn,
           Public Health Nurse

     Film: "Age of Turmoil"

APPENDIX E.

FAMILY HEALTH MAINTENANCE DEMONSTRATION

Reading Shelf

PUBLIC AFFAIRS PAMPHLETS, 22 East 38 Street, New York 16, New York

- #163. 3 to 6; Your Child Starts to School
- 161. So You Think It's Love!
- 154. How to Discipline Your Children
- 149. How to Tell Your Child About Sex
- 148. Comics, Radio, Movies and Children
- 144. Understand Your Child from 6 to 12
- 141. Enjoy Your Child ages, 1, 2 and 3
- 127. Keeping Up with Teen-Agers

SCIENCE RESEARCH ASSOCIATES, 57 West Grand Avenue, Chicago 10, Illinois

- #5B31. Understanding Sex
- 5B32. Should You Go To College?
- 5B33. How to Live with Parents
- 5B150. What Good is High School?
- 5B151. Why Stay in School?
- 5B152. Understanding Yourself
- 5B153. You and Your Mental Abilities
- 5B154. Discovering Your Real Interests
- 5B155. Dating Days
- 5B156. Choosing Your Career
- 5B158. Getting Along with Others
- 5B510. Growing Up Socially
- 5B511. Looking Ahead to Marriage
- 5B515. Enjoying Leisure Time
- 5B561. How to Solve Your Problems
- 5B567. Where Are Your Manners?
- 5B598. Getting Along with Brothers and Sisters
- 5B702. Facts About Alcohol
- 5B705. What are Your Problems?
- 5B800. Your Behavior Problems
- 5B803. Baby-Sitting
- 5B901. Let's Listen to Youth
- 5B903. Self-Understanding
- 5B906. Helping Children Understand Sex
- 5B910. Emotional Problems of Growing Up
- 5B914. Fears of Children
- 5B915. Helping Youth Choose Careers
- 5B916. Exploring Children's Interests
- 5B919. When Children Start Dating
- 5B922. Your Child and Radio, TV, Comics and Movies
- 5B924. Your Children's Manners

CHILD STUDY PUBLICATIONS. The Child Study Association of America, 132 East 74 Street, New York 21, N. Y.

Packet #1: Early Childhood Packet

296

1. How to Give Your Child a Good Start
2. What Makes A Good Home
3. Discipline Through Affection
4. Emotional Growth in the First Year
6. Your Child and You

Packet #2: School Years' Packet

1. That Dear Octopus, The Family
2. Pre-Adolescents: What Makes Them Tick
3. Helping Brothers and Sisters Get Along
4. Aggressiveness in Children
5. When Children Ask About Sex

Packet #3 (Assorted)

6. Steps in Growing Up: The Middle Years
7. Universal Human Problems: Adolescent Phase
9. Modern Mother's Dilemma
11. There is No Substitute For Family Life
14. Discipline: What Is It?
18. Understanding Children's Fears
16. Jealousy, and Rivalry in Children
26. Television: How To Use It Wisely With Children

BOOKS FOR PARENTS

9. The Parents' Manual (Popular Library)
11. Your Child and You (Fawcett)

PARENT-TEACHER SERIES. Bureau of Publications, Columbia University Teachers College, New York 27, N. Y.

Understanding Young Children
Reading Is Fun
Answering Children's Questions
Discipline
Being a Good Parent
Your Child's Leisure Time
Getting Along in the Family
Children in the Family
Understanding Children's Behavior
A Good School Day

MENTAL HEALTH PUBLICATIONS. The National Association for Mental Health, 1790 Broadway, New York 19, New York

Fundamental Needs of the Child
Some Special Problems of Children
How to Live with Children
Your Child from One to Six
Your Child from Six to Twelve
You Don't Have to be Perfect—Even if You are a Parent
Guiding the Adolescent
This is the Adolescent

APPENDIX E.

MENTAL HEALTH PUBLICATIONS CONT'D.

Discussion Aid for "A Healthy Personality for Your Child"
Strengthening Family Life by Education for Family Living

BOOKLETS FROM THE CATHOLIC VIEWPOINT. Walter R. Engel, 23 East
51 Street, New York 22,
New York

Growing Up
How To Give Sex Instruction
Guidance of Youth (Lord)
Guidance of Parents (Lord)
Listen Son
Mother's Little Helper
Modern Youth and Chastity (Kelly)
Tips for Teens (Burnite)

Selected Detailed Tables

Intake and Loss of Families

By Follow-Up Period.

Follow-up months	STUDY			CONTROL		
	Remain Beginning of period	Lost During period	Percent lost (124=100%)	Remain beginning of period	Lost during period	Percent lost (162=100%)
0 - 6	124	0	0	162	6	3.7
7 - 12	124	2	1.6	156	3	1.9
13 - 18	122	3	2.4	153	6	3.7
19 - 24	119	3	2.4	147	8	4.9
25 - 30	116	3	2.4	139	3	1.9
31 - 36	113	6	4.8	136	11	6.8
37 - 42	107	3	2.4	125	5	3.1
43 - 48[a]	104	15 (2)	12.1	120	10 (7)	6.2
49 - 54	89	48	38.7	110	50	30.9
55 - 60	41	41	33.1	60	60	37.0
Total accepted FHMD	124		100.0	162		100.0
Total terminated HIP & FHMD		22	18.0		49	30.2
Total completed FHMD		102	82.0		113	69.8

[a] From this period on, losses are families completed FHMD, except for figure in ( ) which indicates families terminated HIP.

APPENDIX F.

Utilization of FHMD staff by age and sex of family member

Staff Member	Follow-up year	Study[a]				Control[b]			
		Adult		Child		Adult		Child	
		Male	Female	Male	Female	Male	Female	Male	Female
Family doc- tor or pe- diatrician	Average	3.3	4.7	4.6	4.3	1.5	1.8	4.3	4.1
	First	4.0	5.5	4.1	4.4	1.4	1.8	4.1	4.2
	Second	3.3	4.7	4.5	4.2	1.5	1.7	4.1	4.2
	Third	3.2	4.2	5.0	4.4	1.5	1.7	4.5	4.0
	Fourth	2.7	4.3	4.8	4.4	1.8	1.8	4.5	3.9
Specialist	Average	1.5	2.3	1.4	1.2	0.9	1.4	0.9	0.8
	First	1.6	3.0	1.0	1.0	0.8	1.6	0.8	0.8
	Second	1.4	2.4	1.3	1.3	0.8	1.3	1.2	0.9
	Third	1.5	1.7	1.6	1.3	0.8	1.5	0.8	0.8
	Fourth	1.3	2.0	1.7	1.1	1.0	1.2	0.8	0.7
Public Health Nurse	Average	1.3	4.0	2.7	3.1				
	First	2.4	5.7	4.5	5.2				
	Second	1.0	4.0	2.5	2.8				
	Third	0.9	3.4	2.2	2.2				
	Fourth	0.8	2.7	1.5	1.7				
Social Worker	Average	1.4	3.7	2.1	1.2				
	First	2.4	4.9	1.3	1.5				
	Second	1.4	4.2	2.5	1.4				
	Third	1.1	3.4	3.0	1.0				
	Fourth	0.9	2.1	1.6	0.9				

[a] Adults refers to parents and children over 13 years of age serviced by family doctor; children refers to those under 13 serviced by pediatrician.

[b] Adults refers to parents and children over 9 years of age serviced by family doctor; children refers to those under 9 serviced by pediatrician.

Incidence of new cases of diseases

	Number of patients		Total incidence		Major diagnoses		Minor diagnoses	
	Study	Control	Study	Control	Study	Control	Study	Control
4-year total								
cases	505	602	4165	3709	284	266	3881	3443
per person average			2.06	1.54	0.14	0.11	1.92	1.43
First year								
cases	523	644	1321	1119	100	78	1221	1041
per person average			2.52	1.74	0.19	0.12	2.33	1.62
Second year								
cases	513	619	1016	893	63	67	953	826
per person average			1.98	1.44	0.12	0.11	1.86	1.33
Third year								
cases	508	589	1005	871	60	63	945	808
per person average			1.98	1.48	0.12	0.11	1.86	1.37
Fourth year								
cases	476	555	823	826	61	58	762	768
per person average			1.73	1.49	0.13	0.11	1.60	1.38

Four-year annual average rate of new diagnoses per 100 members by physician service and diagnosis. (S=Study; C=Control)

Diagnosis (international statistical classification of diseases)	Total services				Routine physical examination				Nonroutine service			
	Major		Minor		Major		Minor		Major		Minor	
	S	C	S	C	S	C	S	C	S	C	S	C
Total new diagnoses	14.0	11.0	192.2	143.1	3.9	1.7	59.0	16.8	10.1	9.3	133.2	126.3
Infective and parasitic	0.2	(0.04)	8.0	8.1	0.2	0	2.4	0.5	0	(0.04)	5.6	7.6
Neoplasms, malignant	0.4	0.3	--	--	0.1	0	--	--	0.3	0.3	--	--
" benign & unspecified	--	--	3.7	1.8	--	--	2.0	0.7	--	--	1.7	1.1
Allergic, endocrine, meta-bolic	0.3	0.3	10.5	5.3	0.3	(0.04)	7.9	2.5	0	0.3	2.6	2.8
Blood and blood-forming organs	0.6	0.9	--	--	0.2	0.4	--	--	0.4	0.5	--	--
Mental psychoneurotic per-sonality disorders	0.1	0	6.2	3.3	0	0	4.1	1.2	0.1	0	2.1	1.1
Nervous system and sense organs	0.6	0.4	24.1	19.1	0.2	0.2	5.1	1.1	0.4	0.2	19.0	18.0
Circulatory system	1.1	0.3	6.0	3.7	0.8	0.2	3.6	1.0	0.3	0.1	2.4	2.7
Respiratory system	0.1	0.5	73.6	55.8	0	0.1	15.5	3.9	0.1	0.4	58.1	51.9
Digestive system	1.3	1.1	9.4	3.9	0.2	0.2	1.8	0.6	1.1	0.9	7.6	3.3
Genito-urinary system	2.5	1.4	3.2	2.4	0.8	0.2	1.3	0.7	1.7	1.2	1.9	1.7
Complications of pregnancy, childbirth, puerperium	0.5	0.3	--	--	0	0	--	--	0.5	0.3	--	--
Skin and cellular tissue	--	--	14.1	13.1	--	--	3.9	1.4	--	--	10.2	11.7
Bones and organs of move-ment	2.2	2.5	10.7	4.8	0.6	0.2	6.9	1.5	1.6	2.3	3.8	3.3
Congenital malformations	0.8	0.5	--	--	0.4	0.2	--	--	0.4	0.3	--	--
Certain diseases of early infancy	0.1	0.2	--	--	0.1	(0.04)	--	--	0	0.2	--	--
Symptoms, senility, ill-defined conditions	--	--	8.2	10.9	--	--	3.8	1.5	--	--	4.4	9.4
Accidents, poisonings, violence	3.3	2.4	14.1	10.8	0.1	(0.04)	0.7	0.2	3.2	2.4	10.9	10.6

Annual average: study 505; control 602

Initial and final ratings of physical condition evaluation of
study-family members by family doctor or pediatrician

		Final rating			
Initial rating	Total	Excellent	Good	Fair	Poor
Total	489	94	337	49	9
Excellent	82	21	56	5	0
Good	175	45	118	11	1
Fair	218	28	159	28	3
Poor	14	0	4	5	5

Percent of initial rating

	Final rating			
Initial rating	Excellent	Good	Fair	Poor
Total	19.2	68.9	10.0	1.9
Excellent	25.6	68.3	6.1	0
Good	25.7	67.4	6.3	0.6
Fair	12.8	73.0	12.8	1.4
Poor	0	28.6	35.7	35.7

Initial and final ratings of housing evaluation of study-family members by public health nurse

Initial rating	Total	Final rating			
		Excellent	Good	Fair	Poor
Total	473	206	177	85	5
Excellent	107	67	35	5	0
Good	148	57	68	23	0
Fair	189	64	68	52	5
Poor	29	18	6	5	0

Percent of initial rating

Initial rating	Final rating			
	Excellent	Good	Fair	Poor
Total	43.6	37.4	18.0	1.0
Excellent	62.6	32.7	4.7	0
Good	38.5	46.0	15.5	0
Fair	33.9	36.0	27.5	2.6
Poor	62.1	20.7	17.2	0

Initial and final ratings of personal adjustment evaluation
of study-family members by social worker

Initial rating	Total	Final rating			
		Excellent	Good	Fair	Poor
Total	447	36	226	180	5
Excellent	78	17	41	20	0
Good	255	16	140	99	0
Fair	109	3	45	59	2
Poor	5	0	0	2	3

Percent of initial rating

Initial rating	Final rating			
	Excellent	Good	Fair	Poor
Total	8.1	50.5	40.3	1.1
Excellent	21.8	52.6	25.6	0
Good	6.3	54.9	38.8	0
Fair	2.8	41.3	54.0	1.8
Poor	(0)	(0)	(40.0)	(60.0)

EVALUATION OF FAMILY MEDICAL HISTORY
BY family doctor or pediatrician

STUDY

	Excellent	Good	Fair	Poor	Study (FINAL)	Control (FINAL)
Poor	0	1	1	48	50	22
Fair	0	15	157	8	180	97
Good	4	206	44	5	259	165
Excellent	14	5	0	0	19	40
					508	324

FINAL EVALUATION

Excellent   Good   Fair   Poor
   18   227   202   61

INITIAL EVALUATION

CHANGE FROM INITIAL TO FINAL EVALUATION

CHANGE	NUMBER	PERCENT
No change	425	83.7
Improved	62	12.2
Deteriorated	21	4.1
TOTAL	508	100.0

306

EVALUATION OF PHYSICAL CONDITION
BY family doctor or pediatrician

S T U D Y

FINAL EVALUATION	Excellent	Good	Fair	Poor		FINAL Study	Control
Poor	0	1	3	5		9	8
Fair	5	11	28	5		49	73
Good	56	118	159	4		337	170
Excellent	21	45	28	0		94	80
						489	331

Excellent Good Fair Poor
82   175   218   14

I N I T I A L   E V A L U A T I O N

CHANGE FROM INITIAL TO FINAL EVALUATION

CHANGE	NUMBER	PERCENT
No change	172	35.2
Improved	241	49.3
Deteriorated	76	15.5
TOTAL	489	100.0

307

EVALUATION OF NUTRITION
BY Public Health Nurse

S T U D Y

	Excellent	Good	Fair	Poor		Study	Control
Poor	0	0	0	0		–	1
Fair	0	18	29	I		48	39
Good	50	125	36	0		211	190
Excellent	89	79	17	0		185	95
						444	325

FINAL

FINAL EVALUATION

Excellent Good Fair Poor
139   222   82   1

I N I T I A L   E V A L U A T I O N

CHANGE   FROM   INITIAL   TO   FINAL   EVALUATION

CHANGE	NUMBER	PERCENT
No change	243	54.7
Improved	133	30.0
Deteriorated	68	15.3
TOTAL	444	100.0

308

APPENDIX F.

EVALUATION OF HOUSING
BY Public Health Nurse

S T U D Y

F I N A L

					Study	Control

Poor

| 0 | 0 | 5 | 0 |

5   10

Fair

| 5 | 23 | 52 | 5 |

85   128

Good

| 35 | 68 | 68 | 6 |

177   110

Excellent

| 67 | 57 | 64 | 18 |

206   73
473   329

Excellent   Good   Fair   Poor
107   148   189   29

I N I T I A L   E V A L U A T I O N

FINAL EVALUATION

CHANGE FROM INITIAL TO FINAL EVALUATION

CHANGE	NUMBER	PERCENT
No change	187	39.5
Improved	218	46.1
Deteriorated	68	14.4
TOTAL	473	100.0

309

EVALUATION OF RECREATIONAL ADJUSTMENT
BY Public Health Nurse

S T U D Y

| | | | | | FINAL | |
					Study	Control
Poor	0	0	0	0	-	-
Fair	8	13	6	1	28	28
Good	82	82	26	0	190	89
Excellent	193	43	12	0	248	209
					466	326

FINAL EVALUATION

Excellent Good Fair Poor
283 138 44 1

I N I T I A L   E V A L U A T I O N

CHANGE FROM INITIAL TO FINAL EVALUATION

CHANGE	NUMBER	PERCENT
No change	281	60.3
Improved	82	17.6
Deteriorated	103	22.1
TOTAL	466	100.0

310

EVALUATION OF SLEEP AND REST
BY Public Health Nurse

S T U D Y

					Study	Control
				F I N A L		
Poor	0	0	0	0	0	0
Fair	10	22	12	2	46	30
Good	47	65	23	1	136	88
Excellent	169	83	37	0	289	210
					471	328

FINAL EVALUATION

Excellent   Good   Fair   Poor
226   170   72   3

I N I T I A L   E V A L U A T I O N

CHANGE FROM INITIAL TO FINAL EVALUATION

CHANGE	NUMBER	PERCENT
No change	246	52.2
Improved	146	31.0
Deteriorated	79	16.8
TOTAL	471	100.0

EVALUATION OF EDUCATIONAL ACHIEVEMENT
OF SCHOOL AGE CHILDREN

BY Public Health Nurse

STUDY

FINAL EVALUATION

	Excellent	Good	Fair	Poor	FINAL Study	Control
Poor	0	0	1	0	1	2
Fair	1	2	4	0	7	4
Good	4	19	6	0	29	21
Excellent	75	23	2	0	100	114
					137	141

	Excellent	Good	Fair	Poor
	80	44	13	-

INITIAL EVALUATION

CHANGE FROM INITIAL TO FINAL EVALUATION

CHANGE	NUMBER	PERCENT
No change	98	71.6
Improved	31	22.6
Deteriorated	8	5.8
TOTAL	137	100.0

EVALUATION OF PERSONAL ADJUSTMENT
BY Social Worker

S T U D Y

FINAL EVALUATION

	Excellent	Good	Fair	Poor	FINAL Study	Control
Poor	0	0	2	3	5	2
Fair	20	99	59	2	180	94
Good	41	140	45	0	226	180
Excellent	17	16	3	0	36	41
					447	317

Excellent Good Fair Poor
78   255   109   5

INITIAL   EVALUATION

CHANGE   FROM   INITIAL   TO   FINAL   EVALUATION

CHANGE	NUMBER	PERCENT
No change	219	49.0
Improved	66	14.8
Deteriorated	162	36.2
TOTAL	447	100.0

EVALUATION OF OCCUPATIONAL ADJUSTMENT
OF FATHERS
BY Social Worker

S T U D Y

						F I N A L	
						Study	Control
Poor	0	0	0	0		0	1
Fair	0	7	4	0		11	5
Good	12	25	5	1		43	17
Excellent	32	18	5	0		55	47
						109	70
	Excellent	Good	Fair	Poor			
	44	50	14	1			

FINAL EVALUATION (vertical axis label)

I N I T I A L   E V A L U A T I O N

CHANGE FROM INITIAL TO FINAL EVALUATION

CHANGE	NUMBER	PERCENT
No change	61	56.0
Improved	29	26.6
Deteriorated	19	17.4
TOTAL	109	100.0

314

EVALUATION OF FAMILY RELATIONSHIP

OF SPOUSES

BY Social Worker

S T U D Y

	Excellent	Good	Fair	Poor		Study	Control
Poor	0	0	0	0		0	1
Fair	7	16	15	0		38	10
Good	19	34	11	0		64	50
Excellent	6	1	0	0		7	9
						109	70
	32	51	26	-			

FINAL EVALUATION

F I N A L

I N I T I A L   E V A L U A T I O N

CHANGE FROM INITIAL TO FINAL EVALUATION

CHANGE	NUMBER	PERCENT
No change	55	50.5
Improved	12	11.0
Deteriorated	42	38.5
TOTAL	109	100.0

315

EVALUATION OF FAMILY RELATIONSHIP
OF CHILDREN AND FATHERS

BY Social Worker

S T U D Y

						FINAL	
						Study	Control
Poor	1	1	2	0		4	0
Fair	15	33	11	3		62	22
Good	52	67	12	1		132	110
Excellent	10	9	1	0		20	37
						218	169
	Excellent	Good	Fair	Poor			
	78	110	26	4			

FINAL EVALUATION (left axis label)

I N I T I A L   E V A L U A T I O N

CHANGE FROM INITIAL TO FINAL EVALUATION

CHANGE	NUMBER	PERCENT
No change	88	40.4
Improved	26	11.9
Deteriorated	104	47.7
TOTAL	218	100.0

316

EVALUATION OF FAMILY RELATIONSHIP

OF CHILDREN AND MOTHERS

BY Social Worker

S T U D Y

F I N A L

						Study	Control
Poor	0	0	5	0		5	3
Fair	16	59	20	8		103	29
Good	21	51	19	0		91	103
Excellent	18	7	1	0		26	38
						225	173

FINAL EVALUATION

Excellent Good Fair Poor

55   117   45   8

I N I T I A L E V A L U A T I O N

CHANGE FROM INITIAL TO FINAL EVALUATION

CHANGE	NUMBER	PERCENT
No change	89	39.6
Improved	35	15.5
Deteriorated	101	44.9
TOTAL	225	100.0

317

APPENDIX F.

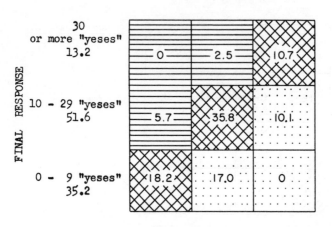

CORNELL MEDICAL INDEX
INITIAL vs FINAL RESPONSE
OF 159 PARENTS

FINAL RESPONSE

30
or more "yeses"
13.2

0 ═══ 2.5 ═══ 10.7

10 - 29 "yeses"
51.6

5.7 ═══ 35.8 ═══ 10.1

0 - 9 "yeses"
35.2

18.2 ═══ 17.0 ═══ 0

0 - 9 "yeses" 10 - 29 "yeses" 30 or more "yeses"
100%   23.9   55.3   20.8

I   N   I   T   I   A   L   RESPONSE

8.2   Deteriorated (greater number "yeses" at Final)

64.7   No change (same number "yeses" at Final)

27.1   Improved (smaller number "yeses" at Final)
100.0%

318

Number of hospital admissions per 100 members per year.[a]

Follow-up year.	STUDY				CONTROL			
	All	Father	Mother	Child	All	Father	Mother	Child
4 - year annual average	8.4	5.6	17.8	5.5	6.1	3.9	12.0	4.5
First	8.0	4.8	20.2	4.0	6.2	2.5	12.1	5.2
Second	8.4	6.8	17.6	5.1	6.5	5.4	11.6	4.6
Third	8.7	5.2	17.2	6.5	5.1	3.6	10.2	3.5
Fourth	8.4	5.6	15.9	6.5	6.7	3.9	14.1	4.7

[a] Including all hospitalizations at Montefiore, plus non-Montefiore hospitalizations for tonsillectomy and delivery.

Number of operations per 100 members per year.

Follow-up year.	STUDY				CONTROL			
	All	Father	Mother	Child	All	Father	Mother	Child
4 - year annual average	4.4	3.7	6.7	3.8	3.0	1.4	3.9	3.4
First	4.8	3.2	8.9	3.6	3.3	1.3	3.8	3.9
Second	4.7	5.9	6.7	3.3	3.1	2.0	2.7	3.7
Third	3.9	2.6	4.3	4.3	2.4	0.7	3.6	2.5
Fourth	4.2	2.8	6.5	3.8	3.4	1.6	5.5	3.4

Number of operations per 100 admissions as percent of admissions with operations.

Follow-up year.	STUDY				CONTROL			
	All	Father	Mother	Child	All	Father	Mother	Child
4 - year annual average	52.7	65.4	37.3	68.3	49.7	36.4	32.4	75.4
First	59.5	66.7	44.0	90.9	52.5	50.0	31.6	76.5
Second	55.8	87.5	38.1	64.3	47.5	37.5	23.5	80.0
Third	45.5	50.0	25.0	66.7	46.7	20.0	35.7	72.7
Fourth	50.0	50.0	41.2	58.8	51.4	40.0	38.9	71.4

Average length of stay (days) per yearly hospital admission.[a]

Follow-up year.	STUDY				CONTROL			
	All	Father	Mother	Child	All	Father	Mother	Child
4 - year annual average	6.3	6.9	6.8	5.2	5.3	8.1	6.2	3.0
First	4.7	3.5	6.2	2.0	5.8	8.0	8.3	2.5
Second	7.3	10.5	6.4	6.8	5.1	7.8	5.8	2.9
Third	7.7	5.8	8.4	7.5	6.0	13.2	5.1	3.9
Fourth	5.3	6.7	6.5	3.6	4.3	4.0	5.4	2.9

a Including all hospitalizations at Montefiore, plus non-Montefiore hospitalizations for tonsillectomy and delivery.

Number of hospital admissions per year.

Follow-up year.	STUDY				CONTROL			
	All	Father	Mother	Child	All	Father	Mother	Child
4 - year annual average	169	26	83	60	147	22	68	57
First	42	6	25	11	40	4	19	17
Second	43	8	21	14	40	8	17	15
Third	44	6	20	18	30	5	14	11
Fourth	40	6	17	17	37	5	18	14

APPENDIX G

Publications from the Family Health Maintenance Demonstration

Cherkasky, M., "Family Health Maintenance Demonstration," in Research in Public Health (New York: Milbank Memorial Fund, 1952).

The Family Health Maintenance Demonstration (New York: Milbank Memorial Fund, 1954).

Freidson, E., "Specialties Without Roots: The Utilization of New Services," Human Organization, 18:112-116 (Fall 1959).

----- Patients' Views of Medical Practice (New York: Russell Sage Foundation, 1961).

----- and G. Silver, "Social Science in Family Medical Care," Public Health Reports, 75:489-493 (June 1960).

McKenzie, Miriam T., "Flexibility and Mental Health: A TAT Study," unpublished dissertation (New York University, 1961).

Schlossman, Howard H., "Transference in Medical Team-Family Research: The Family Health Maintenance Demonstration," Amer. J. Orthopsychiat., 31:612-621 (July 1961).

Shapiro, Irving, Changing Child-Rearing Attitudes Through Group Discussion, Ph.D. dissertation (Columbia, 1954),

----- "Is Group Parent Education Worthwhile?" University Microfilms Pub. #10,801, Ann Arbor, Mich. Marriage and Family Living, 18:154-161 (May 1956).

Silver, George A., "Beyond General Practice: The Health Team," Yale J. Bio. Med., 31:29-39 (September 1958).

----- "Family Health Maintenance," Pub. Hlth Rep. vol. 71, #10 (October 1956).

----- "Family Health Maintenance: A Perspective On The Ailing Family," in Iago Galdston, ed., The Family A Focal Point in Health Education (New York: New York Academy of Medicine, 1961), pp. 135-159.

----- "A Family Health Service as A Teaching Program", J. med. Educ., 33:600-604 (August 1958).

----- "Planning for Family Medical Service," Proc. Roy. Soc. Med., 54:449-452 (June 1961).

----- and C. Stiber, "The Social Worker and the Physician," J. med. Educ., 32:324-330 (May 1957).

BIBLIOGRAPHY

Ackerman, N. W., *The Psychodynamics of Family Life* (New York: Basic Books, 1958).

Adams, W. R., "The Psychiatrist in an Ambulatory Clerkship for Comprehensive Medical Care in a New Curriculum," *J. med. Educ.*, 33:211–220 (March 1958).

Alexander, F., and T. M. French, *Studies in Psychosomatic Medicine* (New York: The Ronald Press, 1948).

Allport, Gordon W., "The Trend in Motivational Theory," *Amer. J. Orthopsychiat.*, 23:107–119 (January 1953).

———— *The Nature of Prejudice* (New York: Doubleday & Company 1958).

Altschule, M. D., "Ideas of XVIIIth Century British Medical Writers about Anxiety," *New Engl. J. Med.*, 248:646–648 (April 9, 1953).

———— "Physiologic Data Bearing on the Clinical Problem of Anxiety," *N.Y. St. J. Med.*, 56:864–871 (March 15, 1956).

"American Board of Internal Medicine," in "Requirements for Certification," *JAMA*, 168:661–664 (October 4, 1958).

AJPH, editorial, "A Theoretical Model of Health," 48:1530–1532 (November 1958).

American Medical Directory, AMA *Report of the Committee on Preparation for General Practice, mimeographed* (Chicago, May 20, 1958).

American Psychiatric Assn. (Report of the Committee on Medical Education) "An Outline for a Curriculum for Teaching Psychiatry in Medical Schools," *J. med. Educ.*, 31:115–128 (February 1956).

APHA, *Basic Principles of Healthful Housing*, 2nd ed. (New York, 1954).

———— *An Appraisal Method for Measuring the Quality of Dwellings* (New York, 1946).

Baehr, George, "Health Insurance Plan of Greater New York," *JAMA*, 143:637–640 (June 17, 1950).

Bakst, H. J., and E. F. Marra, "Experience with Home Care for Cardiac Patients," *AJPH*, 45:444–450 (April 1955).

Basowitz, H., H. Persky, S. J. Korchin, and R. R. Grinker, *Anxiety and Stress* (New York: McGraw-Hill, 1955).

Beck, Flora, "Towards a Philosophy of Social Care," *Lancet*, 273:797–799 (October 1957).

Bellak, Leopold, *The TAT and CAT in Clinical Use* (New York: Grune & Stratton, 1954).

Bernard, Claude, *An Introduction to the Study of Experimental Medicine* (New York: The Macmillan Co., 1927).

Bieber, I., "Pathological Boredom and Inertia," *Amer. J. Psychother.*, 5:215–225 (April 1951).

———— "Critique of Kinsey Report on Women," *Journal of Brooklyn State Hospital Psych. Forum*, vol. 7 (May 1954).

Binger, Carl, *The Doctor's Job* (New York: Norton, 1945).

Boehm, W. W., "The Role of Psychiatric Social Work in Mental Health" in Rose, *Mental Health and Mental Disorder.*

Borsky, P. N., and O. K. Sagen, "Motivations Toward Health Examinations," *AJPH*, 49:514–527 (April 1959).

Bowlby, J., *Maternal Care and Mental Health* (Geneva: WHO, 1952).

——— "Application of Recent Research to Health Visiting," *J. roy. sanit. Inst.*, 73:596–598 (September 1953).

Brodman, K. et al., "The Cornell Medical Index," *JAMA*, 140:530–534 (June 11, 1949).

——— et al., "The Cornell Medical Index Health Questionnaire: As a Diagnostic Instrument," *JAMA*, 145:152–157 (January 20, 1951).

——— A. J. Erdmann, I. Lorge, C. P. Gershenson, H. G. Wolff, and B. Cables, "Evaluation of Emotional Disturbances: Cornell Medical Index Health Questionnaire, part III," *J. clin. psychol.*, 8:119–124 (April 1952).

Brown, E. L., *Nursing For the Future* (New York: Russell Sage Foundation, 1948).

Brown, J. A. C., *The Social Psychology of Industry* (London: Penguin, 1954).

"Building America's Health," vol. 3 (Washington: Government Printing Office, 1952).

Burgess, E. W., and L. S. Cottrell, Jr., "The Prediction of Adjustment in Marriage," *American Sociological Review*, 1:737–751 (October 1936).

Cabot, Richard, *Social Work* (Boston: Houghton Mifflin Company, 1919).

Cannon, Ida, *On the Social Frontier of Medicine* (Cambridge, Mass.: Harvard University Press, 1952).

Cannon, Walter, *The Wisdom of the Body* (New York: W. W. Norton & Company, 1932).

Carter, Richard, *The Doctor Business* (New York: Doubleday & Company, 1958).

Caudill, W., and B. H. Roberts, "Pitfalls in the Organization of Interdisciplinary Research," *Human Organization*, 10:12–15 (Winter 1951).

Cavan, Ruth S., *The American Family* (New York: Thomas Y. Crowell Company, 1953).

Cherkasky, M., "The Montefiore Hospital Home Care Program," *AJPH*, 39:29–30 (February 1949).

——— "The Family Health Maintenance Demonstration" in *Research in Public Health* (New York: Milbank Memorial Fund, 1952).

Chodoff, Paul, "A Re-Examination of Some Aspects of Conversion Hysteria," *Psychiatry*, 17:75–81 (February 1954).

Clark, D. A., and K. G. Clark, *Organization and Administration of Group Medical Practice* (Boston: Edward A. Filene Good Will Fund, 1941).

Clarke, A. D. B., and A. M. Clarke, "Vagaries of Intelligence," *Lancet*, 265:869–870 (October 24, 1953).

Clausen, J. A., and M. L. Kohn, "The Ecological Approach in Social Psychiatry," *Amer. J. Sociology*, 60:140–151 (September 1954).

Cobb, S., S. King, and E. Chen, "Differences Between Respondents and Non-Respondents in a Morbidity Survey Involving Clinical Examination," *J. chron. Dis.*, 6:95–108 (August 1957).

324

Cooley, Charles H., *Human Nature and The Social Order and Social Organization* (Glencoe, Ill.: The Free Press, 1956).

"Cooperation in Health Examination Surveys," *Health Statistics* (Washington: Government Printing Office, June 1960).

Cottrell, L. S., Jr., "Roles and Marital Adjustment," *American Sociological Society*, 27:107–115 (May 1933).

Creak, Mildred, "Parents and Children," *Lancet*, 267:236–238 (July 31, 1954).

Cumming, Margaret Elaine, and John Hamilton Cumming, *Closed Ranks: An Experiment in Mental Health Education* (Cambridge, Mass.: Harvard University Press, 1957).

Cunningham, J. M., "Problems of Communication in Scientific and Professional Disciplines," *Amer. J. Orthopsychiat.*, 22:445–456 (July 1952).

Curtis, Homer, "The 'Normal' Prenatal Patient's Attitude Toward Pregnancy," in *The Promotion of Maternal and Newborn Health* (New York: Milbank Memorial Fund, 1955).

Cust, G., "The Epidemiology of Nocturnal Enuresis," *Lancet*, 275:1167–1170 (November 29, 1958).

Daily, E., "Medical Care Under the Health Insurance Plan of Greater New York," *JAMA*, 170:272–276 (May 16, 1959).

Davidson, W., "A Brief History of Infant Feeding," *J. Pediat.*, 43:74–87 (July 1953).

Davis, Kingsley, "Mental Hygiene and the Class Structure" (1938), reprinted in Rose, *Mental Health and Mental Disorder.*

Davis, Michael, *Medical Care for Tomorrow* (New York: Harper & Brothers, 1955).

Davis, W. A., and R. J. Havighurst, *Father of the Man* (Boston: Houghton Mifflin Company, 1947).

"Definition of a Medical Social Work Position" (New York: National Association of Social Workers, March 1956).

Densen, P. N., "Broadening the Significance of Vital Statistics Through Special Studies," mimeographed address, American Statistical Association (December 30, 1952).

Dicks, H. V., "Strains Within the Family," *Report of the 1954 Conference National Ass'n for Mental Health* (London, March 25, 1954).

———— "The Predicament of the Family in the Modern World," *Lancet*, 268:295–297 (February 5, 1955).

Dongray, Madge, "Social Work in General Practice," *Brit. med. J.*, 2:1220–1223 (November 15, 1958).

Drever, James, *A Dictionary of Psychology* (London: Penguin, 1952).

Dublin, T. D., and M. Fraenkel, *A Demonstration Project in Family Health Maintenance*, mimeographed (New York: Dept. of Prev. Med. and Community Health, Long Island Coll. of Med., 1948).

Dubos, R., *The Mirage of Health* (New York: Harper & Brothers, 1959).

Dürkheim, Emile, *Suicide* (Glencoe, Ill.: The Free Press, 1951).

Dwyer, T. F., and N. Zinbey, "Psychiatry for Medical School Instructors," *J. med. Educ.*, 32:331–338 (May 1957).

Eaton, Joseph, "Social Processes of Professional Team Work," *American Sociological Rev.*, 16:707–713 (October 1951).

———— and R. Weil, *Culture and Mental Disorders* (Glencoe, Ill.: The Free Press, 1955).

The Elements of a Community Mental Health Program (New York: Milbank Memorial Fund, 1956), pp. 19, 57–68.

Elsom, K. A., S. Schor, T. W. Clark, K. O. Elsom, and J. P. Hubbard, "Periodic Health Examination," *JAMA*, 172:5–10 (January 2, 1960).

Engel, George, "Homeostasis" in R. R. Grinker, ed., *MidCentury Psychiatry* (Springfield, Ill.: Charles C. Thomas, 1953), pp. 33–59.

Environment and Health, Federal Security Agency (Washington: Government Printing Office, 1951).

Expert Committee on Nursing (Third Report), *WHO Tech. Report Series* #91 (Geneva: WHO, 1954).

The Family Health Maintenance Demonstration (New York: Milbank Memorial Fund, 1954).

Faris, R. E. L., *Social Disorganization* (New York: The Ronald Press, 1955), chapter 10.

Fleming, W. L., "Teaching a Family Physician's Approach by a Dept. of Preventive Medicine," *JAMA*, 161:711–713 (June 23, 1956).

Flexner, A., *Medical Education in the U.S. and Canada*, Bull. No. 4, Carnegie Found. for the Advancement of Teaching (New York, 1910).

Foote, N., and L. Cottrell, *Identity and Interpersonal Competence* (Chicago: University of Chicago Press, 1955).

Foster, G. M., *Problems in Intercultural Health Programs* (New York: Social Science Research Council, 1958).

Freidson, Eliot, "Client Control and Medical Practice," *The American Journal of Sociology*, 45:374–382 (January 1960).

——— "The Organization of Medical Practice and Patient Behavior," *American Journal of Public Health*, 51:43–52 (January 1961).

——— *Patients' Views of Medical Practice* (New York: Russell Sage Foundation, 1961).

——— "Specialties Without Roots: The Utilization of New Services," *Human Organization*, 18:112–116 (Fall 1959).

——— and G. Silver, "Social Science in Family Medical Care, *Public Health Reports*, 75:489–493 (June 1960).

Freud, Anna, "Psychoanalysis and Education," *Psychoanalytic Study of the Child*, vol. IX (New York: International Universities Press, 1954).

——— and D. T. Burlingham, *War and Children* (New York: International Universities Press, 1944).

Fromm, Erich, "Individual and Social Origins of Neuroses" in Rose, *Mental Health and Mental Disorder*.

Gaffin and Associates, *What Americans Think of the Medical Profession* (Chicago: AMA, n.d.).

Gantt, W. H., "Experimental Basis for Neurotic Behavior," *Psychosomatic Medicine*, Monograph vol. III, nos. 3, 4 (New York, 1944).

Gerard, R. W., "Anxiety and Tension," *Bull. N.Y. Acad. Med.*, 34:429–444 (July 1958).

Ginsburg, Ethel L., *Public Health is People* (New York: Commonwealth Fund, 1950).

Glaser, K., and L. Eisenberg, "Maternal Deprivation," *Pediatrics*, 18:626–642 (October 1956).

Goffman, Erving, *The Presentation of Self in Everyday Life* (Edinburgh: University of Edinburgh, 1956).

—— "The Moral Career of the Mental Patient," *Psychiatry*, 22:123–141 (May 1959).

Goldmann, Franz, "Potentialities of Group Practice of Medicine," *Conn. med. J.*, 10:289–294 (April 1946).

Gordon, Gerald, "Industrial Psychiatry," *Industr. Med. Surg.*, 21:585–588 (December 1952).

Goss, Mary E. W., "Physicians in Bureaucracy," Ph.D. dissertation (Columbia University, 1959), L.C. Card #Mic 59-2845.

Graham, Saxon, "Socio-Economic States, Illness and the Use of Medical Services," *Milbank mem. fd quart.*, 35:58–66 (January 1957).

Greenberg, M., O. Pellitteri, and J. Barton, "Frequency of Defects in Infants Whose Mothers Had Rubella During Pregnancy," *JAMA*, 165:675–680 (October 12, 1957).

Grinker, R., and J. P. Spiegel, *Men Under Stress* (Philadelphia: Blakiston, 1945).

Grundy, F., and J. M. Mackintosh, *The Teaching of Hygiene and Public Health in Europe* (Geneva: WHO, 1957).

Hall, Oswald, "The Informal Organization of Medical Practice in an American City," unpublished Ph.D. dissertation (University of Chicago, 1944).

—— "The Stages of a Medical Career," *Amer. J. Sociol.*, 53:327–336 (March 1948).

—— "Types of Medical Careers," *Amer. J. Sociol.*, 55:243–253 (November 1949).

Halliday, J. L., *Psychosocial Medicine* (New York: W. W. Norton & Company, 1948).

Hamilton, Walton, in *Medical Care for the American People* (Chicago: University of Chicago Press, 1932).

Harvey, W. A., "Changing Syndromes and Culture," *Int. J. soc. Psychiat.*, 2:165–171 (Winter 1956).

Health and Demography (Washington: Government Printing Office, 1956).

Health Insurance Plan, *Health and Medical Care in New York City* (Cambridge, Mass.: Harvard University Press, 1957).

—— "1957 Annual Statistical Report," mimeographed (New York, 1958).

—— "Utilization Experience by Contractor Groups," mimeographed (New York, 1959).

Health Manpower Source Book (Washington: Government Printing Office, 1959), section 9, Physicians, Dentists, Nurses.

Henderson, L. J., "Physician and Patient as a Social System," *New Engl. J. Med.*, 212:819–823 (May 2, 1935).

Herbolsheimer, H., and B. L. Ballard, "Multiple Screening in Evaluation of Entering College and University Students," *JAMA*, 166:444–453 (February 1, 1958).

Hill, Reuben, *Families Under Stress* (New York: Harper & Brothers, 1949).

Hinkle, L. E., Jr., and H. G. Wolff, "Health and the Social Environment" in *Explorations in Social Psychiatry*, ed. Leighton, Clausen, and Wilson (New York: Basic Books, 1957).

—— "Ecologic Investigations of the Relationship Between Illness, Life Experiences and the Social Environment," *Ann. intern. Med.*, 49:1373–1388 (December 1958).

Hollingshead, A. B., and F. C. Redlich, *Social Class and Mental Illness* (New York: John Wiley & Sons, 1958).

Howells, J. G., and J. Layng, "Separation Experience and Mental Health," *Lancet,* 269:285–288 (August 6, 1955).

Hubbard, J. P., ed., *The Early Detection and Prevention of Disease* (New York: Blakiston, 1957).

Hughes, Everett, *Men and Their Work* (Glencoe, Ill.: The Free Press, 1958).

Hughes, E. C., H. M. Hughes, and I. Deutscher, *20,000 Nurses Tell Their Story* (Philadelphia: J. B. Lippincott, 1958).

Hume, C. W., "The Strategy and Tactics of Experimentation," *Lancet,* 273:1049–1052 (November 23, 1957).

Hunt, G. H., and M. Goldstein, *Medical Group Practice in the United States,* Federal Security Agency (Washington: Government Printing Office, 1951).

Hunter, Floyd, *Community Power Structure* (Chapel Hill: University of North Carolina Press, 1954).

Hyman, H. H., and P. B. Sheatsley, "Some Reasons Why Information Campaigns Fail," from *Public Opinion Quarterly,* 1947; quoted in Maccoby, Newcomb, and Hartley, *Readings in Social Psychology* (3rd ed., New York: Henry Holt & Company, 1948).

Ingalls, T. H., and F. R. Philbrook, "Monstrosities Induced by Hypoxia," *New Engl. J. Med.,* 259:558–564 (September 18, 1958).

Jahoda, Marie, *Evaluation in Mental Health* (Washington: Government Printing Office, 1955).

———— *Current Concepts of Positive Mental Health* (New York: Basic Books, 1958).

Joint Commission on Mental Illness & Health (Second Annual Report) (Cambridge, Mass., 1958).

Jones, Ernest, *The Life and Work of Sigmund Freud* (New York: Basic Books, 1955).

JAMA, editorial, "Woe and Work," 168:1377 (November 8, 1958).

Journal of Medical Education, "Symposium on Extramural Facilities in Medical Education," 28:9–53 (July 1953).

Kanev, I., *Aspects of Social Security in Israel* (Tel Aviv: Histadrut Economic and Social Research Institute, 1960).

Kardiner, Abram, *The Psychological Frontiers of Society* (New York: Columbia University Press, 1945).

Kark, S. L., "The Future: Health Service Among Rural Bantu," *S. Afr. med. J.,* 16:197–198 (May 23, 1942).

———— "Health Center Service — A South African Experiment in Family Health and Medical Care" in *Social Medicine,* ed. E. H. Cluver (Johannesburg, South Africa: Central News Agency, 1951).

———— and I. Cassel, "The Pholela Health Center," *S. Afr. med. J.,* 26:101–104, 132–136 (February 9, 16, 1952).

Kasius, Cora, ed., *Principles and Techniques of Social Case Work* (New York: Family Service Association, 1950).

Katz, Elihu, and Paul F. Lazarsfeld, *Personal Influence* (Glencoe, Ill.: The Free Press, 1955).

Kaufman, M. R., "The Problem of Psychiatric Symptom Formation," *J. Mich. med. Soc.,* 57:71–76 (January 1958).

Kindschi, L. G., "The Role of the Preceptor in the University of Wisconsin Preceptor Program," *J. med. Educ.,* 34:649–653 (July 1959).

Kluckhohn, Clyde, *Mirror for Man* (New York: McGraw-Hill, 1949; Premier Reprint, 1957).

—— and H. A. Murray, eds., *Personality in Nature, Society and Culture* (New York: Knopf, 1949).

Kohn, M. L., and J. A. Clausen, "Social Isolation and Schizophrenia," *American sociol. Rev.*, 20:265–273 (June 1955).

—— "Parental Authority Behavior and Schizophrenia," *Amer. J. Orthopsychiat.*, 26:297–313 (April 1956).

Koos, E. L., *Families in Trouble* (New York: King's Crown Press, 1946).

—— "Metropolis — What City People Think of Their Medical Services," *AJPH*, 45:1551–1557 (December 1955).

Kraus, H., "Role of Social Case Work in American Social Work," in Kasius, *Principles and Techniques of Social Case Work.*

Lancet, editorial, "Routine Medical Examination," 274:948, 949 (May 3, 1958).

—— annotation, "Psychotherapy in General Practice," 271:1340 (December 29, 1956).

—— special article, "Contribution of Social Work to Medical Care," 1:1194 (June 5, 1959).

Landis, C., and M. M. Bolles, *Personality and Sexuality in the Physically Handicapped Woman* (New York: Harper & Brothers, 1942).

—— et al., *Selective Partial Ablation of the Frontal Cortex* (New York: Columbia Greystone Associates, Paul B. Hoeber, 1949).

Lange, J., *Crime and Destiny* (New York: Boni, 1930).

Lapouse, R., and M. Monk, "An Epidemiologic Study of Behavior Characteristics of Children," *AJPH*, 48:1134 (September 1958).

Leavell, H. R., and E. G. Clarke, *Textbook of Preventive Medicine* (New York: McGraw-Hill, 1953).

Leavy, S. A., and L. Z. Freedman, "Psychoneurosis in Economic Life," *Social Problems*, 4:55–66 (July 1956).

Leighton, Dorothy C., "The Distribution of Psychiatric Symptoms in a Small Town," *Amer. J. Psychiat.*, 112:716–723 (March 1956).

Lemkau, Paul, *Mental Hygiene in Public Health* (New York: McGraw-Hill, 1949).

—— B. Pasamanick, and Marcia Cooper, "The Implications of the Psychogenetic Hypothesis for Mental Hygiene," *Amer. J. Psychiat.*, 110:436–442 (December 1953).

Leone, L. P., "The Changing Needs of People," *AJPH*, 47:32–38 (January 1957).

Levy, David, *Maternal Overprotection* (New York: Columbia University Press, 1943).

Lewin, Kurt, "Frontiers of Group Dynamics," *Human Relations*, I:35 (June 1947), quoted in A. K. Cohen, *Delinquent Boys* (Glencoe, Ill.: The Free Press, 1955).

Lilienfeld, A., "Prevention and Control of Chronic Disease," *AJPH*, 49:1135–1140 (September 1959).

Ling, E. M., J. A. Purser, and E. W. Reese, "Incidence and Treatment of Neuroses in Industry," *Brit. med. J.*, 2:159–167 (July 5, 1950).

Linton, Ralph, *Culture and Mental Disorders* (Springfield, Ill.: Charles C Thomas, 1956).

McCann, Mary, and M. F. Trulson, "Long-Term Effective Weight Reducing Programs," *J. Amer. diet. Assn.*, 31:1108–1110 (November 1955).

McKenzie, Miriam T., "Flexibility and Mental Health: A TAT Study," unpublished dissertation (New York University, 1961).

McKinnon, N. E., "Cancer Mortality Trends in Different Countries," *Canad. J. publ. Hlth*, 41:230–240 (June 1950).

—— "Cancer of the Breast: The Invalid Evidence for Faith in Early Diagnosis," *Canad. J. publ. Hlth*, 42:218–223 (June 1951).

—— "Downward Trend in Breast Cancer Mortality?," *Lancet*, 2:1086–1087 (November 29, 1952).

Mackintosh, J. M., *Housing and Family Life* (London: Cassell, 1952).

MacMahon, B., "Statistical Methods in Medicine," *New Engl. J. Med.*, 253:646–652, 688–693 (October 13, 20, 1955).

Mann, K. J., "An Experiment in Community Health within the Framework of a University Hospital," *Report of the VIIIth International Hospital Congress* (London, May 1953).

Maslow, A. H., "The Authoritarian Character Structure," *J. Social Psych.*, 18:402 (November 1943), quoted in Rose, *Mental Health and Mental Disorder*, chapter 31.

Mead, Margaret, ed., *Cultural Factors and Technical Change*, UNESCO (New York: Mentor, 1955).

Menninger, Karl, *Love Against Hate* (New York: Harcourt, Brace & Company, 1942).

Menninger, William with Martin Mayman, "Psychological Homeostasis and Organismic Integrity," mimeographed notes (January 1, 1956, Topeka, Kansas), based on material published previously as "Psychological Aspects of the Organism Under Stress," Part I, *J. Amer. psychoanal. Ass.*, 2:67–106 (January 1954); "The Homeostatic Regulatory Function of the Ego," Part II, 2:280–310 (April 1954); "Regulatory Devices of the Ego Under Major Stress," *Int. J. Psychoanalysis*, Part IV, pp. 412–420 (1954).

Merton, Robert K., "Manifest and Latent Functions," chapter I, and "The Self-Fulfilling Prophecy," chapter XI in *Social Theory and Social Structure* (Glencoe, Ill.: The Free Press, 1957).

Munroe, R. L., *The Schools of Psychoanalytic Thought* (New York: Dryden, 1955).

Murphy, Gardner, *Personality* (New York: McGraw-Hill, 1937).

Neubauer, P. B., "The Technique of Parent Group Education" in *Parent Group Education and Leadership Training* (New York: Child Study Association 1953).

New England Journal of Medicine, editorial, "Fifty Years of Social Service," 259:404 (August 21, 1958).

Osler, William, "The Home in Its Relation to the Tuberculosis Problem," *Med. News* (N.Y.), 83:1105–1110 (December 12, 1903).

Parkin, R. C., and O. L. Peterson, "The Role of the Preceptorship in Medical Education," *J. med. Educ.*, 34:644–648 (July 1959).

Parran, Thomas, "A Career in Public Health," *Pub. Hlth Rep.* (Wash.), 67:930–943 (October 1952).

Parsons, T., and R. Bales, *Family, Socialization and Interaction Process* (Glencoe, Ill.: The Free Press, 1955).

Paterson, Jane, "The Almoner's Contribution to Medical Teaching," *The Almoner*, Part I, 3:163–177 (August 1950); Part II, 3:201–206 (September 1950).

Peabody, Francis, *The Care of the Patient* (Cambridge, Mass.: Harvard University Press, 1928), reprinted from *JAMA* 88:877–882 (March 19, 1927).

Pearse, I. H., "The Peckham Experiment," *Eugen. Rev.*, 37:48–55 (July 1945).

—— and L. H. Crocker, *Biologists in Search of Material* (London: Faber and Faber, 1938), pp. 52–91.

—— and L. H. Crocker, *The Peckham Experiment* (London: Allen and Unwin, 1943).

Phillips, H. T., and Eva J. Salber, "Some Social Aspects of Pediatrics," *S. Afr. med. J.*, 29:499–503 (May 21, 1955).

Piaget, Jean et al., *The Moral Judgment of the Child* (London: Routledge and Kegan Paul, 1950).

Pollack, H., C. F. Consolizio, and G. J. Isaac, "Metabolic Demands as a Factor in Weight Control," *JAMA*, 167:216–219 (May 10, 1958).

Pomrinse, S. D., and M. S. Goldstein, "Report of the 1959 Survey of Group Practice," presented at Annual Meeting of *APHA*, mimeographed (November 2, 1960).

Pond, M. A., "How Does Housing Affect Health," *Pub. Hlth Rep.*, 61:665–672 (May 10, 1946).

—— "The Influence of Housing on Health," *Marriage and Family Living*, 19:154–159 (May 1957).

Potter, S., and J. Handy, "Observations in a 'Control' Group of Patients in Psychosomatic Investigations," *New Engl. J. Med.*, 255:1067–1071 (December 6, 1956).

"Preventive Use of Psychotherapy in Childhood," *Bull. N.Y. Acad. Med.*, 32:33–56 (January 1956).

Rapaport, David, M. M. Gill, and R. Schafer, *Diagnostic Psychological Testing* (Chicago: Year Book Publishers, 1945–1946).

Reader, G. G., "Comprehensive Medical Care," *J. med. Educ.*, 28:34–39 (July 1953).

—— "Organization and Development of a Comprehensive Care Program," *AJPH*, 44:760–765 (June 1954).

—— L. Pratt, and M. C. Mudd, "What Patients Expect from Their Doctors," *Mod. Hosp.*, 89:88–94 (July 1957).

Reed, R., and B. Burke, "Collection and Analysis of Dietary Intake Data," *AJPH*, 44:1015–1026 (August 1954).

Reid, D. D., "The Design of Clinical Experiments," *Lancet*, 267:1293–1296 (December 25, 1954).

Riesman, David, *The Lonely Crowd* (New Haven: Yale University Press, 1950).

Roberts, K., *Solo or Symphony* (New York: Medical Adm. Service, 1946).

Rodman, Hyman, "On Understanding Lower Class Behavior," *Social and Economic Studies*, 8:441–450 (December 1959).

Roe, Anne, *The Psychology of Occupations* (New York: John Wiley & Sons, 1956), part II.

Roemer, Milton I., "A Program of Preventive Medicine for the Individual," *Milbank mem. Fd Quart.* 23:209–226 (July 1945).

Roethlisberger, F. J., and W. J. Dickson, *Management and the Worker* (Cambridge, Mass.: Harvard University Press, 1939).

331

Rogers, C. R., and R. F. Dymond, *Psychotherapy and Personality Change* (Chicago: University of Chicago Press, 1954).

Rose, Arnold, ed., *Mental Health and Mental Disorder* (New York: W. W. Norton & Company, 1955).

Rosen, George, "Origins of Medical Specialization," *Ciba Symposia*, 22:1125–1156 (September, October, November 1949).

—— *A History of Public Health* (New York: M.D. Publications, 1958).

Safford, F. K., Jr., "Health Center for Preventive Medicine, Recreation and Education," *Architectural Record*, 83:66–71 (February 1938).

Saunders, L., *Cultural Differences and Medical Care* (New York: Russell Sage Foundation, 1954).

Schlossman, Howard H., "Transference in Medical Team-Family Research: The Family Health Maintenance Demonstration," *Amer. J. Orthopsychiat.*, 31:612–621 (July 1961).

Scott, Richard, "Edinburgh University General Practice Teaching Unit," *J. med. Educ.*, 31:621–634 (September 1956).

Shapiro, Irving, "Is Group Parent Education Worthwhile?," *Marriage and Family Living*, 18:154–161 (May 1956).

—— *Changing Child-Rearing Attitudes Through Group Discussion*, Ph.D. dissertation (Columbia, 1954), University Microfilms Pub. #10, 801, Ann Arbor, Mich.

Sheehan, M. W., "The Family as a unit for Public Health," in *The Family as a Unit of Health* (New York: Milbank Memorial Fund, 1949).

Shryock, R. J., "The Origins and Significance of the Public Health Movement in the U.S.," *Ann. med. Hist.*, New Series, 1:645–665 (November 1929).

—— *The Development of Modern Medicine* (New York: Alfred A. Knopf, 1947).

—— *Medicine and Society in America* (New York: New York University Press, 1960).

Sigerist, Henry E., *American Medicine* (New York: W. W. Norton & Company, 1934).

—— "The Beginnings of American Medicine," *Therapeutic Notes*, 62:73–76 (March 1955).

—— "The Place of the Physician in Modern Society," *Proc. Amer. Phil. Soc.*, 90:275–279 (September 1946).

Silver, George A., "Beyond General Practice: The Health Team," *Yale J. Bio. Med.*, 31:29–39 (September 1958).

—— "Family Health Maintenance," *Pub. Hlth Rep.* vol. 71, no. 10 (October 1956).

—— "Family Health Maintenance: A Perspective on the Ailing Family," in Iago Galdston, ed., *The Family, A Focal Point in Health Education* (New York: New York Academy of Medicine, 1961), pp. 135–159.

—— "A Family Health Service as a Teaching Program," *J. med. Educ.*, 33:600–604 (August 1958).

—— "Planning for Family Medical Service," *Proc. Roy. Soc. Med.*, 54: 449–452 (June 1-961).

—— M. Cherkasky, and J. Axelrod, "An Experience with Group Practice," *New Engl. J. Med.*, 256:785–791 (April 25, 1957).

—— and C. Stiber, "The Social Worker and the Physician," *J. med. Educ.*, 32:324–330 (May 1957).

———— M. Cherkasky, and H. Weiner, "The Home Care Program in a General Hospital," in *Frontiers in General Hospital Psychiatry*, L. Linn, ed. (New York: International Universities Press, 1961).

Simmons, Ozzie, *Social Status and Public Health* (New York: Social Science Research Council, 1958).

Smith, Geddes, *Psychotherapy in General Medicine* (New York: Commonwealth Fund, 1946).

Spence, J., W. S. Walton, F. J. W. Miller, and D. M. Court, *A Thousand Families in Newcastle-Upon-Tyne* (London: Oxford University Press, 1954).

Spiegel, John, "Homeostatic Mechanisms Within the Family," in *The Family in Contemporary Society* (New York: New York Academy of Medicine, 1958), pp. 70–94.

Spitz, René, "Unhappy and Fatal Outcomes of Emotional Deprivation and Stress in Infancy" in *Beyond the Germ Theory*, ed. Iago Galdston (New York: New York Academy of Medicine, 1954).

Spock, B. M., *Baby and Child Care* (New York: Pocket Books, Inc., 1957).

Statistical Abstract of the United States (Washington: Government Printing Office, 1951).

Stearns, Genevieve, "The Nutritional State of the Mother Prior to Conception," *JAMA*, 168:1655–1659 (November 22, 1958).

Swan, C., A. L. Tostevin, B. Moore, H. Mayo, and G. H. B. Black, "Congenital Defects in Infants Following Infectious Diseases During Pregnancy," *Med. J. Aust.*, 2:201–210 (September 11, 1943).

Sydenstricker, Edgar, *Health and Environment* (New York: McGraw-Hill, 1933).

Taylor, J. A., "A Personality Scale of Manifest Anxiety," *J. abnorm. soc. Psychol.*, 48:285–290 (April 1953).

Titmuss, R., *Essays on The Welfare State* (London: Allen and Unwin, 1958).

Tomkins, S. S., and B. J. Tomkins, *The Thematic Apperception Test* (New York: Grune & Stratton, 1947), chapters 6, 7, 10.

———— and J. B. Miner, *The Picture Arrangement Test* (New York: Springer Publishing Company, 1957).

Townsend, Peter, *The Family Life of Old People* (London: Routledge and Kegan Paul, 1957).

Trowbridge, M., Jr., "Extramural Preceptorships," *New Engl. J. Med.*, 258:691–695 (April 3, 1958).

Tureen, Louis L., "The Role of the Psychiatrist in a Prepaid Group Medical Program," *AJPH*, 49:1373–1378 (October 1959).

Vertue, H. St. H., "Chlorosis and Stenosis," *Guy's Hosp. Rep.*, 104:329–348 (1955).

Vital Statistics — Special Reports, vol. 46, 1956 and 1957 (Washington: Government Printing Office, 1956, 1957).

"Volume of Physicians' Services," *Health Statistics* (Washington: Government Printing Office, August 1960).

Warner, W. L., M. Meeker, et al., *Social Class in America* (Chicago: Science Research Association, 1949).

Watts, Alan W., "Asian Psychology and Modern Psychiatry," *Amer. J. Psychoanalysis*, 13:25 (1953), reprinted in C. F. Reed, I. E. Alexander, and

S. S. Tomkins, *Psychopathology: A Source Book* (Cambridge, Mass.: Harvard University Press, 1958).

Weiskotten, H. G., and M. E. Altenderfer, "Trends in Medical Practice," *J. med. Educ.*, 27: Part 2 (September 1952).

—— "Trends in Specialization," *JAMA*, 160:1303–1305 (April 14, 1956).

—— "Trends in Medical Practice," *J. med. Educ.*, 31: Part 2 (July 1956).

—— W. S. Wiggins, M. E. Altenderfer, M. Gooch, and A. Tipner, "Trends in Medical Practice," *J. med. Educ.*, 35:1071–1121 (December 1960).

Weisman, A. D., and E. P. Hackett, "Psychosis After Eye Surgery," *New Engl. J. Med.*, 258:1285–1289 (June 26, 1958).

Wescoe, W. C., "Preceptors as General Educators in Medicine," *J. med. Educ.*, 31:598–604 (September 1956).

"What Are the Facts About Mental Illness in the U.S.?" (Washington: National Mental Health Comm., 1955).

What Makes for Strong Family Life (New York: Community Service Society, n.d.).

Williamson, G. S., "Peckham," *Lancet*, 250:393–395 (March 16, 1946).

Wilner, D. M., R. P. Walkley, M. N. Glasser, and M. Tayback, "Study of the Effects of Housing Quality on Morbidity" presented at APHA meeting November 11, 1957.

—— R. P. Walkley, T. C. Pinkerton, M. Tayback, "Housing as an Environmental Factor in Mental Health," *APHA*, 50:55–63 (January 1960).

Winkelstein, L. B., "Hypnosis, Diet and Weight Reduction" *N.Y. St. J. Med.*, 59:1751–1756 (May 1, 1959).

Witmer, H. L., and R. Kotinsky, *Personality in the Making* (New York: Harper & Brothers, 1952).

Zubin, J., "Failures of the Rorschach Technique," *J. project. Techn.*, 18:303–315 (September 1954).

NOTES

CHAPTER I. Beginnings

1. In 1948, Bailey Burritt wrote in a memorandum to the Health Maintenance Committee of the Community Service Society, "One of the greatest economic and social losses to individuals, their families, and the nation is the failure to maintain a robust, vigorous state of health." He ascribed the failure to lack of application of existing knowledge of preventive measures. Burritt obviously reflected the motivation of the sponsors of the Demonstration. So did Cherkasky, who, as first director of the Family Health Maintenance Demonstration, spelled out a similar policy in an early Milbank conference. (Cherkasky, "The Family Health Maintenance Demonstration," 1952).

2. Sydenstricker, *Health and Environment*, pp. 127, passim.

3. Koos, *Families in Trouble*; Hill, *Families Under Stress*; Faris, *Social Disorganization*.

4. Dramatic presentation of these numbers in graphic form can be found in Health Information Foundation bulletins "Progress in Health Services" and Metropolitan Life Insurance Company "Statistical Bulletins." Comparable presentations in verbal form are in Louis Dublin's *The Facts of Life* (New York: Macmillan, 1954). Basic data can be found in the "Statistical Abstract" (Department of Commerce) for various years and the periodic publications of the National Office of Vital Statistics, particularly the recent ones.

5. Pearse, "The Peckham Experiment," 1945; Pearse and Crocker *The Peckham Experiment*, 1943. At the end of 3 years the investigation concluded: "(1) Examination of the man-in-the-street by modern scientific methods disclosed disorders of a pathological nature not anticipated by us nor by the families themselves. (2) Such disorders when discovered at this early stage, were easier to treat and adjust than in a more advanced or chronic stage. (3) If individuals after their 'cure' remained in the environment in which they had been living, those disorders were prone to recur. This last was a very serious finding. It meant clearly that *periodic overhaul accompanied by early treatment of disorder was of little use if unaccompanied by measures to modify the environment in which the disorders had arisen.*"

6. Recreation as such never appealed to Americans as an aspect of public health or preventive medicine activity. Safford, "Health Center," tried to interest health departments in Peckham-type recreation–health centers without success.

7. See Pearse and Crocker, *"Biologists in Search of Material."*

8. See Kark, "Health Service Among Rural Bantu," and "Health Center Service." Sidney Kark has left South Africa and is now engaged in a some-

what similar program based on a health center for new immigrants in Jerusalem, Israel — Kiryat Hayovel — under the auspices of Hadassah, The Hebrew University Medical School, and the World Health Organization. Mann, "An Experiment in Community Health."

9. For example, it is with nostalgic regret that I read the statistics of the Pholela Health Center (Kark and Cassel, "Pholela") because the very crudest type of public-health statistics demonstrated the effectiveness of the program. The crude mortality rate between 1942 and 1950 was brought down from 38.3 per thousand to 13.6 per thousand; the infant mortality rate was reduced from 27.5 percent to 10 percent. In the more sophisticated Bronx crude mortality was already below 10 per thousand at that time, and infant mortality less than 2 percent. Gross measurements of the effectiveness of a program available to the South Africans were not possible for us. Furthermore, health center activities in South Africa were restricted and the broad range of medical care, including the home and hospital service, was not part of their job.

10. Excellent documentation can be found in *Health and Demography*.

11. A staggering amount of responsibility shifts to the doctor with another change, also a result of industrialization and scientific advance — the change in disease prevalance and the kinds of diseases that require attention. Shifting from acute chronic disease as the major cause of death and disability results in increased demand for medical service quantitatively and qualitatively. The doctor has to see people who are less seriously ill, be prepared to do less in physical care, recognize more of socio-economic aspects and look after psychological and emotional aspects, prevent disease at interval stages, and restore the patient to relative social usefulness. The role is more complex, more demanding, and advisory as much as therapeutic.

12. For the historical development of American medical practice and to identify those elements contributing to the present difficulties, see Shryock, "Origins of the Public Health Movement" and *Medicine and Society in America;* Sigerist, *American Medicine* and "Beginnings of American Medicine."

13. The proprietary medical school was a grouping of apprenticeships in which a number of physicians pooled their resources and the income from students to establish medical colleges unconnected with universities. Baltimore had the first proprietary school.

14. *Scientific American* (November 1858): "In New York there is one physician to every 610 inhabitants; in Massachusetts, one to every 605; in Pennsylvania, one to every 561; in North Carolina, one to every 802; in Ohio, one to every 465; in Maine, one to every 884; and in California, one to every 147. We can envy Maine and pity California, for some must swallow physic at a frightful rate in the Golden State." In *Medical Education,* Flexner reports that in communities with as few as 80 people, 3 or 4 physicians were practicing.

15. Abraham Flexner's famous report is given credit for triggering the scientific revolution in medical education; but actually he only facilitated a development already almost fifty years old in laboratory training of physicians. The report did contribute heavily to the subsequent closure of poor schools and the improvement of licensing procedures.

16. For a careful and thorough examination of the growth of specialism

336

in the United States see Rosen, "Origins of Specialization." See also Weiskotten et al., "Trends in medical Practice."

17. The New York Academy of Medicine now subscribes to more than 3000 journals.

18. Hunt et al., "Medical Group Practice"; Pomrinse and Goldstein, "Report of 1959 Survey."

19. Roberts, *Solo or Symphony?*; Clark and Clark, *Organization of Group Medical Practice*; Goldmann, "Potentialities of Group Practice."

20. Silver et al., "An Experience with Group Practice."

21. Health Insurance Plan Groups are scattered through the 5 boroughs of New York City, and Nassau and Columbia counties of New York State.

22. The greatest difficulty in maintaining a satisfactory group structure stems from financial factors. While there is no perfect system of reimbursement, the technique in use in the Montefiore Medical Group seems to favor the best interests of both patient and doctor. An equal responsibility devolves upon the group to arrange for a limited panel, appointment system, and other working conditions to protect the doctor from exploitation.

23. This yearning for a "Golden Age" medical service is reported from other areas of the United States (Koos, "Metropolis," for example). For a patient-oriented description of the role of the doctor of the future, see Sigerist, "The Place of the Physician."

24. A number of social scientists have underlined the value of this message for the success of public health programs. See Foster, *Intercultural Health Programs*, and Simmons, *Social Status*.

25. There are now over 2,000,000 people helping to provide medical care (paramedical workers), as compared with some 225,000 physicians in the United States. ("Building America's Health," pp. 135.) Of this number of physicians, only 160,000 are in community practice. So that there are more than 12 paramedical people for every doctor.

26. For descriptions of new courses, see *Journal of Medical Education, 1953.* "Symposium"; and Reader, "Comprehensive Care Program," 1954. For curriculum modification see Wescoe, "Preceptors"; Fleming, "Family Physician's Approach"; and Trowbridge, "Preceptorships." For modification of psychiatric teaching to include family practice, see American Psychiatric Association, "Outline For A Curriculum"; Adams, "The Psychiatrist in an Ambulatory Clerkship"; and Dwyer and Zinbey, "Psychiatry for Medical School Instructors." For preceptorships, see Parkin and Peterson, "Role of the Preceptorship"; and Kindschi, "Wisconsin Preceptor Program." For general practitioner reorientation, see Smith, *Psychotherapy in General Medicine.*

CHAPTER II. Problems of Emotional Health and Treatment

1. Cherkasky, "Family Health Maintenance."

2. Bowlby, "Application of Recent Research to Health Visiting."

3. Merton, *Social Theory and Social Structure*, pp. 158, 159.

4. Piaget et al., *Moral Judgment of the Child*, pp. 335 ff.

5. Kluckhohn and Murray, *Personality.*

6. See Glaser and Eisenberg, "Maternal Deprivation"; R. Spitz quoted in Creak, "Parents and Children"; and, of course, Bowlby. We have to make the additional assumption that there is such a thing as psychological

injury. For a discussion of this as a possible source of neurosis see Lemkau et al., "Psychogenetic Hypothesis."

7. Bowlby, "Application of Recent Research to Health Visiting." This is not an unreasonable assumption in the light of known physical factors impeding physical development. See Swan et al., "Congenital Defects," and Greenberg et al., "Frequency of Defects," for the rubella influence in pregnancy; and Ingalls and Philbrook, "Monstrosities Induced by Hypoxia," where it was shown that in mice, exact knowledge of the moment of pregnancy during which oxygen was reduced enabled the investigator to predict the precise defect!

8. See Kohn and Clausen, "Social Isolation and Schizophrenia"; Landis and Bolles, *Personality and Sexuality*; and Eaton and Weil, *Culture and Mental Disorders*.

9. Cottrell, "Roles and Marital Adjustment." See also Dicks, "Strains Within the Family" and "The Predicament of the Family." Compare also Ezekiel, "The fathers have eaten of the sour grapes and the children's teeth are set on edge."

10. We tried to avoid conclusions about "normal" sexuality and restricted ourselves to "satisfactory" sexuality in marriage partners. Sexual contacts outside of marriage were considered evidence of an unsatisfactory relationship, just as sex contacts between unmarried people were considered unhealthy because of existing social taboos. And of course, open, active sexuality in young children were considered unhealthy because it transgressed the prevailing cultural pattern of restraint of sexuality in young people.

11. Horsley Gantt, "Experimental Basis for Neurotic Behavior," has shown (in dogs) that neurotic sexual behavior patterns are related to and derive from the establishment of neurosis in childhood. In that case, sexual behavior reflects the neurotic personality. Linton, *Culture and Mental Disorders*, cities a South Sea Island culture in which neurotic expressions center about food rather than sexual deprivation because there isn't any such there. Again, however, the neurosis is established in childhood, the deviant adult behavior a result.

12. A recent book, Arnold Rose, ed., *Mental Health and Mental Disorder* (1955) brings together a large number of papers from the field of sociology bearing on this subject. See particularly chapter 22 (William Sewell on infant training), chapter 23 (Arnold Greene on middle-class values), and chapter 37 (Kingsley Davis on class in general).

13. Linton, *Culture and Mental Disorders*.

14. Erich Fromm, "Individual and Social Origins of Neuroses," makes a subtle distinction between what society imposes and what happens when society becomes what the majority of the individuals in it are. He talks of the "socially patterned defect." Where pinta is prevalent in a very high percentage of the population, people *without* this disease may be considered sick. Would one be permitted to introduce penicillin to "cure" the "well" people?

15. Anna Freud, "Psychoanalysis and Education." David Levy, in *Maternal Overprotection*, considers the necessity for limiting the *parental* role.

16. Fashions in child-rearing do change, and the pendulum swings from permissiveness to rigidity. It must be kept in mind that *both* types of handling were deemed "good" for the child in their time, *both* were con-

sidered expressions of affection, in their time. Tenderness is not a novel contribution of this age or of modern psychiatrists.

17. Even the World Health Organization is backtracking on this definition and devising health "indicators" in *three* categories, only one of which is personal health. (*AJPH*, "A Theoretical Model of Health.") In discussing this change the editor, whose approach is similar to that attempted in this book, writes: "adequate performance of physiological and psychological functions as well as estimates of the total efficiency of the organism."

18. Health in terms of social functioning must be considered in the light of what society demands of the individual and how the individual measures up to these expectations. See Riesman, *The Lonely Crowd,* and Witmer and Kotinsky, *Personality in the Making.*

19. Compare Bernard, *Experimental Medicine,* and Cannon, *The Wisdom of the Body,* on the steady state and homeostasis. Dr. William Menninger has developed an excellent elaboration on this theme in "The Concept of Psychological Homeostasis" (1954 and 1956). Engel, "Homeostasis," has contributed the concept of health as the phase of successful adjustment.

20. R. Ross and E. Van den Haag, *Fabric of Society* (New York: Harcourt, Brace, 1957), p. 11.

21. See W. Trotter, *Instincts of the Herd in Peace and War* (New York, Macmillan, 1919), p. 89; and Witmer and Kotinsky, *Personality in the Making.* Jahoda, writes in *Current Concepts of Positive Mental Health*: "It is generally accepted that the term, normality, covers two different concepts: normality as a *statistical* frequency concept and normality as a normative idea of how people ought to function. To believe that the two connotations always coincide leads to the assertion that whatever exists in a majority of cases is right by virtue of its existence." In "Asian Psychology," Watts extends the view eastward: ". . . for Oriental psychology, 'normalcy' could never be a standard of mental health — where normalcy means the ways of thinking and feeling, the conventions and life goals acceptable to the majority of persons in a particular culture." Only Boehm, in "Psychiatric Social Work," takes an affirmative position: "Mental health is a condition and level of social functioning which is socially acceptable and personally satisfying" (italics author's).

22. A great deal of nonsense is written about this probably because so little accurate information is available. Many children have tics, bite their nails, masturbate, suffer from nightmares, display varying degrees of aggressive behavior. Lapouse and Monk, "Epidemiologic Study of Behavior Characteristics," studying the universality of these presumably unhealthy behavior characteristics found only 35 percent of the children observed showed no symptoms. It is possible that these symptoms should be regarded not as precursors of neurosis or indicative of potential psychiatric disorder but simply as transient developmental phenomena. On the other hand, Cust in "Epidemiology of Nocturnal Enuresis" ties together bed-wetting with emotional troubles and difficulties in school. In a recent symposium all the child psychiatrists agreed with this notion of high incidence of disturbance in apparently normal children, but they thought disturbances may be evidence of serious developmental problems too. How is the parent to know when a symptom or sign is to be ignored and when symptoms are to be taken care

of by the physician? Well, one of the ways is to wait and see whether it persists ("Preventive Use of Psychotherapy"). This counsel would satisfy a few parents and irritate many. Another way is to have an agency appraisal — on assumption that the parents should go for advice and guidance in *every case,* and *early!* This counsel is unlikely to satisfy any more than the first, but it would frighten more parents.

23. Taylor, "A Personality Scale"; Landis et al., *Selective Partial Ablation.*

24. The term has been in use in English since 1525. Not only psychiatry, since Freud's painstaking formulations but philosophy and literature have a stake in anxiety as an abnormal manifestation. See Auden "The Age of Anxiety" (New York: Random House, 1947). Altschule, "Ideas of XVIIIth Century Medical Writers," points out that Eighteenth-century England gave us the expression "Age of Anxiety" for that time. Titmuss, *Essays on the Welfare State,* quotes Benjamin McCreedy who wrote in 1837: "The Americans are an anxious, careworn people."

25. See Basowitz et al., *Anxiety and Stress;* Altschule, "Physiological Data"; Dürkeim, *Suicide;* and Merton, *Social Theory and Social Structure.*

26. While H. Frankfort et al., *Intellectual Adventure of Ancient Man* (Chicago: Univ. of Chicago, 1946) describe movingly the anxiety of Egyptians as expressed in their literature of 4000 years ago, Gerard, "Anxiety and Tension," takes issue with those who would broaden the concept of anxiety to extend it to other times and other cultures, believing that less civilized people have no "projection of apprehension," and that danger to them is either imminent or nonexistent.

27. For example, there must be no obvious friction between parents and there should be loving affection between parents and children. The children should have no hostility toward the parents, no difficulty in school, and no obvious defects of a psychological nature.

28. In our implicit assumptions we might go so far as to say that removing oneself from a family pattern or failing to form a family, is to miss an important part of development or of living and that this militates against such a person being healthy. In our evaluations, the measure of the closeness of the attachment of family members was a measure of the healthy functioning of the individuals: antagonisms and conflict represented unhealthy functioning.

29. *What Makes for Strong Family Life,* published by the Community Service Society. See also Davis and Havighurst, *Father of the Man,* who point out that the parent in each social class is preparing his child for the kind of life approved and desired by *his* social class.

30. Parsons and Bales, *Family.*

31. See Parsons and Bales *Family;* Dicks, "The Predicament of the Family"; and Burgess and Cottrell, "The Prediction of Adjustment in Marriage."

32. Bowlby, in "Application of Recent Research": "Our relationships with friends and acquaintances and professional colleagues are in great measure coloured by our relationships within our families — and that the very first relationship we make — that with our mothers — is the most important of all."

33. Howells and Layng, "Separation Experience," add that frequent

separations for fairly long periods are most damaging, and that these occur most commonly with inadequate parents. So the fact of separation may be less a source of traumatic deprivation than the inadequacy of parental love which it compounds.

34. Creak, "Parents and Children." Halliday, *Psychosocial Medicine,* bewails the excessive concern with cleanliness that public health has engendered.

35. The parents of American children are fortunate to have avoided social catastrophes like famine and revolution, but the Second World War had a hand in molding their parents. (Roe, *The Psychology of Occupations.* left its imprint on the children now growing up, and the Great Depression

36. B. Bettelheim has described this function as "in-service education of parents." I like to think that this is the role of the Family Health Maintenance Demonstration, or even, of health education in general: providing an in-service educational program for parents.

CHAPTER III. Aims and Methods of the Study Design

1. Grundy and Mackintosh, *The Teaching of Hygiene and Public Health in Europe,* p. 40.
2. Cherkasky, "Family Health Maintenance," p. 194.
3. Dublin and Fraenkel, *A Demonstration Project in Family Health Maintenance,* p. 13.
4. Dublin and Fraenkel, visualizing a community health program rather than a family sample, in their report had noted a similar approach: "(1) The initial health inventory. (2) The development of a specific health maintenance schedule as a result of this, a program for prevention as well as for curative services. (3) Periodic evaluation. (4) Health education."
5. See R. Kasius, "Are the Records Suitable?" in *The Family Health Maintenance Demonstration.*
6. H.I.P., *Health and Medical Care in New York City.*
7. Roethlisberger and Dickson, *Management and The Worker.*
8. Dr. Fertig suggested, and perhaps this could be incorporated in a future study, that alternate study and control families be selected only from those agreeing to participate (*Family Health Maintenance Demonstration,* p. 226). This would obviate the doubt about the nonparticipants in the control group being similar to the nonparticipants in the study group.
9. *Ibid.,* p. 231.
10. Cobb, King, and Chen, "Differences Between Respondents and Non-Respondents."
11. See Kasius, "Are the Records Suitable?," for a balanced review of the possibilities and problems involved in the scorings.
12. A limited analysis of character (description, rating, and comparability) appears in McKenzie, "Flexibility and Mental Health: A TAT Study." Mrs. McKenzie was the psychologist associated with the Demonstration for the whole of its existence.
13. Hume, "The Strategy and Tactics of Experimentation."
14. MacMahon, "Statistical Methods in Medicine."
15. Reid, "The Design of Clinical Experiments."
16. *Family Health Maintenance Demonstration,* p. 234.
17. P. Densen, "Broadening the Significance of Vital Statistics."

CHAPTER IV. Service and Research in Operation

1. Within a short time the physicians abandoned this introductory visit. We felt that it was not consistent with the layman's view of the doctor and might affect the doctor-patient relationship unfavorably.

2. *Diagnostic Psychological Testing*, by Rapaport et al., provided the basis for this decision. Any interpretation and use reflecting on the tests or their authors and any difficulties occasioned were of our own doing, and I hasten to absolve Dr. Rapaport of any responsibility. See also J. Zubin, "Failures of Rorschach Technique," and Tomkins and Tomkins, *The Thematic Apperception Test*.

3. Tomkins and Tomkins, *The Thematic Apperception Test*, and Bellak, *The TAT and CAT in Clinical Use*.

4. Tomkins and Tomkins, *The Thematic Apperception Test*, p. 109. Bellak makes this same point.

5. Tomkins and Tomkins, *The Thematic Apperception Test*, p. 266.

6. See also Rogers and Dymond, *Psychotherapy and Personality Change*, for an effort to analyze the variables in the TAT. Our fruitless search for certainty in this important area of comparison (personality structure and sources of emotional difficulty) underlines a valuable field of research inadequately tilled. The standardization of psychological tests on average families or on population cross sections has been inadequate. The vogue for standardization of college students and institution inmates seems to me almost without value. For the future, I would like to have available a carefully standardized, easily applicable, and rapidly scored test as a psychological support to interview and observation. While such a test of personality does not yet exist, Tomkins and Miner in *The Picture Arrangement Test* have made an interesting and perceptive start.

7. Brodman et al., "Evaluation of Emotional Disturbances."

8. For a complete description of the Cornell Medical Index and its use see Brodman et al., "The Cornell Medical Index Health Questionnaire," 1951. Other publications on standardizing the test and its widespread use will be found in various journals. An earlier review, Brodman et al., "The Cornell Medical Index," 1949, may be helpful.

9. Clarke and Clarke, "Vagaries of Intelligence."

10. Reed and Burke, "Collection and Analysis of Dietary Intake Data."

11. Pollack et al., "Metabolic Demands as a Factor in Weight Control."

12. Stearns, "The Nutritional State of the Mother," with particular reference to the work of Dugald Baird in Aberdeen on the effect of social class and nutrition on pregnancy performance.

13. Pond, "The Influence of Housing on Health." For similar views, see Wilner et al., "Study of the Effects of Housing Quality on Morbidity," and "Housing as an Environmental Factor in Mental Health."

14. For an analysis of the need for such data see *Environment and Health*, 1951 and for a thoughtful analysis, Mackintosh, *Housing and Family Life*.

15. See APHA, *Basic Principles of Healthful Housing*, and *An Appraisal Method* from which our form was developed.

16. See J. A. C. Brown, *The Social Psychology of Industry*.

17. Leavy and Freedman, "Psychoneurosis in Economic Life." For a

more critical view, see JAMA, "Woe and Work," and Gordon, "Industrial Psychiatry."

18. Roe, *The Psychology of Occupations*, part II, pp. 43 ff.

19. This may be an appropriate place to thank the Board of Education for its valiant efforts to obtain for our nurses and other team members access to school records and interviews with teachers and school nurses. I say efforts advisedly, because the Board of Education (and the Interdepartmental Committee on Health Problems in the Schools which includes the Health Department), being an imperfect bureaucracy, does not have iron-clad control over borough supervisors and school principals. Occasional principals were uncooperative, although we tried to explain that we were in a position to give as well as receive information. The vast majority of teachers and principals in the public schools were very cooperative. We are very appreciative of their help and that of the parochial schools which in general were quite cooperative.

20. Bieber, "Pathological Boredom and Inertia."

CHAPTER V. The Roles of the Team Members

1. Cunningham, "Problems of Communication in Scientific and Professional Disciplines."

2. Caudill and Roberts, "Pitfalls in the Organization of Interdisciplinary Research."

3. Cherkasky, "The Montefiore Hospital Home Care Program."

4. Eaton, "Social Processes of Professional Teamwork."

5. A general discussion of Sir Charles Lock's motivation in initiating the almoner movement is given in the editorial in the *New England Journal of Medicine*, "Fifty Years of Social Service." Richard Cabot's concern with obtaining information and assistance for carrying out his own job better is summarized in his book *Social Work*. On p. xi he writes: "The unmanageable increase in the number of patients to be treated by the doctor is one of the chief reasons why the home visitor has become necessary. In the old days and in country practices, especially, it was doubtless possible for the doctor to follow the lives of his patients individually as acquaintances and through many years to watch the growth and development of families, to know their members as a friend and not merely in a professional capacity." Ida Cannon's *On the Social Frontier of Medicine* brings to life the excitement and satisfactions of those days.

6. Kraus, "Role of Social Case Work," defines medical social work as, "The 'helping relationship' combined with the use of psychoanalytic concepts of human behavior," in Kasius, *Principles and Techniques*. For a recognition of the difference between the British and American views on the role of the social worker see the *Lancet*, "Contribution of Social Work to Medical Care," and "Definition of a Medical Social Work Position."

7. Silver and Stiber, "The Social Worker and The Physician."

8. See M. Davis, *Medical Care for Tomorrow*. On p. 671 he writes: "It should be apparent that medical social work is in one aspect a corrective to certain overspecializations in medicine." Also see Dongray, "Social Work in General Practice;" *Journal of Medical Education*, "Symposium on Extramural Facilities in Medical Education"; Paterson, "The Almoner's Contribu-

tion to Medical Teaching"; and Richard Scott, "Edinburgh University General Practice Teaching Unit."

9. See Allport "The Trend in Motivational Theory."

10. Information obtained from the Social Service Exchange.

11. The interrelatedness of the generations in the origin and fixation of personal problems was strikingly apparent in these formulations. As Mrs. Stiber, the social worker who participated throughout the program, expressed it: "old wounds rankle and old ties bind."

12. For an outline of the diagnostic and therapeutic responsibilities, see Silver and Stiber, "The Social Worker and The Physician."

13. Nursing can be said to begin with the Hippocratic apprentice who remained behind to look after the master's patients. Nursing training begins with Pastor Fliedner in the early nineteenth century. Public health nursing had its inception in the health educational need brought on by poverty and urbanization of the peasantry. See Rosen, *A History of Public Health*, pp. 374–382, and Osler, "The Home in Its Relation to the Tuberculosis Problem." For a different view of the origin of public health nursing, see Sheehan, "The Family As a Unit for Public Health."

14. "The house is the temple of family life. Its soundness is closely interlocked with the family health." (Mackintosh, *Housing and Family Life*, p. ix.)

15. The philosophic base for the emphasis on group meetings as a health education device stems largely from Kurt Lewin. See especially "Frontiers of Group Dynamics."

16. The Appendix contains: A list of various types of group meetings and discussion leaders; topics of general meetings; lists of films shown; lists of pamphlets distributed; the reading shelf. It was our very strong feeling that pamphlets of themselves are useless health education devices. Pamphlets may promote awareness, but they cannot give any insight. The human contact is what makes the difference in the promotion of health. And so, each of the workers in the program, in a discussion related to family health or to a medical service, or to some other family need, used the pamphlet in *conjunction* with the discussion, or in response to a question asked by the patient and never simply as an instrumental on its own.

17. Many adult subjects portrayed parental figures in their picture interpretations as opposed to the emancipation of their children from parental control. Parents were often shown as punitive, untrustworthy, and failing to provide needed recognition and affection.

18. See Smith, *Psychotherapy in General Medicine*, and a description of the "anticipatory guidance" activities of health departments in Lemkau, *Mental Hygiene in Public Health*, chapter V, and Ginsburg, *Public Health is People*.

19. A British view is expressed in *Lancet*, "Psychotherapy in General Practice." Watts divides psychiatry into three grades: "rapport," simply offering a friendly ear; assessment of emotional disorder and psychotherapy; and recognizing and treating mental illness. The first is every doctor's job; the second what every family doctor should be trained to do; and the third, the psychiatrist's job.

20. See Chapter X on action taken by families after revelations, but without direction from the team; *Lancet*, "Psychotherapy in General Practice"; and Henderson, "Physician and Patient as a Social System."

21. Dr. Carol Creedon.

22. His findings are reported in *Patients' Views of Medical Care,* 1961.

23. A good deal of social medicine is an effort to inculcate in medical students ideas of the differences between people and their attitudes so that they will look and listen and not simply assume understanding between themselves and patients. See footnote 20.

24. E. Hughes, *Men and Their Work.* Oswald Hall's very perceptive analysis of the types of medical careers is most helpful in considering health-team organization. If the distribution of colleague types and missionary types exceeds the competitive ones by a significant proportion there will be no dearth of qualified candidates for group practice and health team organization. See "The Informal Organization of Medical Practice in an American City," and "The Stages of a Medical Career." Goss, "Physicians in Bureaucracy."

CHAPTER VI. Reactions to Health-Team Service

1. The late Dr. Joseph Mountin, a heroic model of a public health doctor and social medicine pioneer, made a statement about public health that is equally applicable to medical practice: "an applied technology resting on the joint pillars of natural science and social science. Until both the pillars of natural and social science are strong, the arch of public health will not be firm." Quoted by Parran in "A Career in Public Health."

2. Even the care available for patients in the Montefiore Medical Group is not yet available to all Americans, but it is potentially available and within the framework of existing practice.

3. Recently a woman wrote, "The doctor . . . showed enough interest in your problems — so that you were confident in his skills as a doctor and secure in his concern for your welfare . . . If it were possible to maintain our Family Health Maintenance Demonstration care on a private basis — we would feel it worthwhile to drop HIP and use this service on a fee paying basis."

4. The Group's specialists were surprised by this table. In *their* opinion the Family Health Maintenance Demonstration physician was more apt to refer patients. There is no good explanation for this altered perception; the Demonstration doctor feels it may be due to the fact that he always called personally to refer a patient.

5. Included in family-doctor services are the annual physical examination, which every Demonstration patient obtained, but only 40 percent of the control patients received. Also, preventive services and educational visits as part of the research inflate the number of family-doctor services to study families.

6. The argument is often used that in group practice with prepayment, where no economic barrier to specialist referral exists, patient pressure and physician load will dictate unnecessary and undesirable referrals. The implication is that the family doctor is "demoted" in group practice. The contrary can apparently be true. It would seem to be rather a function of physician time, that the physician will not slough responsibility nor will the patient press for specialist care, when the family doctor gives adequate time.

7. Hughes et al., *20,000 Nurses Tell Their Story.*

8. Silver and Stiber, "Social Worker and The Physician."

9. For example, the nurse found that the husband in a lower-class family had been home a week with a "cold." She asked why the doctor hadn't been called and was told that he didn't want to bother the doctor.

10. See Hughes, *Men and Their Work*; Hughes et al., *20,000 Nurses Tell Their Story*; and Brown, *Nursing For the Future*.

11. Modern training of public health nurses encourages the "polyvalent" or secondary practitioner approach. For developing countries this experience is rich and valuable. See Expert Committee on Nursing, published by WHO, in which less highly skilled (subprofessional nurses) workers are recommended to assist the public health nurse! In the United States professional leaders of nursing recognize and describe such a larger professional role for modern nurses (Leone, "The Changing Needs of People").

12. "Class" is used to categorize families in terms of the occupation of the family head. In very general terms, upper middle class includes proprietary, managerial, and professional occupations; lower middle class refers to lower professionals and skilled workers; and lower class to semi-skilled and unskilled workers. The scale is modified from Warner, *Social Class in America*.

13. See K. Davis, "Mental Hygiene"; Hollingshead et al., *Social Class and Mental Illness*; Cavan, *The American Family*.

14. Rodman, "On Understanding Lower Class Behavior."

15. The family histories of the majority of the study families show marks of the Depression. It is mentioned frequently in discussions of childhood, of family relations, of choice of job. A number of the adults in the study group when they were children must have seen relief investigators ("social workers") in action — perhaps even experienced the humiliation of justifying the family's basic needs to a case worker. Most relief investigators were social workers by title and by courtesy only. It is possible that they were responsible for an unfortunate perception of the social worker's role, in addition to the unhappy association. If not the relief investigator, perhaps a hospital clinic "case worker" was encountered and became part of the bitter personal or social experience of the Depression generation. These "social workers" were (not by their own choice) barriers to money, food, shelter, medical care, summer camp — barriers to be overcome. They were to be endured, hopefully without hatred, but certainly without gratitude.

16. It should be emphasized that every effort was made to explain the function of the social worker and give her status as a member of the team. In the family conference, her role was described and if a suggestion was made for social-work follow-up, the team recommended this to the family. In further contacts with the doctor and nurse, when such a family had had a referral to the social worker, the referral was pressed. Failure in utilization cannot be ascribed to patients' ignorance of social-work function.

17. Measured in terms of correlation coefficients. While the data do not conform to usual requisites for the coefficient of correlation, nevertheless the coefficient does give a rapid idea of the degree of correspondence.

18. Since nurse and social worker had access to each other's notes in the common record and discussed cases in the regular weekly conferences, each had an opportunity to be influenced by the other and each had information on the other's ideas and judgments.

19. The whole of the story is not found simply in social class, acceptance

by families, or reaction to rejection of role by the families. Many writers on personality and the social role of the individual have commented that personality may be treated as a mirror in which other people's views of you are reflected. Perhaps the social worker in some way reacted to the reflection, in interpreting her role in the Demonstration. See Cooley, *Nature and the Social Order*; Kluckhohn and Murray, *Personality*; Sullivan, quoted in Goffman, *Presentation of Self*; Murphy, *Personality*; and Merton, "The Self-Fulfilling Prophecy."

20. The description of role and behavior stems from observations made by 3 different social workers in this program. Clearly more experiences with more social workers in daily medical practice will be necessary to elucidate the special or general nature of these observations. Statistical assessment of the agreement between the 2 sets of nurses and social workers showed that nurse A and social worker A responded to their evaluations in the same way that nurse B and social worker B did.

21. In recent years, the American Academy of General Practice has pressed hard for such a family practitioner, both in medical-school training and hospital experience.

CHAPTER VII. Changes in the Health of Demonstration Families

1. We assume that good housing is important to good health, although experts have been unsuccessful in proving this statistically.

2. The defect of a research design in which duration of the experiment is a factor should be emphasized here. Four years may or may not be long enough to see the changes that can occur in children (certainly more plastic and more likely *to* change) or the end results of intervention.

3. Our impression as to whether the family improved or not and the family's impression as to whether the program was helpful do not necessarily correspond. Close to 100 percent of the families thought that participation in the program was helpful to them.

4. From the observations of nurse and social worker, the way in which parents treated children was not related to the children's difficulties. Children treated permissively did not have fewer problems than more strictly treated children. Unfortunately, this item was not marked separately and numerical data in support of this thesis are lacking. Adults who related stressful childhood experience as a result of economic difficulties or immigration to a new country did not seem to show any more psychological difficulties than those who did not.

5. Francis Bacon. *The Advancement of Learning*.

CHAPTER VIII. Utilization of Services

1. In the first year or so of The British National Health Service, there was a great demand for service, a "backlog," not repeated in succeeding years. (Titmuss, *Essays on the Welfare State*.)

2. A professional service means a face-to-face contact, prearranged or scheduled at the request of the patient or team member, not including group educational meetings. Telephone calls, casual informal contacts, and group educational visits are not counted, although they provided important and sometimes crucial professional channels for services. However, since they were not always noted in the daily log, inclusion of some would have been

misleading. Besides, no data from other sources would have been comparable.

3. Prepayment is often opposed on the grounds that it leads to overuse and overuse equals abuse. Another argument is that used by Freud (Jones, *The Life and Work of Sigmund Freud,* 1958) that direct payment of client to practitioner is a necessary condition for effective treatment.

4. "Volume of Physicians' Services," and H.I.P., "1957 Annual Statistical Report."

5. Tables on hospitalization and hospital utilization are included in the Appendix. Since we had no knowledge of the quantity of outside utilization of hospitalization by control families, I decided to pass over the comparison or discussion as part of the text. Briefly, the tables seem to indicate higher hospital admission rates and higher operation rates for study-family parents. Length of stay is about the same for study and control families. For study-family children, admission rates are higher, but operative rates are not, and length of stay is greater for study than control children. These findings may be a function of better case finding. Bakst observed that patients on Home Care, with long-standing heart disease had twice as many admissions as those followed in routine out-patient fashion. (Bakst and Marra, "Experience with Home Care for Cardiac Patients.")

6. This need not be true, of course, since the parent may use the child as a "presenting symptom" in getting to see the doctor. Maybe the demotion of the pediatrician to "consultant" and the more apparent dominant role of the internist as family doctor played a part in this.

7. "Less" does not mean "better" either. A child who suffered from a character disorder with lack of sphincter control had been diagnosed previously as cerebral palsy with feeblemindedness. After long discussions with the mother, frequent visits to the doctor, and a series of specialized examinations, it was demonstrated that the difficulty was primarily an emotional one! The child was put under treatment along with the parents. The difference in future social prospects for a presumed feebleminded child with cerebral palsy and those for an emotionally disturbed child are enormous. One is the equivalent of a life sentence to prison, the other profoundly hopeful.

8. These evaluation areas were selected as characteristic of the evaluation performed by the particular professional worker and could be considered typical of the functional relationship.

9. The general decline of utilization continued. A check of high and low utilizers 2 years after the Demonstration ended and they had returned to the Medical Group for care, indicated little change in the pattern. High utilizers continue to use more services, low utilizers less.

10. Younger Jewish parents would seem to use more services than older ones, which is curious. The very high rate of utilization in Israel is well known. See Kanev, *Aspects of Social Security in Israel.*

11. It should be remembered that an unknown quantity of utilization of physicians existed outside the framework of the Demonstration. We have a clue from the study of patient satisfaction that about a third of the families sought some medical care outside the Group in addition to using Group and Demonstration services. How much outside service, precisely, was used, is unknown, but the distribution by class was exactly the same as in the Dem-

onstration. In other words, adding in non-Demonstration physician use would have augmented, not altered, this pattern.

12. See Hinkle and Wolff, "Health and the Social Environment" and "Ecologic Investigations"; Freud and Burlingham, *War and Children*; and Graham, "Socio-Economic Status."

13. Again, the small numbers make it difficult to extract class and education as influences in the ethnic area. The statement is tentative.

14. As New York City has not fluoridated the drinking water, credit for improvement must be ascribed to the Demonstration.

CHAPTER IX. Symptoms, Illness, and Family Life

1. Pearse and Crocker, *The Peckham Experiment*.

2. Leighton, "The Distribution of Psychiatric Symptoms in a Small Town."

3. As emotional problems, the data included physician's and social worker's diagnoses.

4. The remainder of families, "other religions" and "no religion" had the highest proportion with emotional problems, 16 out of 22 or 72.7 percent.

5. The helpful, cooperative Demonstration families deserve a better fate than to have their difficulties exposed in this summary fashion so as to lead the reader to consider them horribly unique. They are not; among the control families we find similar "sordid" details.

6. The word "coping" is commonly used to describe the personal activity here intended, i.e., putting up with difficulties, making do, adjusting without fuss, compensating. See Goffman, "The Moral Career of the Mental Patient"; Clausen and Kohn "The Ecological Approach In Social Psychiatry"; and Foote and Cottrell, *Interpersonal Competence*.

7. See Lange, *Crime and Destiny*.

8. Krause, "Role of Social Case Work."

9. Grinker and Spiegel, *Men Under Stress*.

10. The emphasis in both medicine and social work on illness and disease is frustrating. Serious evidence of emotional difficulty may yield no defect in functioning. The key word is *functioning*, not symptomatology. In functioning mechanisms there may be periods of compensation and periods of decompensation. A family no longer coping is decompensated, but this too may be only an interval stage.

11. Potter and Handy ("Observations in a 'Control' Group", in assessing the emotional state of psychiatric patients in order to explore emotional *causes* of mental breakdown, selected a group of patients with physical illness, who turned out to have the same variety of social difficulties and emotional problems as the psychiatric cases.

12. It would be very helpful if there were a simple chemical test for this adaptation mechanism. With such a diagnostic test, research would be far simpler, strenuous justifications unnecessary.

13. I am indebted to Charlotte G. Schwartz for this viewpoint.

14. Some support for this position may be drawn from the investigations of world-wide mental disease prevalence which indicate that the psychoses have a fairly uniform prevalence all over the world — about 6 percent of the population at any given time (Eaton and Weil, *Culture and Mental*

Disorders — a percentage far lower than that of emotional difficulties. The latter would seem to vary quantitatively and qualitatively from place to place (Kardiner, *The Psychological Frontiers of Society*) and from generation to generation and may be subject to cultural influences. Chodoff, "A Re-Examination of Some Aspects of Conversion Hysteria," 1954, examines the curious disappearance of conversion hysteria in our time; Vertue, "Chlorosis and Stenosis," the disappearance of chlorosis; and Harvey, "Changing Syndromes and Culture," describes many other changing diagnoses and symptoms.

CHAPTER X. Family and Team Interaction

1. Roe, *The Psychology of Occupations*. Since many industrial jobs today with union coverage, pensions, and seniority, are indistinguishable from civil service jobs, it would be a mistake to consider our patients in the Demonstration different from the bulk of the working population.

2. Compare Thoreau's "The mass of men lead lives of quiet desperation."

3. Precise information on the number of couples who used particular contraceptive methods could not be obtained. The impression remains that withdrawal was fairly commonly used, possibly because of religious objection to other forms of contraception. Invariably there was associated tension between the spouses when this method was used, and this tension would be overtly expressed in sexual terms. In one family the wife had gone so far as to be fitted with a diaphragm, whose use she believed would ease this tension. But she could not bring herself to use it, and "felt bad" about it.

4. For example, 60 percent of Catholic families sent their children to parochial school.

5. Alexander and French, *Studies in Psychosomatic Medicine*.

6. Sexuality requires both a cultural and sexual role definition. In some cultures the wife is expected to initiate sex activity; it is the husband's job to satisfy her. In others the woman is expected to be passive; the man must take the initiative, and the woman's satisfaction is a secondary consideration. Class also seems to influence role. Sexual difficulties may arise from a failure to fulfill these male/female roles; or, failure to fulfill an expected role may be evidence of family difficulty.

7. This may point up the fact there is never one localized problem, nor ever simply one individual in a family who has a problem. Whether this is because of a "contagion," or because to be healthy many people must be in a healthy environment, is not certain. Family members may be visualized as embedded in a matrix, and vibration at any point in the matrix is transmitted to all parts of it. In that case it might be said that a disturbed person in a family means a disturbed family.

8. The amount of information available in the schools was limited. In 1950, for example, in looking at school nursing records, only one record showed a teacher-nurse conference for 150 Demonstration children. The fact that this conference was held is important; the fact that the rest of the children did not have such conferences on their behalf is even more important. In the parochial schools, the teacher-nurse conferences did not exist.

CHAPTER XI. Preventive Medicine and Health Promotion

1. See Leavell and Clarke, *A Textbook of Preventive Medicine,* for "levels of prevention."

2. The routine of the preventive examination was based on Roemer, "A Program of Preventive Medicine for the Individual."

3. Herbolsheimer and Ballard, "Multiple Screening"; Hubbard, *The Early Detection and Prevention of Disease.*

4. McKinnon, "Cancer Mortality," "Cancer of the Breast," and "Downward Trend in Breast Cancer Mortality?"

5. Hubbard, *The Early Detection and Prevention of Disease.* The group Roberts describes falls into categories similar to those in our findings and those of Peckham: 13½ percent could be described as entirely healthy, 37½ percent with a significant disease.

6. All but one of the individuals in the study families was examined annually during the 4 years of observation. Cooperation in health examinations is rarely of this order; see "Cooperation in Health Examination Surveys."

7. A recent paper from the University of Pennsylvania Diagnostic Clinic on the results of periodic examinations on executives (a selected older group) bears this out (Elsom et al., "Periodic Health Examination").

8. A study of the Montefiore Medical Group in 1959, in which a sample of charts was surveyed indicated that only a little over 20 percent of the group obtained an annual physical examination, although all are entitled to one. Borsky and Sagen ("Motivations Toward Health Examinations") point out that "cooperators" in a health-examination project tend to be more interested in health matters generally and more knowledgeable.

9. In "Routine Medical Examination," the *Lancet* takes a fairly strong position against the routine examination. The editor argues that few disorders can be detected in the normal individual, that early diagnosis does not always lead to successful cure, that chronic disorders are dealt with in the later, symptomatic, stages, and that it is enormously expensive to carry on periodic examinations in addition to providing medical service. He brings up the psychological point that "the system must, for many people, mean more thoughts about illness and more anxiety."

10. We do not wish to discourage the routine examination of certain groups in the population with special problems or high incidence of specific illnesses. And there are other people for whom it is helpful to know that nothing important is wrong, so that the sneaking worry about cancer may be dissipated. For these people any number of examinations at their own request may have to be done.

11. See Neubauer, "The Techniques of Parent Group Education."

12. Of course the problem is more complicated than this. An important motivation for learning about health or medical care lies in the degree of an individual's preoccupation with his own body processes or the possibility of illness in himself which he may suspect or fear. See Merton's thoughtful presentation on latent functions in *Social Theory and Social Structure.*

13. Ernest Osborne, "Democracy Begins In The Home," Public Affairs Pamphlet #192, 1953.

14. *A Healthy Personality For Your Child,* Children's Bureau, Federal Security Agency, Social Security Administration, Pamphlet #337, 1952, based on the Mid-Century White House Conference on Children.

15. The effect of group meetings is difficult to isolate since individual contacts with team members were frequent, and the exchange of experiences, so important a part of group meetings, may have occurred anyhow.

16. Shapiro, *Changing Child-Rearing Attitudes Through Group Discussion.*

17. Our failure to show progress in weight control was not unique (McCann and Trulson, "Long-Term Effective Weight Reducing Programs"), and we may have to consider more modern methods of obesity control. Hypnosis is currently recommended (Winkelstein, "Hypnosis, Diet and Weight Reduction"), and may turn out to be effective.

18. See Shapiro, *Changing Child-Rearing Attitudes Through Group Discussion* and "Is Group Parent Education Worthwhile?"

19. It is not too far-fetched to assume that the use of health education by groups is based on the same principle that determines how they select a doctor or use medical service. For a discussion of community selection mechanisms see Katz and Lazarsfeld, *Personal Influence,* and Townsend, *The Family Life of Old People.* For an analyses of power relations, see Hunter, *Community Power Structure.*

CHAPTER XII. Family Health Maintenance

1. See Margaret Mead's discussion of validation of physician's right to treat in *Cultural Factors and Technical Change,* p. 231, and Freud's comment quoted in Jones, *Life and Work of Sigmund Freud,* vol. 2, p. 210.

2. Personal communications from Dr. R. S. Aaron and Dr. E. Glogau Estrin, paraphrased. The sharing of responsibility by internist and pediatrician, dictated by the nature of the program was a weakness which probably could be resolved in a larger program.

3. See also Hughes et al., *20,000 Nurses Tell Their Story,* for survey information on popular attitudes toward social workers.

4. "Anticipatory Guidance" in health department nursing programs (Ginsburg, *Public Health is People; Elements of a Community Mental Health Program*) increasing mental hygiene emphasis in public health nursing, and social-work consultants as part of public health nursing departments.

5. The experience of Cumming and Cumming, *Closed Ranks,* does not make one sanguine about changing popular attitudes toward mental illness.

6. The fact that the team members were able to transmit to each other their differing viewpoints on family members, and to the individual family member the *meaning* of family events, was an important contribution to team operation. This information regarding behavior and attitudes, exchanged in team conferences, was said by the psychiatrist to be greater than would come up in analysis of an individual in several years of psychoanalysis.

7. This learning and helping was not altogether one-sided. The team members looked at the psychiatrist in a similar clinical fashion. They felt that he was learning at their expense, and that at the termination of the program he was better qualified to do a consultative job than in the beginning. The education consisted mostly in forceful demonstration to him that the symptoms of conflict occurred in "normal," *functioning* individuals and families, so that the concepts "sick" and "well" were irrelevant. The psychiatrist could not assume that the problems were necessarily cries of dis-

tress, as they must be interpreted when patients apply for treatment in a psychiatrist's office.

8. There were about 6,500 practicing psychiatrists in the United States and another 2,000 in other jobs, according to the National Mental Health Commission, 1955. Recent membership figures of the American Psychiatric Association run over 11,000 (1960).

9. Psychiatric training of an unspecified duration, but a part of the 18-month residency, is recommended by the Committee on Preparation for General Practice of the American Medical Association (mimeographed report dated May 20, 1958).

10. Tureen, "Role of the Psychiatrist in a Prepaid Group Medical Program."

11. Home Care for psychiatric patients is a beginning step in this direction. See proposals by Silver et al., chapter 16 in *Frontiers in General Hospital Psychiatry*, ed. L. Linn (New York: International Universities Press, 1961).

12. See Grundy and Mackintosh, *The Teaching of Hygiene and Public Health in Europe*, for a description of the introduction of public health into medical education, an analogous situation and the possible sources of improper emphasis particularly pp. 28 ff.

CHAPTER XIII. Social Science Research in the Family
Health Maintenance Demonstration

1. *Perceived* rather than *actual* utilization is the emphasis here, for until we know the context of actual utilization, we do not know its meaning. The quantity of utilization is irrelevant for present concerns when we find that a patient uses the Family Health Maintenance Demonstration for routine services, but a "private" doctor for anything believed serious, or when we find that a patient will use the social worker for aid in getting into low-cost housing but not for counseling.

2. For further data on this survey see Eliot Freidson, "The Organization of Medical Practice and Patient Behavior."

3. For more extensive discussion of this see Eliot Freidson, "Client Control and Medical Practice."

4. See Eliot Freidson, "Specialties Without Roots: The Utilization of New Services."

5. The entire study upon which this report was based may be found in Eliot Freidson, *Patients' Views of Medical Practice*.

INDEX